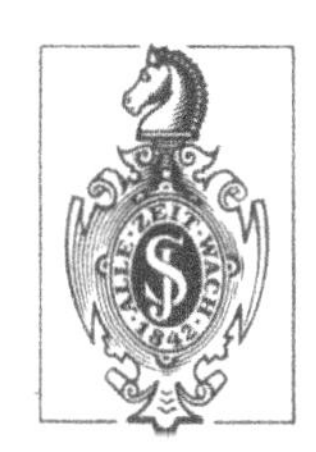

Springer-Verlag France S.A.R.L

Brigitte Martin

Atlas of Scrotal Ultrasound

Preface by Professor H. Hricak

with 710 Figures

Springer-Verlag France S.A.R.L

Brigitte Martin, M.D.
Service de Radiologie de l'Hôpital Saint-Antoine
184, rue du Faubourg Saint-Antoine
75571 Paris Cedex 12

Diagrams of illustrations by Marc Donon

Title of the original French edition: Atlas d'échographie scrotale.

ISBN 978-3-642-85683-9 ISBN 978-3-642-85681-5 (eBook)
DOI 10.1007/978-3-642-85681-5

Originally published by Springer-Verlag Paris in 1992
Softcover reprint of the hardcover 1st edition 1992

ISBN 978-3-642-85683-9

2918/3917/543210. Printed on acid free paper.

Preface

Ultrasonography is an established technique used as an adjunct to the physical examination in the evaluation of scrotal diseases. This book provides the reader with a comprehensive overview of testicular diseases and the appearance of these diseases on ultrasonography.

Dr. Martin is one of the leading investigators who early recognized the value and enthusiastically pursued the capability of ultrasound for the diagnosis of scrotal diseases. Her experience has been gathered over several years, so the richness and depth of description of the panoply of scrotal diseases is indeed comprehensive. The detailed description of the technique should provide practical value for the practitioner. The description of the embryology, epidemiology, anatomy and disease processes represents a comprehensive treatise on ultrasound imaging of the scrotum. The sonographic findings are illustrated with high quality images reflecting the author's long-term experience.

The book is intended to be a complete guide to practical ultrasound applications of testicular diseases for the physicians in training, general radiologists, and ultrasound specialists. The contents integrate the essential clinical characteristics of the various diseases (symptoms, physical findings, epidemiology) with information concerning their diagnosis and treatment. Based on extensive personal experience, the author succeeds brilliantly in providing a comprehensive insight into the problems of testicular diseases.

Professor H. Hricak
Urology and Radiology
UCSF, San Francisco

Preface of the french edition

Genital and more specifically scrotal ultrasound has from now on a significant role to play in the examination of the male urogenital system, as demonstrated by this superbly illustrated atlas.

So one must stipulate that in 1992 a clinical examination of the scrotal contents must if possible be completed by an ultrasound examination. However, this stipulation must be tempered according to whether the context of examination is either an acute or chronic one.

In the acute stage of an emergency, whether confronted or not with presence of a swollen injured scrotum, making a primary clinical diagnosis right away is more important than any of the imaging examinations. Therefore, the slightest suspicion of torsion of the testis, whether based on either medical history or physical examination, is an emergency which must lead to immediate exploratory surgery. Surgery is indicated irregardless of the result of an ultrasound examination even if it was obtained under satisfactory conditions given the nature of the emergency. Furthermore, following a scrotal traumatic injury, existence of a large distended scrotum must lead without delay to surgery which will permit evacuation of the hematoma, an evaluation of lesions, and reparation of the testicle.

Indubitably, when satisfactory technical requirements are met for scrotal ultrasound and if it will not cause in the least a delay in surgery, it must be encouraged to be performed. In fact, it permits learning of the ultrasound semiology for these types of lesions through comparison of clinical, anatomical and ultrasound information.

In cases other than emergencies, the value of scrotal and genital ultrasound is manifestly evident such as in the following situations :

– in the surveillance of an acute orchiepididymitis during which ultrasound permits the discovery in time of a developing abcess or even an infectious testicle, or in the context of the prostate where it may check on the condition of the deep genital tracts,

– in the finding of supporting evidence, even revelation in clinically normal testicles, of existence of tumors of the testicle,

– in the verification of testicular integrity when a hydrocele of the tunica vaginalis exists.

Finally, to be sure, testicular ultrasound is an integral part of the battery of examinations performed in the conditions of intersexuality, unpalpable testicle, and male infertility.

One must lastly insist upon the routine use of testicular ultrasound in patients complaining of testicular pain whose clinical examination evidences no anomalies in external genitalia. This pathological context is frequently encountered, preoccupies patients, and frustrates clinicians. Testicular ultrasound is here of primordial importance. Exceptionally it can evidence lesions susceptible to explain pain, but most often it demonstrates an indemn testicle and envelopes which allows reassuring of the patient. Put into the patient's medical records, with this respect it has an unquestionnable legal interest with regard to medical care.

Thus, in completing a careful clinical examination of external genitalia, genital ultrasound results in diagnostic precision, but in no way and under no pretext can be substituted for the rigorous discipline of careful examination of the scrotal contents.

Professor L. Boccon-Gibod

Foreword

This Atlas of scrotal ultrasound was conceived principally as an aid to the daily clinical practice of Radiologists and Clinicians. The format of the Atlas has been influenced by this aim, namely the order of the chapters and the short text supplemented by the tables and decision-making algorithms. The images form the largest portion of the book. The text of each chapter is deliberately separate from the images. Each image is illustrated by a clearly labelled diagram and detailed description. This layout enables the reader to refer to the book to a variable level of detail. This may either be a superficial reference to the anotated diagrams, perhaps encompassing the Legends, or a more detailed reference including all the texts of each chapter. This very pragmatic approach has led us to abandon any reference to the bibliography.

Duplex Doppler Ultrasound is not included in this Atlas of imaging for two reasons. The principal reason is that, despite the extreme interest in colour Doppler at the moment, our own experience indicates that in the vast majority of cases a good understanding of conventional ultrasound of the scrotum is sufficient to make the diagnosis and the role of Doppler is limited to confirming it. The second reason is the limited availability of Doppler ultrasound equipment in many places where it is reserved for vascular and abdominal investigations.

The Atlas is divided into eight chapters. The first chapter contains a review of the embryology and ultrasound anatomy essential for the performance of scrotal ultrasound and the understanding of congenital anomalies which the Practitioner may encounter. The following four chapters are concerned with the four major areas of pathology which present to the Clinician and Radiologist ; the acute scrotum, the chronically enlarged scrotum, the clinically normal scrotum with a suspected underlying tumour and infertility. The concluding three chapters deal with the post-operative scrotum, intrascrotal calcifications and cystic structures. These are arranged in the form of gamuts allowing the ultrasonologist to easily make a differential diagnosis when confronted with an intrascrotal calcification or cyst.

The Atlas is mainly concerned with pathology of the adult scrotum, but several ultrasound examinations in infants are included to illustrate some of the congenital anomalies.

It is not possible to conclude this preamble without thanking all those who contributed to the preparation of this work. Firstly I would like to thank those Clinicians who have had confidence in me, particularly Professor L. Boccon-Gibod who provided me with the essential link with a Urologist and Dr. J. Belaisch to whom I owe my training in the still poorly understood field of male infertility.

I would also like to specially thank Professor H. Hricak who particularly wished to preface the English version of this Atlas. All this help and goodwill would not have been enough without the assistance of the Radiology Department where I routinely work at the Saint Antoine Hospital in Paris. A very special thanks to Professor J.M. Tubiana for his encouragement and guidance during the preparation of this book as well as to all the ultrasound unit team with which I use to work.

Finally I would like to express my love and thanks to my family, particularly my husband for all his help despite all the restrictions imposed on us during the preparation of this Atlas.

Table of contents

Embryology; technical notes and ultrasound anatomy

Only a brief resume will be given of the embryology and physiology which is vital for the understanding of the congenital anomalies and pathologies which result from disorders of embryogenesis.

Also, after having considered the practical aspects of scrotal ultrasound, or more broadly genital ultrasound, the details of the anatomy of the scrotum and other organs of the male reproductive system necessary for the performance of this examination will be described.

Review of the embryology

The outlines

Testes

The primitive undifferentiated gonad arises from the genital crest, close to the primitive kidney, during the 3rd-5th weeks of fetal life. It is formed from a medulla which developes into the testis and from a cortex which involutes to form the tunica albuginea. The germinal cells derive from the cloacal endoderm or yolk sac. These colonise the primitive gonad.

Genital tracts

The *Wolffian duct* appears in the 5th week. It is a paired structure from which derive the *body* and *tail of the epididymis*, the *vas deferens*, the *seminal vesicles* and the *ejaculatory ducts*.

It joins up with the mesonephric ducts which become the efferent tubules, connecting the epididymis to the rete testis.

The prostate develops from the urogenital sinus which is situated between the Wolffian and Mullerian ducts.

The penis and scrotum develop from the genital bud and scrotal swelling.

Male differentiation

This occurs under the essential influence of a chromosomal factor attached to the Y chromosome.

- In the 7th week, the germinal cells migrate into the primitive gonad. The medulla, under the influence of the genotype, forms the sexual cords which canalise to produce the seminiferous tubules.

- In the 9th week, the *interstitial cells of Leydig* develop from the mesenchyma. They secrete testosterone which, between the 10th and 20th weeks, stimulates primary sexual differentiation, namely the differentiation of the Wolffian ducts into the genital passages (epididymis, vas deferens, seminal vesicles and ejaculatory ducts). Another hormone, di-hydrotesterone,is also secreted and this promotes the development of the external genitalia (penis and scrotum), the urethra and the prostate.

The *Sertoli cells* differentiate from supporting cells of the sexual cords. These secrete the anti-Mullerian hormone which stimulates the involution of the Mullerian ducts.

- In the seventh month, under the influence of several factors (hormonal, mechanical and epididymal), the testes descend each accompanied by a peritoneal evagination, the peritoneo-vaginal process. This later becomes the future tunica vaginalis around the testis and the peritoneo-vaginal canal higher up, which normally closes at birth. The gubernaculum testis guides this migration, later forming the cremaster muscle in its upper portion and

Table 1. ***Investigation of male pseudohermaphrodism (MPH)***

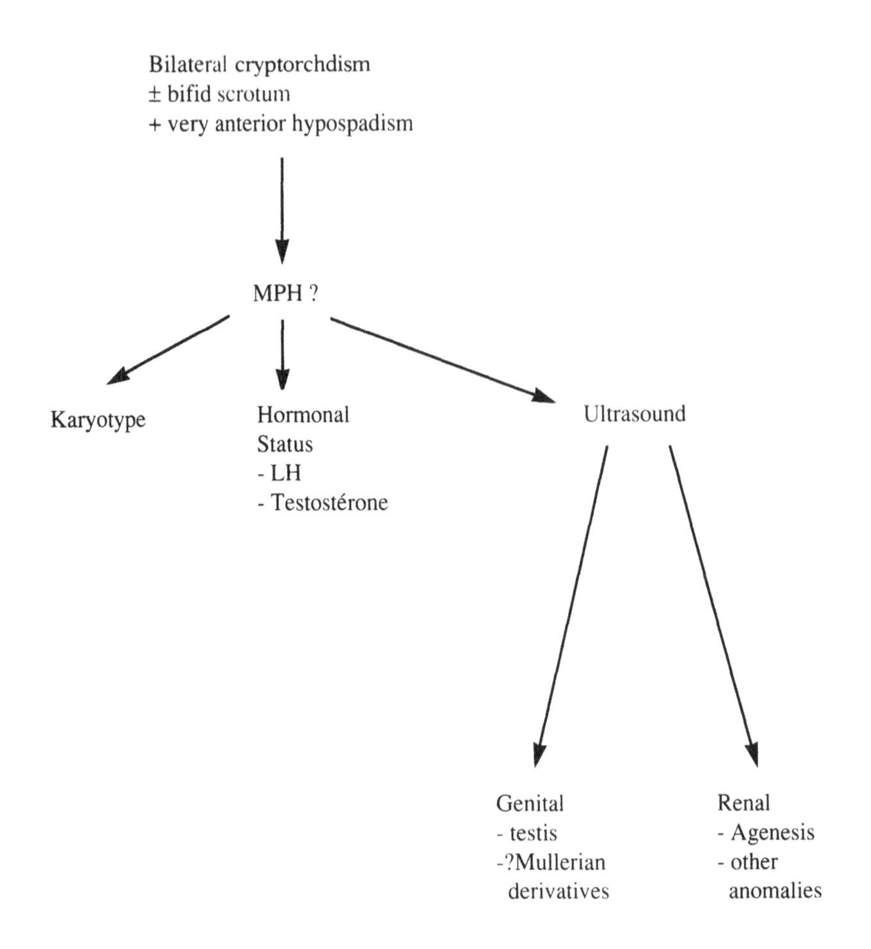

the scrotal ligament in its lower portion.

- By the eighth month, the testes are intra-scrotal.

Congenital anomalies

These result from one or several embryological anomalies. Only those anomalies which may be encountered during scrotal ultrasound examination will be considered here.

Intersex states or ambiguous sex

These consist of an inadequacy or anomaly of sexual differentiation. They form a rare and complex group of conditions.

Male pseudohermaphrodites, defined as insufficient formation of the external genitalia in an XY genotype, are due to 3 types of anomaly (Table 1) :

- *Gonadal dysgenesis* (30%-35%). Due to the close proximity of the primitive kidneys to the primitive gonads, there is often a co-existing renal anomaly.
- *Defective synthesis* of testosterone (5%-10%).
- *Insensitivity to androgens* (60%-70%)

Anomalies of testicular migration: ectopic testis and cryptorchidism

Strictly speaking, an ectopic testis is situated outside the scrotum and outside the normal path of descent, whereas the testis in cryptorchidism is situated outside the scrotum but somewhere along the normal path of descent. In fact the two terms are often interchangeable.

The problem for the Radiologist is to identify the position of undescended and impalpable testes (Table 2).

At the age of one year, approximately 1% of infants born at term still have undescended testes, this figure increasing to 25% in infants born prematurely.

Table 2. ***Undescended and impalpable testes diagnostic algorithm***

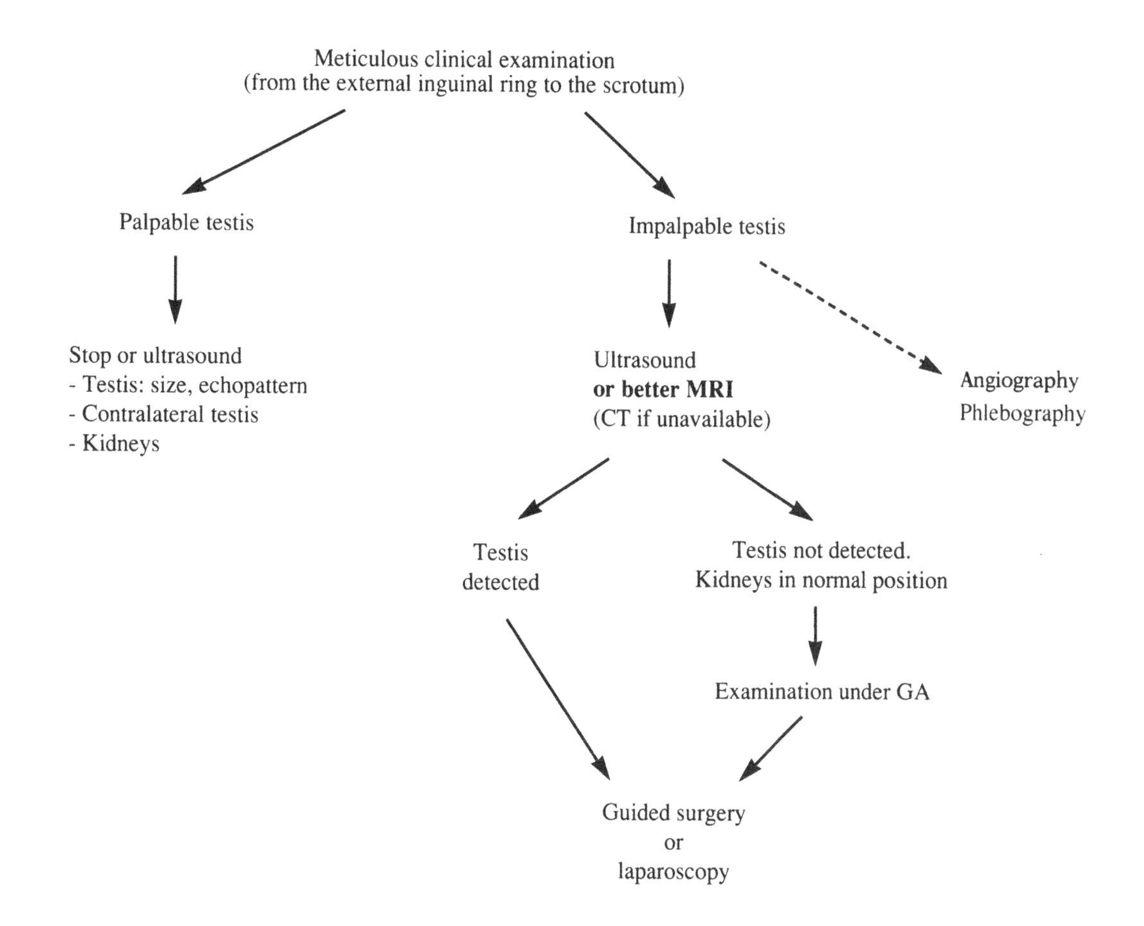

The right testis is most often affected. Ten per cent of cryptorchids are bilateral. The commonest site for an undescended testis is the inguinal ring (80% of cases) (Diagram 1).

Twenty per cent of undescended testes are impalpable. The risk of cancer is 10 - 40 times greater than for a normally situated testis. This risk increases further if the testis is situated higher (intra-abdominal testis).

Ultrasound has proved to be disappointing in the detection of undescended testes with the exception of the inguinal region where the testis is, in fact, also often palpable. MRI is now the investigation of choice.

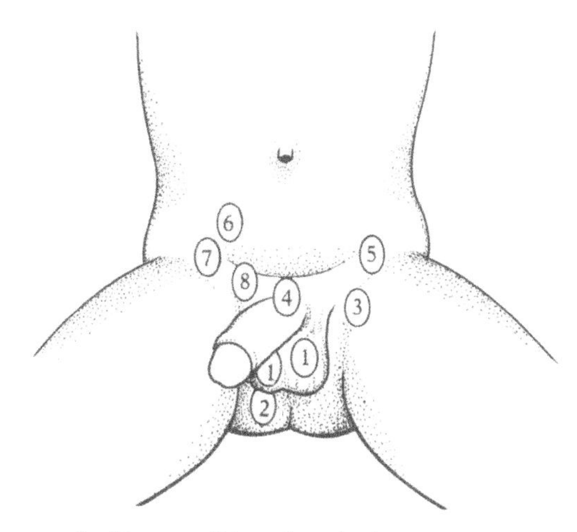

Diagram 1. ***Abnormalities of testicular migration. The different positions of the testis.*** *1* Scrotal (normal position), *2* perineal, *3* femoral, *4* penile, *5* interstitial, *6* abdominal, *7* inguinal, *8* at the external inguinal ring

Miscellanous anomalies

These can affect one or several elements of the scrotal contents:

- *The testis*: Absence bilaterally indicates anorchi-

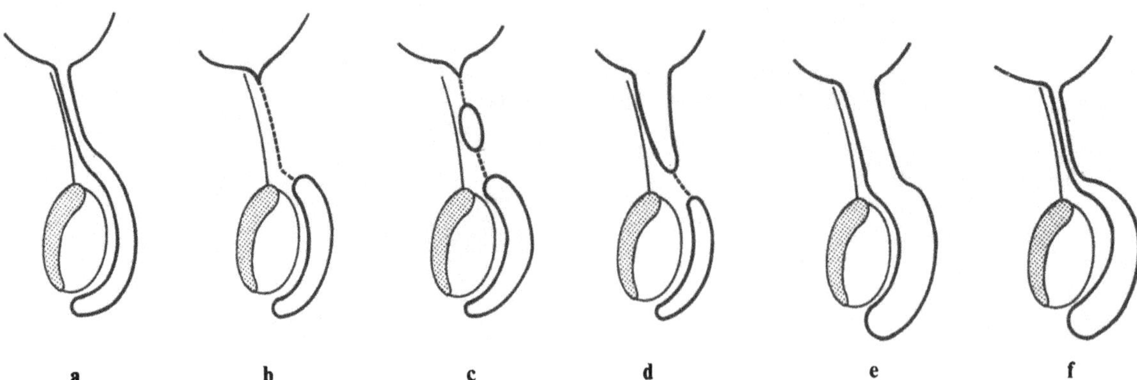

Diagram 2 a-f. ***The normal stages and abnormalities of the embryology of the peritoneo-vaginal process*** (P. Mollard, Precis of Paediatric Urology, Edition Masson, 1984, p 3). **a** A peritoneal evagination, the *peritoneo-vaginal process* accompanies the testis on its migration. **b** Later, the peritoneo-vaginal process closes. **c** Persistence of its middle portion results in a *cyst of the cord.* **d** Persistence of its proximal portion results in an *inguinal hernia.* **e** Sometimes the *hernia* is *inguino-scrotal*, with a wide communication between the peritoneal cavity and vaginal cavity. **f** A persistent narrow communication between the peritoneal cavity and tunica vaginalis constitutes a *communicating hydrocele*

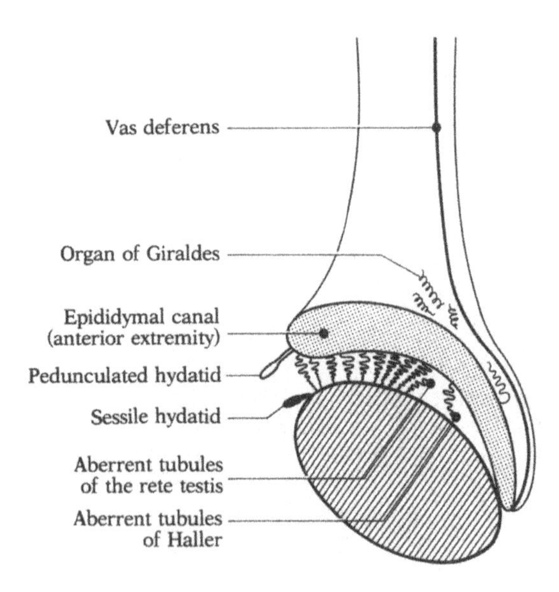

Diagram 3. ***Juxta-testicular embryonic vestiges*** (from Rouvière, Human anatomy Volume11)

dism, unilateral absence is monorchidism. Polyorchidism (greater than 2 testes) is rare but easily diagnosed ultrasonically. Finally, an apparently solitary testis can in fact be due to the fusion of two and is accompanied on each side by an epididymis and vas deferens.

- *The epididymis* and *vas deferens*: anomalies of these structures are often associated with testicular anomalies. Agenesis or hypoplasia, either total or partial, are the commonest. Bilateral agenesis of the vas deferens is an important cause of infertility. An anterior epididymis occurs in 10%-15% of cases. This is important to remember and is easily recognised ultrasonically but can pose diagnostic problems in cases of an acute scrotum (differentiation between epididymitis occuring in an anterior epididymis and torsion).

It is not possible by ultrasound to recognize the absence of just a segment of the excretory ducts (e.g. the body of the epididymis). It is therefore imperative, when such an abnormality is suspected clinically, to examine the renal areas as there are often co-existent renal anomalies.

Anomalies of closure of the peritoneo-vaginal process

These may be associated with anomalies of testicular migration. They are classified as follows (Diagram 2):

- Congenital inguinal hernias (non-closure of the upper portion), or inguino-scrotal (communication between the peritoneal cavity and the processus vaginalis);

- cysts of the cord (failure of closure of the middle portion);

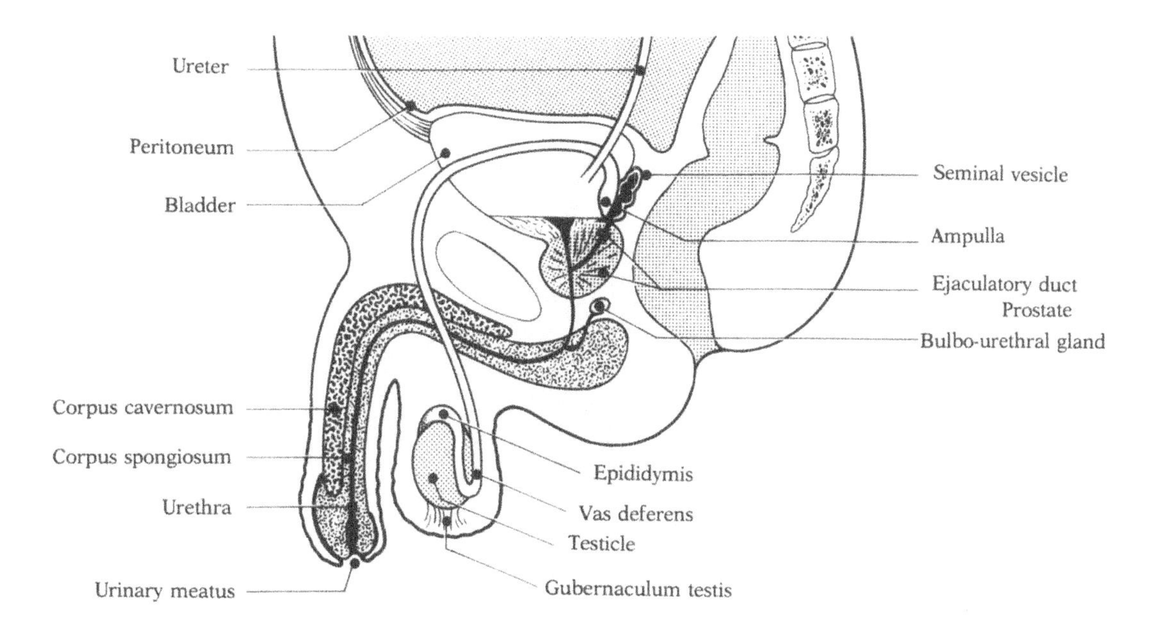

Diagram 4. ***Sagittal section of the true pelvis in the male***
(from Histology by J.P. Dadoune & Co, Editions Flammarion 1990, p 333)

- hydroceles of the tunica vaginalis, extending along the spermatic cord, (persistence of the lower portion);
- communicating hydroceles, a filiform communication persists between the peritoneal cavity and tunica vaginalis.

Dystrophic cysts

This group of cysts is formed from embryological rests (Diagram 3):

- The most frequent is *the sessile hydatid of Morgagni*, a vestige of the uppermost portion of the Mullerian duct situated anteriorly at the epididymo-testicular junction. It is a small rounded structure of a few millimetres diameter, containing fibrous tissue and may be calcified. It may undergo torsion, particularly in children, or become secondarily detached. It is the most frequently encountered vestigial structure in the adult seen on ultrasound.

- *The pedunculated hydatid of Morgagni* is the remnant of the superior aspect of the Wolffian duct overlying the head of the epididymis. This small rounded cystic structure of a few millimetres in size is much less frequently visualised.

The other vestigial elements are rarer and correspond to the fragmented Wolffian canaliculi which are often responsible for cyst formation:

- *The Organ of Giraldes or paradidymis* - Wolffian remnant situated in the cord opposite the head of the epididymis.

- *The Organ of Haller or aberrant canals.* Probably of Wolffian origin, it is an insignificant structure attached to the head or tail of the epididymis.

Ultrasound anatomy

Technique and performance of the examination

It is preferable to perform a complete genital ultrasound which includes a scrotal ultrasound as well as a study of the internal genital organs (prostate, seminal vesicles, ampullae of the vasa deferentia) rather than a scrotal ultrasound alone (Diagram 4). It is therefore important to ask the patient to come with a moderately full bladder.

Examination of the scrotum

- With the patient supine, the scrotum is flattened out by applying gentle traction to the penis towards the umbilicus.

- It is absolutely imperative to select a probe designed for the study of superficial structures, namely of a high frequency (minimum 5 Megahertz, MHz. with a stand-off waterbath, or better 7.5 - 10 MHz.) .

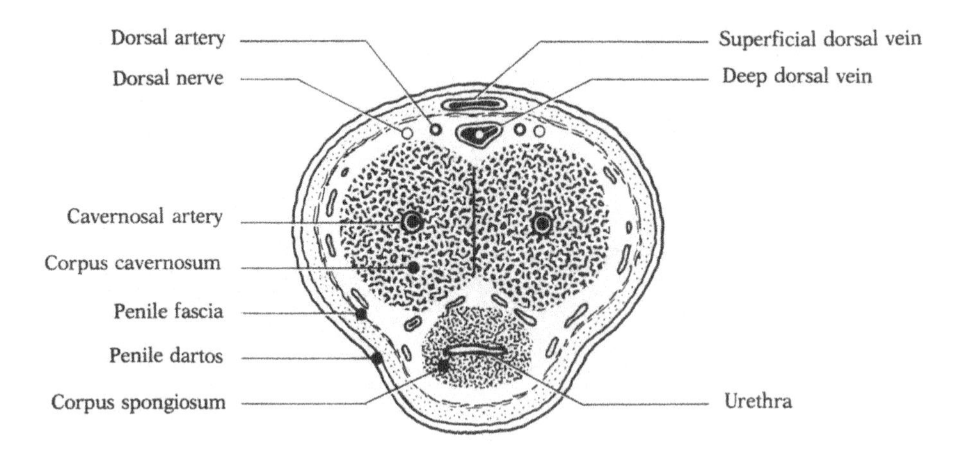

Diagram 5. ***Transverse section of the penis*** (from Rouvière)

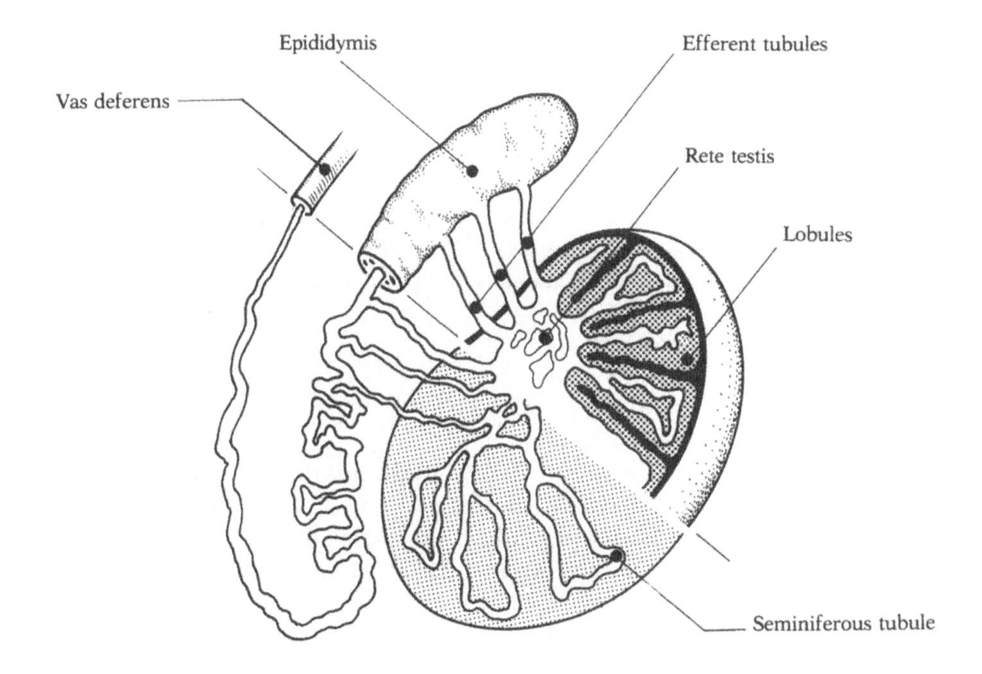

Diagram 6. ***General structure of the testis***

The addition of pulsed or colour Doppler can be of benefit.

- Measurements are compared with the supposedly normal side.

- The examination comprises of :

  • Bilateral examination

  • Methodical analysis and comparison of both sides of the scrotum :

    - The investing layers: thickness, echo pattern;

    - testes : dimensions (length, width, thickness) and volume (by assuming the testis is elliptical);

    - epididymis : head, tail and body;

    - spermatic cords.

Longitudinal sections are the most important and

should include the whole of the scrotum. Transverse scans are complimentary and allow direct comparison of the testes.

- Dynamic manoeuvres (Valsalva manoeuvre, erect and supine scans) are sometimes indicated.

Examination of the pelvis

- Initially this should be performed by a suprapubic approach using a 3.5 or 5 MHz. sector scanner, depending on the size of the patient.
- If an abnormality is detected, further detail may be obtained by a transrectal scan with a biplanar facility.
- The scan should include :
  - the prostate : contour, morphology, weight, echo pattern;
  - seminal vesicles : symmetry, measurements of the bases and extremities, echo pattern;
  - ampullae of the vasa deferentia;
  - finally the bladder and lower ureters.

The testis

This is the male gonad. It is a paired organ with a dual function :

- *Gametogenesis:* the production of spermatazoa occurs in the epithelium of the seminiferous tubules. This epithelium comprises of two types of cells, the *germinal cells* which represent the different stages of spermatogenesis and the *Sertoli cells* the vital support cells.

- *Endocrine function:* the synthesis of several hormones, principally testosterone and other steroids by the Leydig cells which are situated in the interstitial tissue between the seminiferous tubules.

The testes lie in the scrotum below the penis. This consists of the erectile organs, the corpus spongiosum and the two corpora cavernosa which are surrounded by a capsule, the tunica albuginea. The root of the penis is usually visible on longitudinal or oblique sections of the scrotum (Diagram 5).

The testis is ovoid in shape and of variable size, depending on the individual. In our experience, the most sensitive parameter for detecting a small degree of hypotrophy is the maximum width on longitudinal sections, normally 20 mm. or greater. 15-20 mm.indicates hypotrophy, less than 15 mm. is atrophic.

The value of measurements of testicular volume, made possible by recent advances in the software on the scanners, is still in the process of evaluation and needs to be compared with orchidometry. However, it is probable that this parameter will eventually be the measurement of choice.

The testis is enclosed by a tough capsule 1 mm. thick, the *tunica albuginea* with the vessels running over it. In the postero-superior portion of the testis, the capsule thickens and penetrates into the substance of the gland in a triangular wedge to form the *Highmore body.* This structure corresponds to the *'hilum of the testis'* on the ultrasound image, an echogenic linear or triangular region whose visibility is variable depending on the patient and the echogenicity of the adjacent parenchyma. This hilar region represents the confluence of vessels and tubules, since it comprises of the *rete testis* which drains the *straight tubules,* the excretory canals of the lobules, and which are in turn the continuation of the *seminiferous tubules.* The rete testis is attached to the head of the epididymis by the *efferent cones* which are not normally visible ultrasonically unless distended. The lobules are separated by *interlobular septa* which terminate at the level of the Highmore body. These septa are sometimes partially visible when using a 10 MHz. probe (Diagram 6).

The tunica albuginea can also sometimes be partially visualised as an echogenic line in case of an adjacent hydrocele or fibrous plaques. The testicular parenchyma is homogenous and fairly echogenic.

The excretory genital passages

These paired structures carry the spermatazoa from the testis as far as the urinary meatus and consist of the intra-testicular spermatic canal, the efferent tubules or cones, the epididymal canal, the vas deferens and the urethra (Diagram 4).

The epididymis

This is a tube 3-6 mm long, very narrow (less than 1 mm) and convoluted, which covers the supero-posterior border and part of the lateral aspect of the testis. It is divided into 3 segments:

- The *head* (or globus major) at the superior pole of the testis: it is the only portion which is always visible ultrasonically: rounded or triangular, it normally measures less than 12 mm. It has an homogenous echo pattern slightly more echogenic than the testis.

- The *body* : in the absence of any abnormality, this segment is not really visualised on ultrasound and blends with the posterior border of the testis.

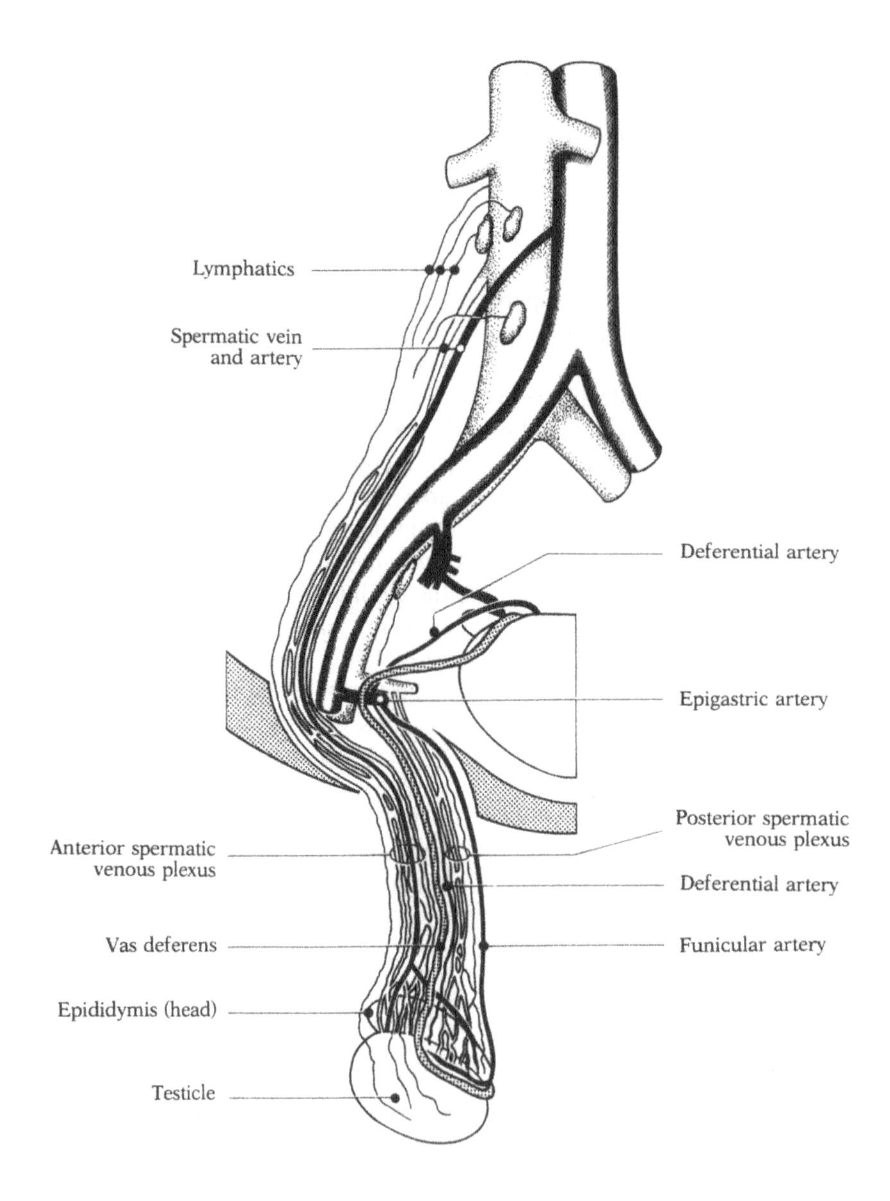

Diagram 7. ***Vessels of the testis and epididymis. Spermatic veins and arteries*** (from Rouvière)

- The *tail* : this is the inferior portion situated below the testis. Its visualisation is variable and is facilitated by the presence of a small hydrocele. Normal diameter is less than 5 mm. and it is slightly echogenic.

The epididymis has two essential functions: *the transport* and *the maturation of spermatozoa* which, initially immobile, acquire their mobility during transit through the epididymis. The patency of the epididymis is confirmed by the presence of *carnitine* (which has a role in the motility of the spermatazoa) in the seminal fluid. Carnitine is therefore a *marker of epididymal function.*

Vas deferens

This is a direct continuation of the epididymis, the junction is called the *epididymo-deferential loop.* It is a thin-walled rectilinear tube, often palpable, 45 cm long and 2-3 mm in diameter. Normally it cannot be

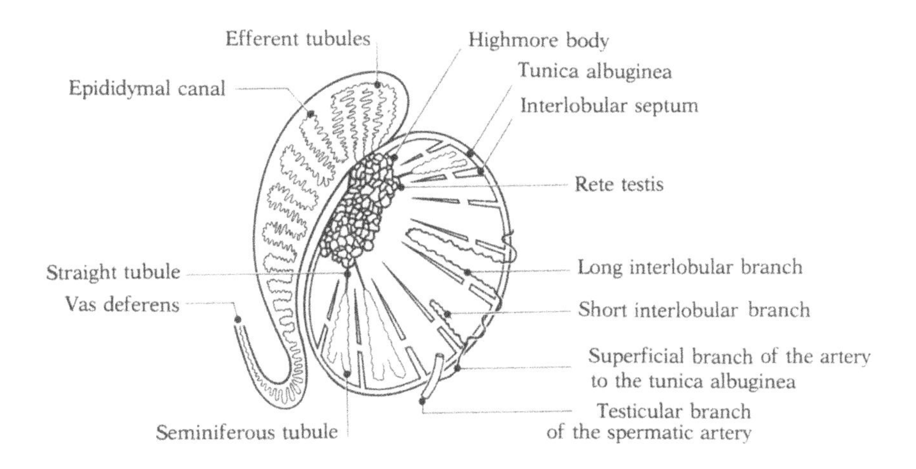

Diagram 8. ***General structure and arterial supply of the testis*** (from Histology by J.P. Dadoune & Co)

distinguished as a separate structure ultrasonically.

Five portions are described: the *epididymo-testicular portion* which is intrascrotal; the *funicular portion* which passes in the spermatic cord, the inguinal, iliac and pelvic portions.

Before entering the prostate, the vas deferens dilates to form the *deferential ampulla.* This can sometimes be visualized by endorectal scanning. It is joined by the seminal vesicle at its termination to form the *ejaculatory duct* which enters the prostate and opens into the prostatic urethra on each side of the prostatic utricle.

The accessory glands

These consist of the *seminal vesicles*, the prostate and bulbo-urethral glands of Cowper.

Only the anatomy of the seminal vesicles will be described. They are paired, saccular and very convoluted organs which contribute to the production of seminal fluid. They are well visualised on ultrasound and have an elongated shape on longitudinal sections with a thicker lateral portion. On transverse section they appear as linear structures at the bases and inverted triangles in their lateral extremities. Their height is variable. In effect they act as reservoirs which empty during ejaculation. Their overall dimensions can vary but are always essentially symmetrical. The height is usually less than 15 mm. Ultrasonically of intermediate echogenicity , they are more hypoechoic when full of fluid and occasionally small fluid-filled pockets can be seen on endorectal scanning.

Among the many substances secreted by the seminal vesicles, *fructose* is used as a marker of function of the vesicles.

The vessels (Diagram 7)

Arteries

- *The spermatic artery* arises from the anterior aspect of the aorta. Having passed through the inguinal canal it divides at the superior pole of the testis into two branches : the testicular artery and the epididymal artery.
- *The testicular artery* divides in the tunica albuginea and interlobular septa into terminal branches which converge towards the Highmore body. This interlobular network is not visible ultrasonically (Diagram 8). By contrast the arteries of the cord and in particular the spermatic artery can be recognized with the help of Doppler.

In addition, each pole receives another vascular supply from the spermatic or epididymal arteries to the superior pole and from the deferential artery to the inferior pole.

- *The epididymal artery* gives an anterior branch to the head of the epididymis and a posterior branch to the body and tail.
- *The deferential artery*, a branch of the hypogastric artery, supplies the vas deferens and also the epididymal tail via anastomoses.

In fact, there are numerous anastamoses in the cord between the spermatic and deferential arteries.

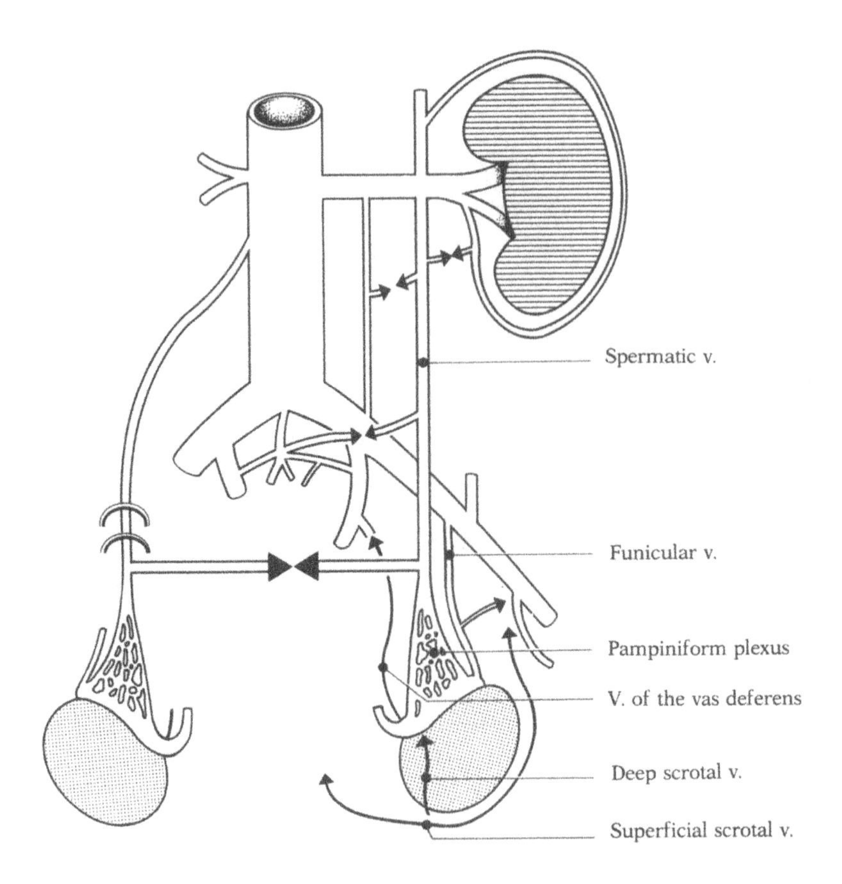

Diagram 9. ***The veins of the testis***

Veins

Within the scrotum there are three venous plexi (Diagram 9):

- *The anterior spermatic venous plexus or pampiniform plexus.* This drains the testis and head of the epididymis and reforms into about 10 veins. They are seen as very fine hypoechoic, linear structures of less than 2 mm behind and above the testis leading into the spermatic cord. If necessary, visualisation can be improved slightly by performing the Valsalva manoeuvre.

- *Posterior spermatic venous plexus or cremasteric plexus* drains the body and tail of the epididymis. It is really more slender and normally not discernible ultrasonically.

- *Scrotal veins* form two networks, one superficial and more importantly, the second which empties into the cremasteric plexus. This can dilate considerably in cases of varicocele.

There are numerous anastomoses between these three systems. The two plexi ascend behind the epididymis and testis into the cord. In the iliac region, the pampiniform plexus forms the spermatic vein which has a different termination on each side, the left draining into the renal vein and the right into the inferior vena cava directly.

The cremasteric plexus empties into the main inferior epigastric vein which in turn drains into the external iliac vein.

The lymphatics

The lymphatic vessels of the testis and epididymis run with the spermatic vessels and empty into the lumbo-aortic lymph nodes from the aortic bifurcation to the renal pedicles. An accessory duct terminates in the external iliac nodes. Normally, they are not visible on ultrasound. By contrast, in cases of chronic or previous parasite infestation, calcified larvae within the lymphatic vessels can outline their course to a lesser or greater extent, especially in the spermatic cords.

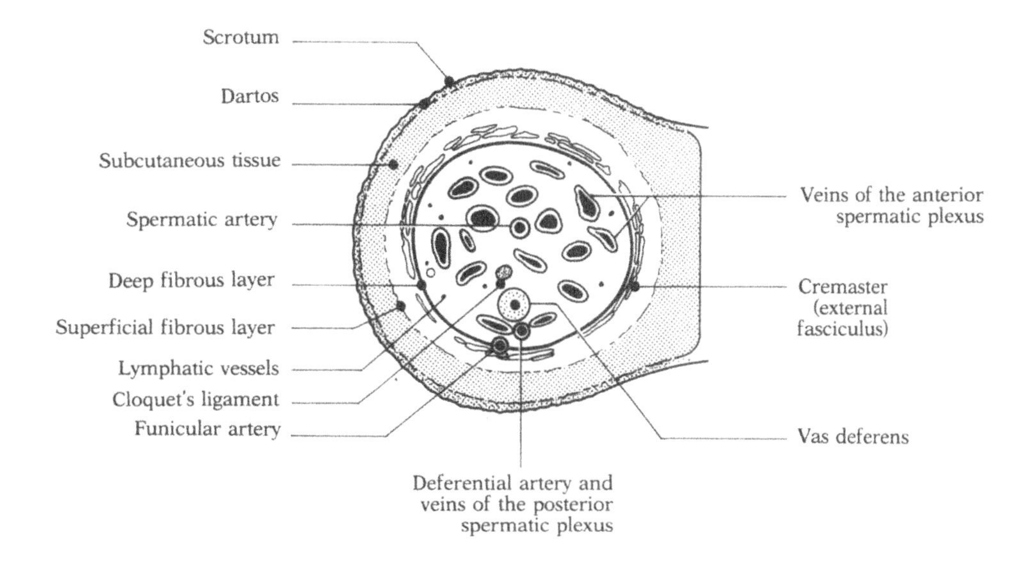

Diagram 10. ***Transverse section of the cord and investing layers*** (from Rouvière)

The spermatic cord (Diagram 10)

This forms the pedicle from which hang the testis and epididymis. It contains all the elements entering or leaving the scrotum, namely the vas deferens, the spermatic and deferential arteries, the spermatic venous plexi, the lymphatic vessels and the ligament of Cloquet (formed by the obliteration of the perito-neo-vaginal canal). These structures are held together by a fatty cellular connective tissue. The latter is responsible for the ultrasonic appearance of the cord : an echogenic structure through which runs fine hypo echoic linear vessels. It is normally less than 1 cm. in diameter.

The nerves

The testis and epididymis are innervated by branches of the *spermatic plexus* formed from the solar plexus. The vesiculo-deferential plexus, formed from the hypo-gastric plexus, supplies the vasa deferentia, seminal vesicles and ejaculatory ducts. They are not visible on ultrasound.

The investing layers of the scrotal sac (Diagram 11)

These form a sac, the *scrotal sac*, situated anterior to the perineum and inferior to the penis. It is suspended below the pubis by a narrowed segment, the *pedicle*. It is divided into two by the *median raphe* which extends posteriorly to the perineum. The layers are in continuity with the different layers of the anterior abdominal wall.

There are seven layers. In the absence of pathology these cannot be distinguished separately ultrasonically and are seen as a band of variable echogenicity (depending on the gain settings) but with a stratified appearance suggesting several superimposed layers. The overall thickeness is generally less than 5 mm. However, this upper limit can be seen in small and high lying scrotums.

From superficial to deep the layers consist of:

- The *skin or scrotum:* this can be of variable thickness explaining the different thicknesses which are encountered. It is seen as a regular echogenic band.

- The *dartos:* covering the deep surface of the scrotum, it essentially consists of muscle fibres more numerous antero-laterally. It blends with the penile dartos superiorly and can sometimes extend posteriorly to form the perineal dartos. It is normally not recognisable as an individual structure.

- The *subcutaneous connective tissue and superficial fibrous layer*.

- The *cremaster* : this striated muscle is composed of two fasciculi; the *external* or *crural fasciculus* is the only one to reach the anterior surface of the testis. It is responsible for the cremasteric reflex which is sometimes elicited by the application of gel onto the scrotum and renders the cremaster more

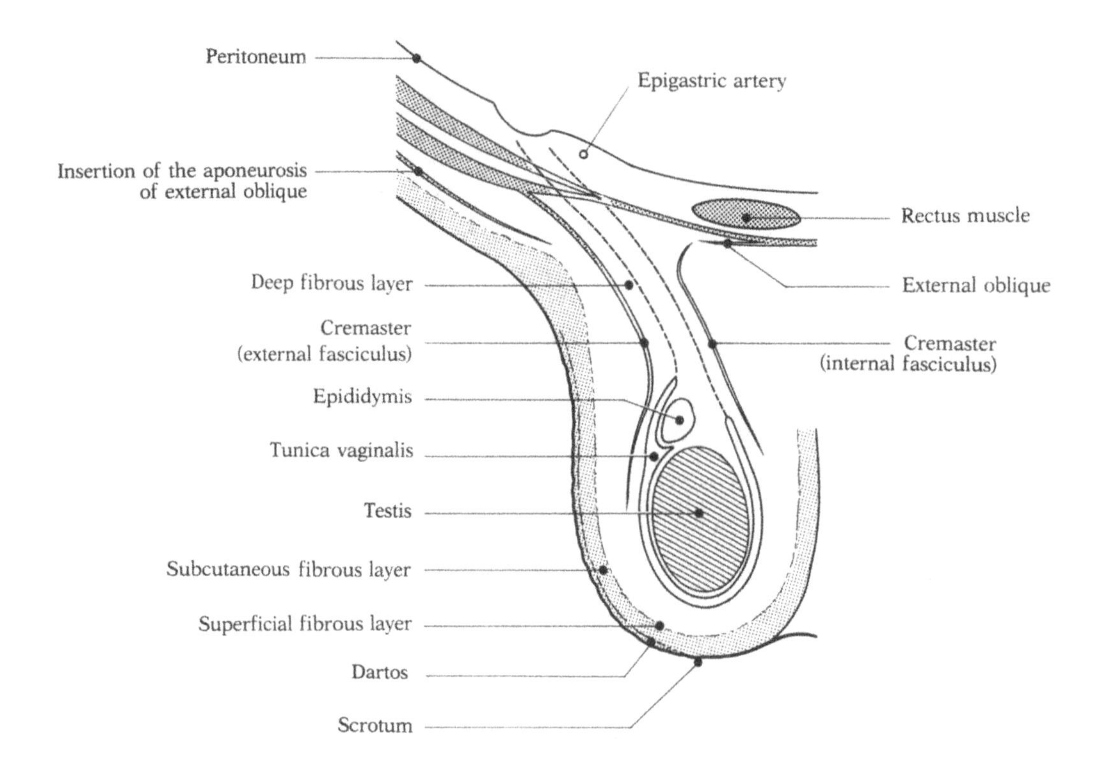

Diagram 11. ***Schematic diagram of the investing layers of the testis and their connections with the different layers of the abdominal wall*** (from Rouvière)

visible ultrasonically. It appears as an echogenic triangular structure with the apex inferiorly and the base superiorly.

- The *deep fibrous layer*. This is an evagination of the transversalis fascia which surrounds the cord, the testis and the epididymis. It is attached inferiorly, around the *scrotal ligament* to the vestige of the gubernaculum testis. This connects the most posterior part of the testis and epididymis to the deep surface of the scrotum. Ultrasonically it is visualised when surrounded by a small amount of fluid.

- The *tunica vaginalis*. This is a peritoneal expansion and is therefore a serous cavity with two layers:

• the *visceral layer*; this leaves uncovered a part of the testis and the epididymis (the medial surface of the testis and the most posterior portions of both). Over the testis it is closely adherent to the tunica albuginea from which it is indistinguishable;

• the *parietal layer* is separated from the fibrous tunica by cellular tissue. It is often visualised ultrasonically in inflammatory conditions. It becomes thickened fairly frequently; fibrous plaques in the form of small echogenic linear structures are also observed. Visualisation is facilitated by the presence of even a small physiological amount of fluid in the tunica vaginalis. This is generally best seen at the two poles of the testes.

Finally, a prolongation of the tunica vaginalis extends between the testis and epididymal head, the *interepididymo - testicular recess* or *fossa*.

Embryology; technical notes and ultrasound anatomy

Testis

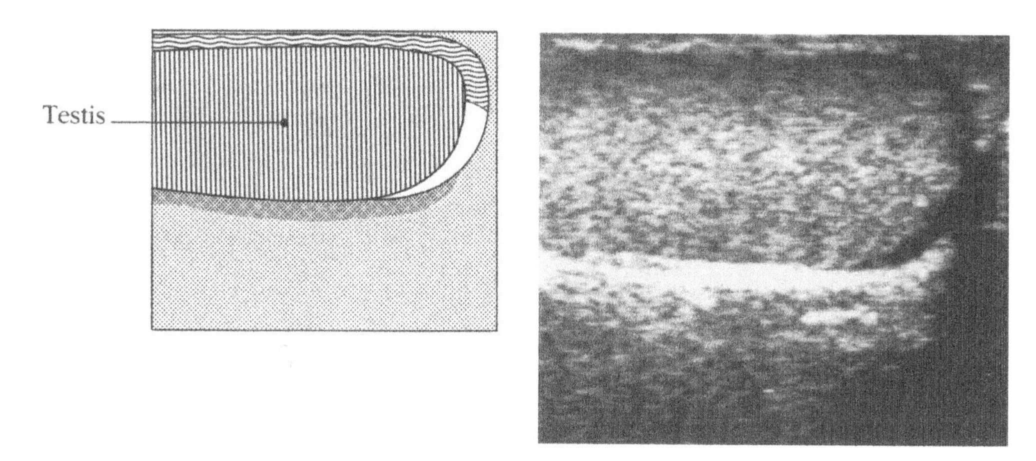

Fig. 1. ***Normal adult testis.*** Sagittal section. Regular oblong shape. Largest width greater than or equal to 20 mm. Testicular parenchyma homogenous and fairly echogenic

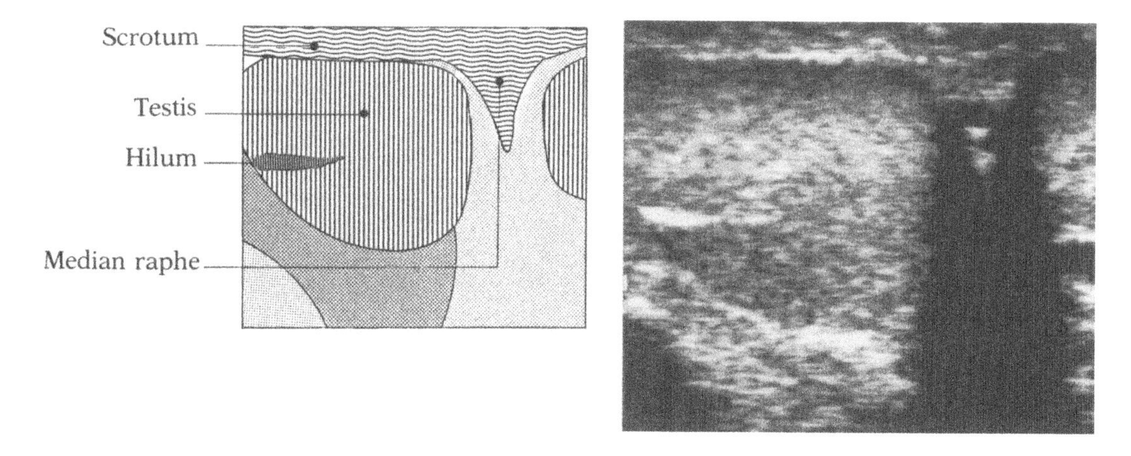

Fig. 2. ***Normal adult testis.*** Transverse section. Testicular hilum corresponding to the Highmore body at the zone demarcated by a regular hyperechoic line, about 1 cm long, running postero-superiorly

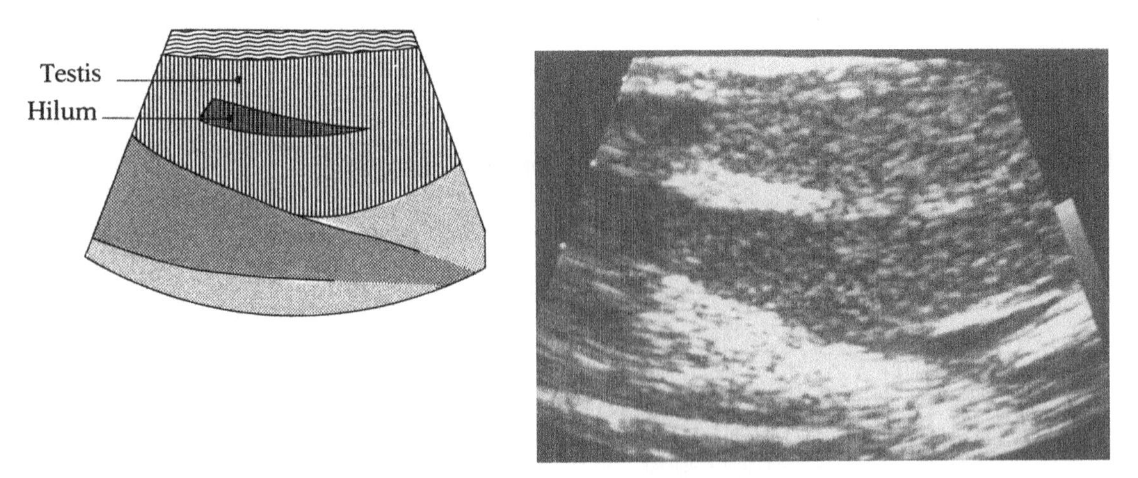

Fig. 3. ***Testicular hilum; morphology.*** Approximately triangular in shape, with apex internally and base externally, due to the tunica albuginea thickening or Highmore body which is set into the parenchyma of the testis

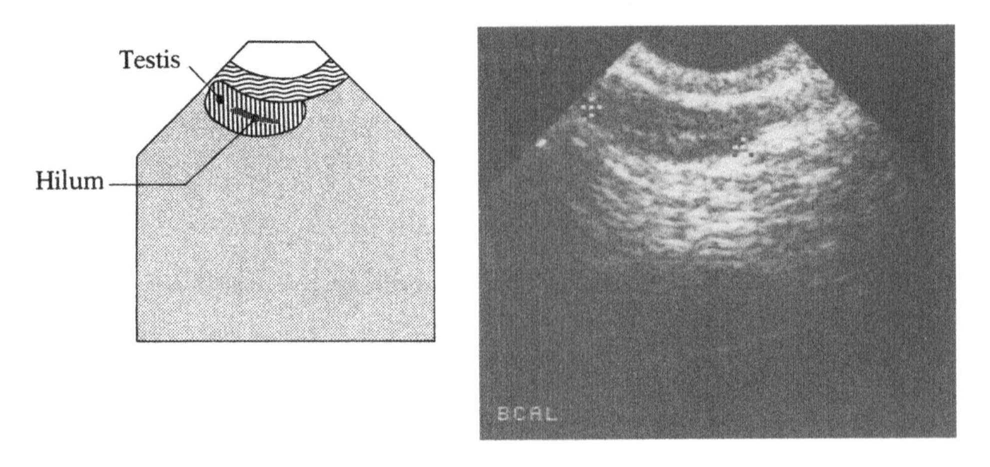

Fig. 4. ***The prepubertal testis.*** Sagittal section. Small hypoechoic testis within which the hyperechoic hilum is well visualised

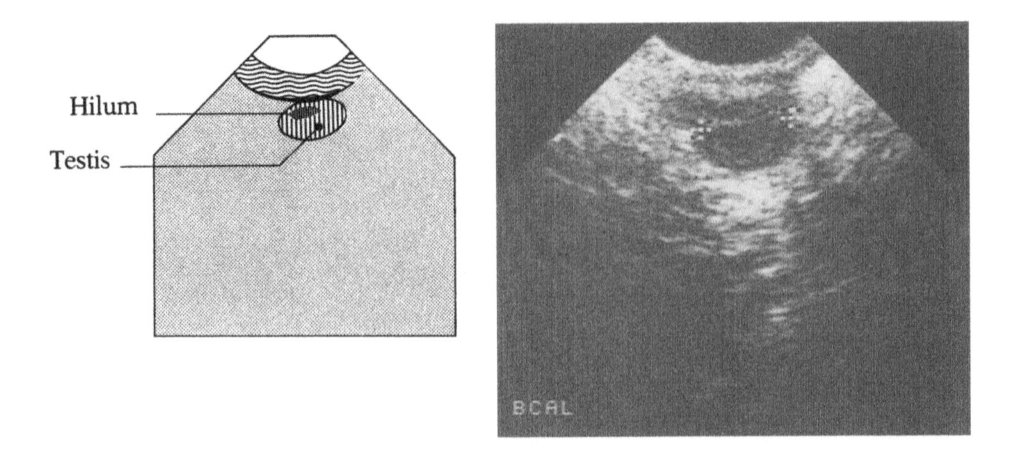

Fig. 5. ***The prepubertal testis.*** Transverse section. The hilum is visible. By contrast the testicular appendages are not identified

Epididymis and tunica vaginalis

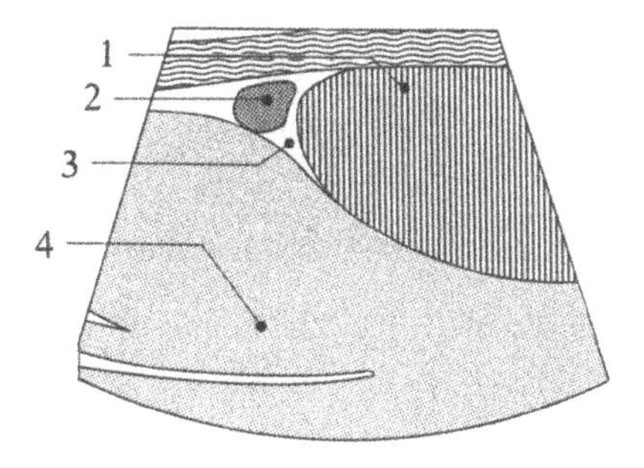

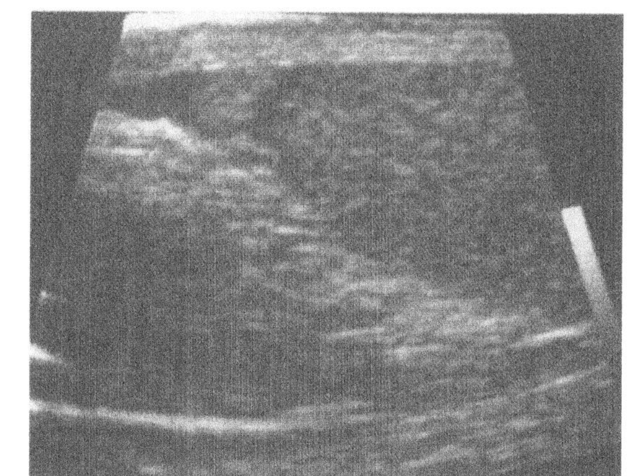

1 Testis
2 Epididymal head
3 Superior interepididymo-testicular recess of the serous layer of the tunica vaginalis
4 Root of the penis

Fig. 6. ***Epididymal head and the antero-superior interepididymo-testicular recess of the tunica vaginalis.*** Sagittal section of superior pole. Rounded head, about 1 cm in size. Homogenous echo pattern, iso- or slightly hyper-echoic compared to the testis. The antero-superior epididymo-testicular fold of the tunica vaginalis is opened out by a small quantity of fluid. Below the testis, the base of the penis is seen

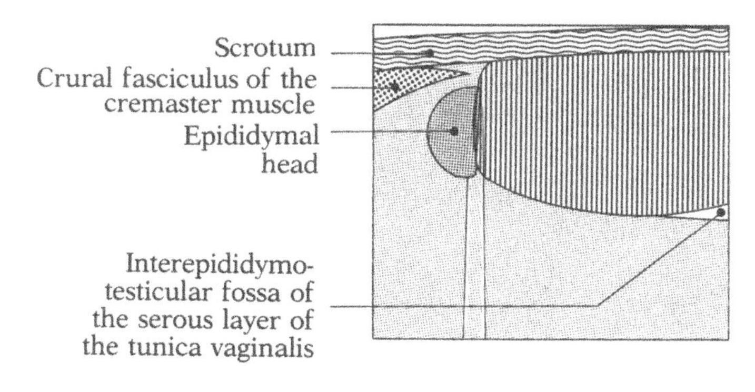

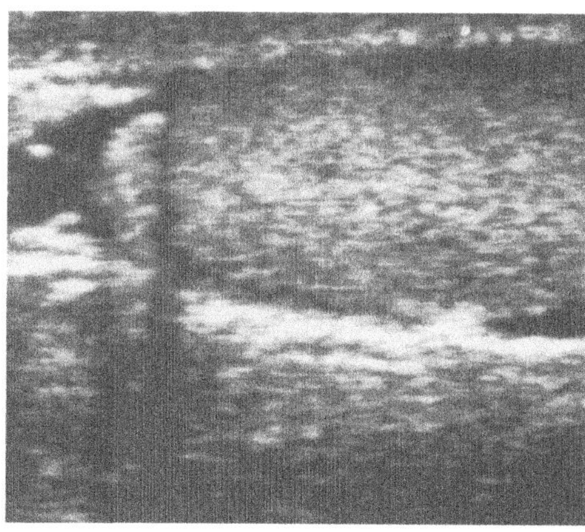

Fig. 7. ***Epididymal head; another view. Interepididymo- testicular fossa of the tunica vaginalis.*** Sagittal section. Normal scrotal thickness with visualisation of the crural fascia of the cremaster muscle. Epididymal head appears triangular. Its junction with the superior pole of the testis is marked by a narrow anechoic band. The interepididymo - testicular fossa is filled with a small amount of fluid between the testis and body of the epididymis

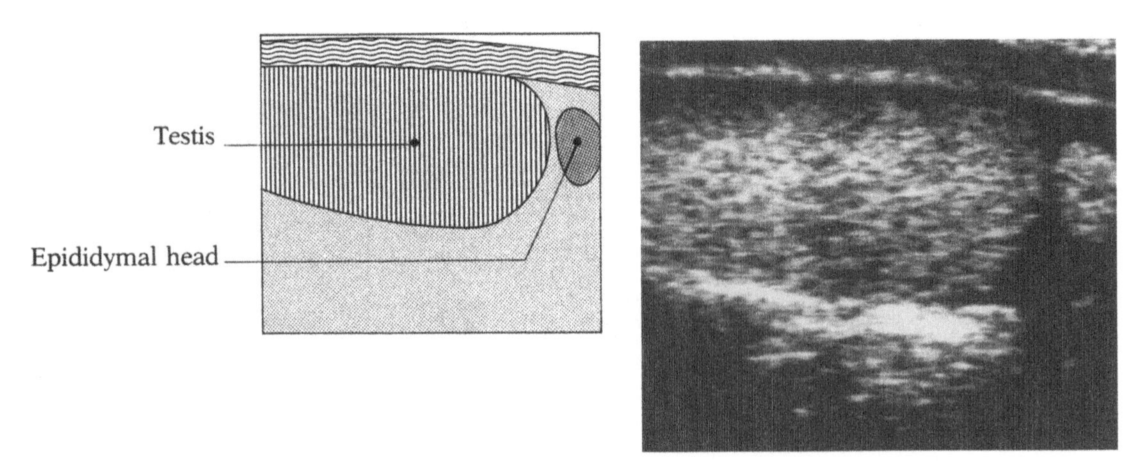

Fig. 8. ***Epididymal variant : antero-inferior position.*** Sagittal section. Epididymal head is morphologically normal but inverted in position (10-15% of cases)

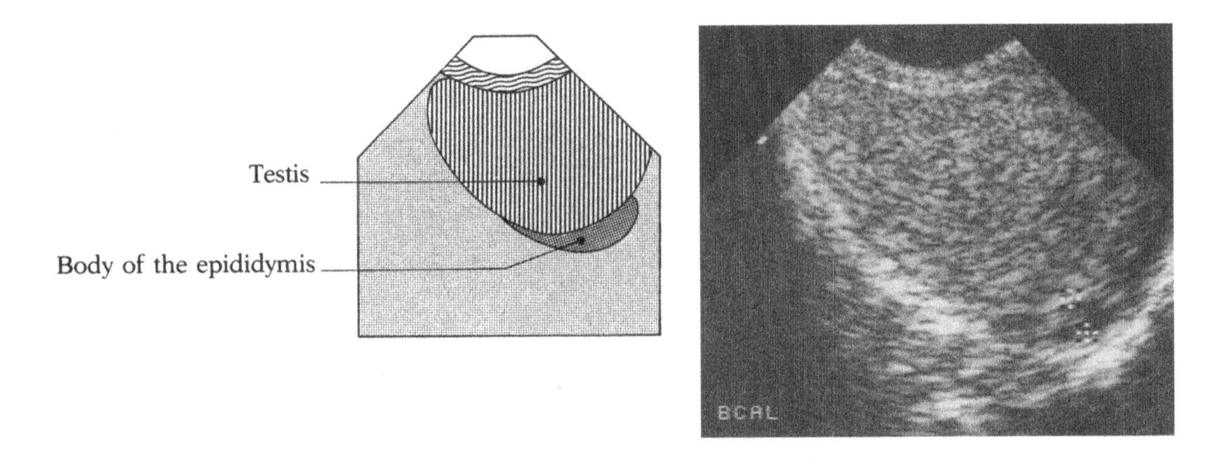

Fig. 9. ***Body of epididymis.*** Sagittal section. A narrow hypo echoic structure of a few millimetres size situated behind the testis, contained within an echogenic border

Embryological vestiges

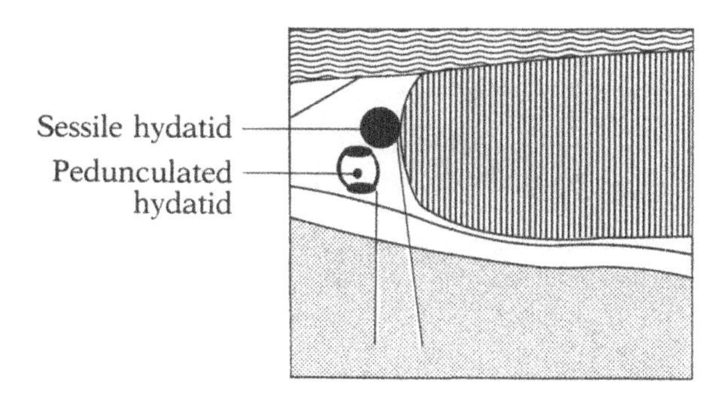

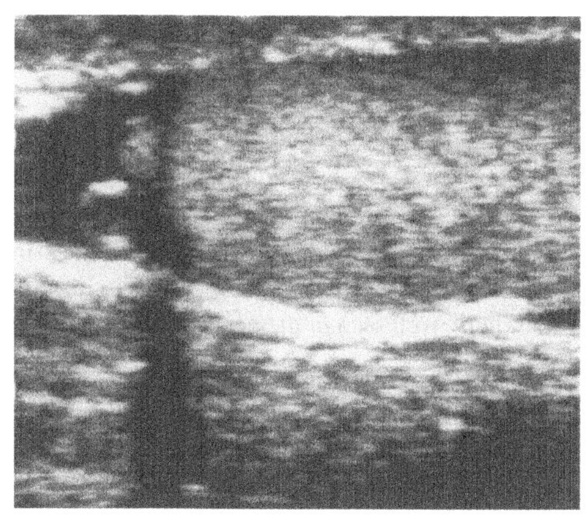

Fig. 10. ***Hydatids of Morgagni.*** Sagittal section. Sessile Hydatid of Morgagni, vestige of the superior extremity of the Mullerian duct, a small fluid-filled structure of a few millimetres in size with variable echogenicity and disappearing at the superior epididymo-testicular junction (due to fibrosis). Pedunculated Hydatid of Morgagni (remnant of the superior extremity of the Wolffian duct), rarer, seen as a small cyst bordered by echoes situated above the head of the epididymis

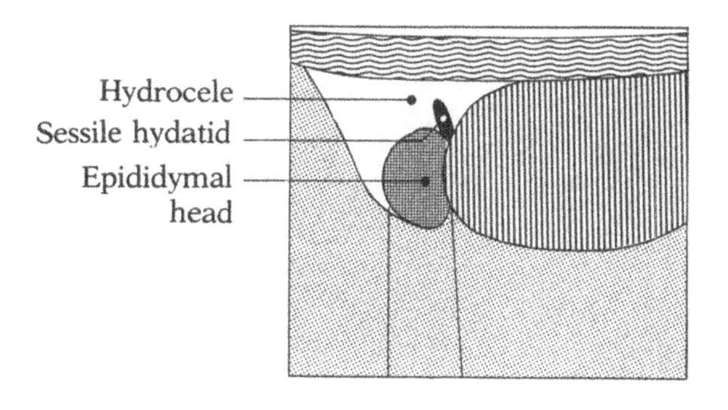

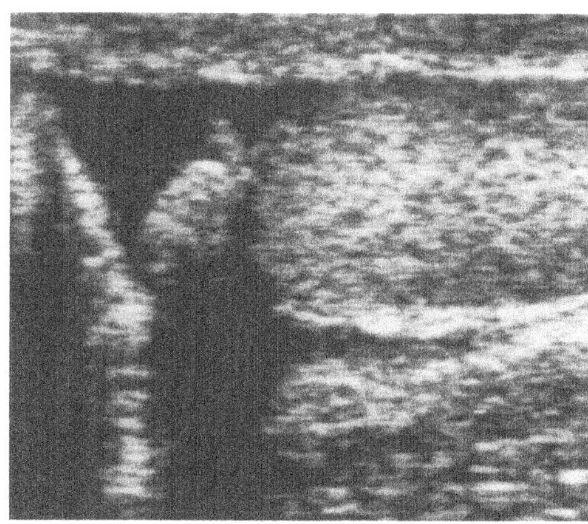

Fig. 11. ***Sessile Hydatid of Morgagni.*** Morphological variant. Sagittal scan. Small hydrocele of the superior pole which surrounds the epididymal head (fibrotic due to resorption) and a sessile hydatid

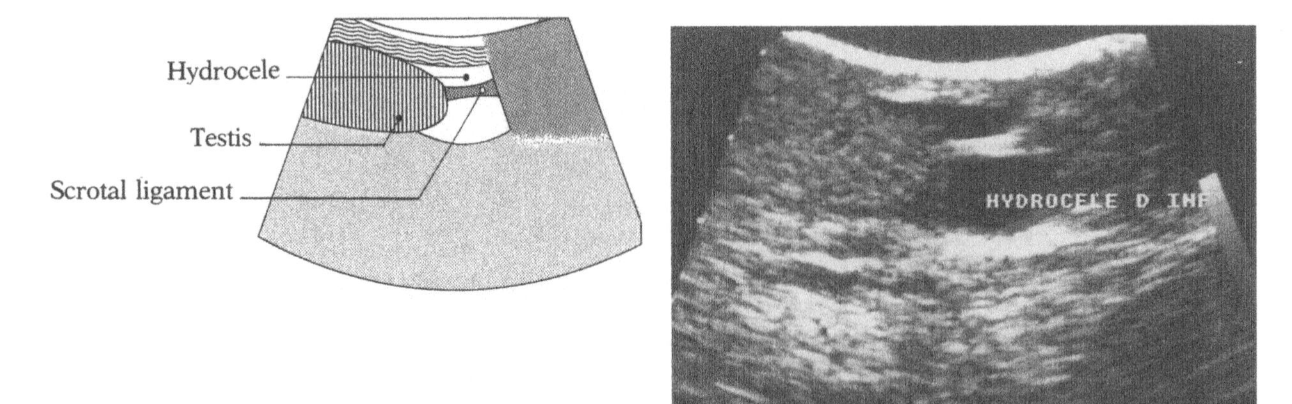

Fig. 12. ***Scrotal ligament.*** Sagittal section of inferior pole. Remnant of the gubernaculum testis and vaginal process. It is a structure made of fibrous connective tissue attaching the inferior pole of the testis and epididymis to the deep surface of the scrotum, well seen in the presence of a hydrocele

Investing layers of the testis

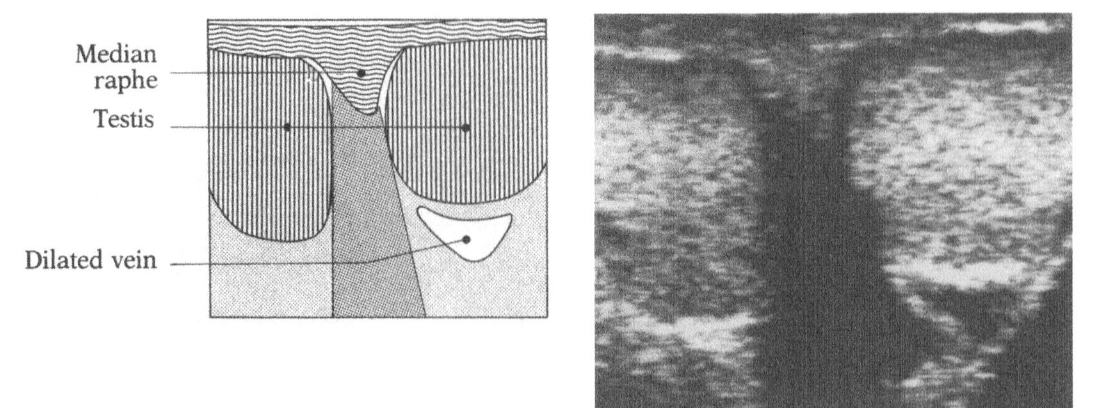

Fig. 13. ***Median Raphe.*** Transverse section comparing the size and echopattern of both testes. The median raphe separates the scrotum into two halves and casts an acoustic shadow behind it. Small left varicocele

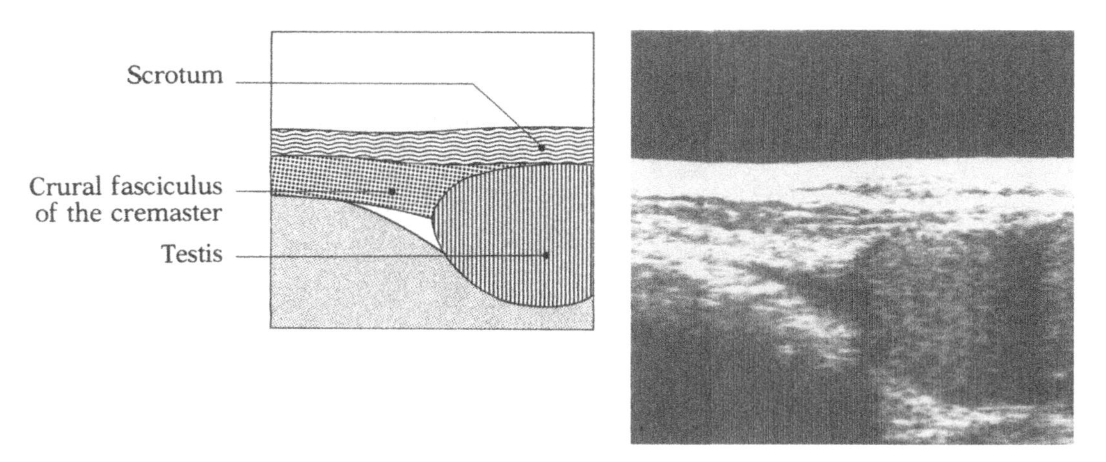

Fig. 14. ***Crural fasciculus of the cremaster muscle.*** Sagittal section of the inguino-scrotal region. The external or crural fasciculus terminates at the level of the testis in the form of a fairly echogenic band, easily identifiable when contracted (cremasteric reflex)

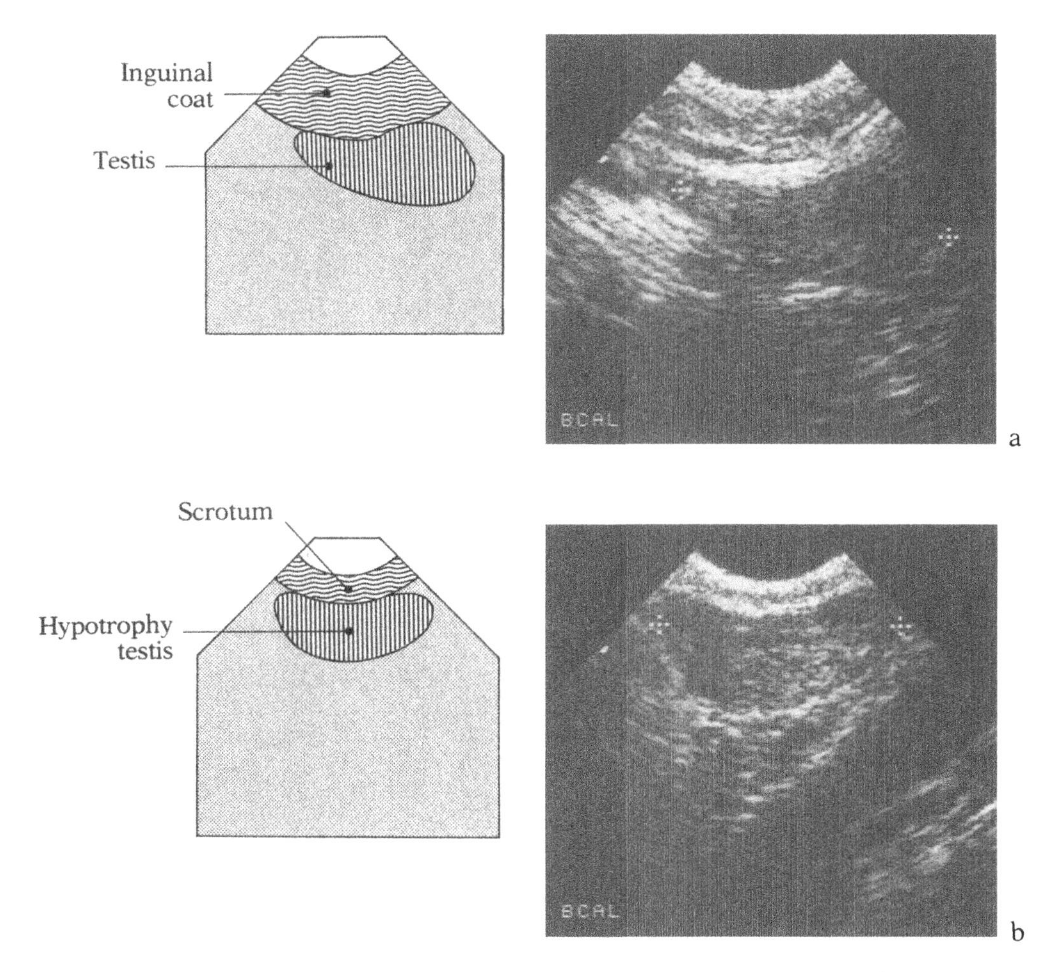

Fig. 15a, b. ***Retractile testis.*** **a** Sagittal section of inguinal region. Inguinal testis, piriform in shape, cramped in the patent peritoneo- vaginal canal. Note the inguinal wall is thicker than the layers of the scrotum. **b** Sagittal section of the scrotum. The testis has been manipulated back into the scrotum. It is of normal echogenicity but of a small volume indicating a degree of testicular hypotrophy

Spermatic cord

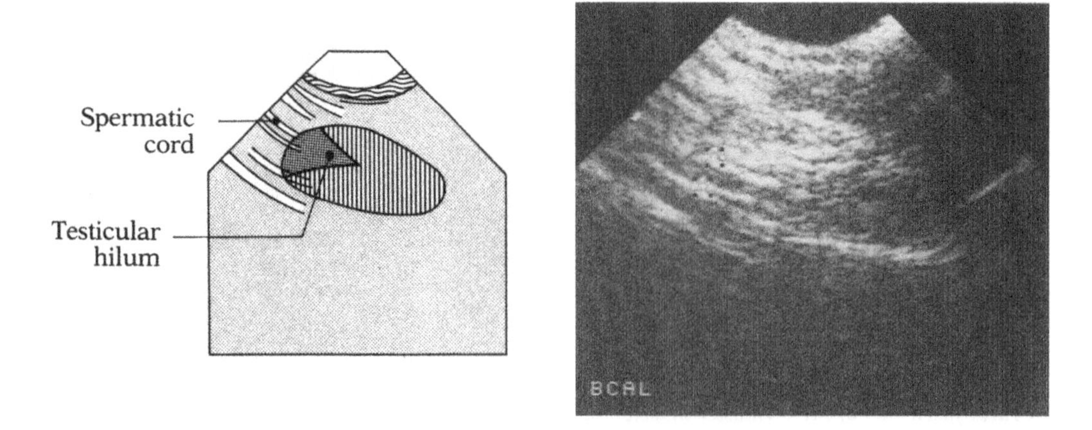

Fig. 16. *Spermatic cord.* Superior oblique section of scrotum. Within a fairly echogenic area due to fibro-fatty tissue are several transonic canals of a few millimetres in size corresponding to the vessels

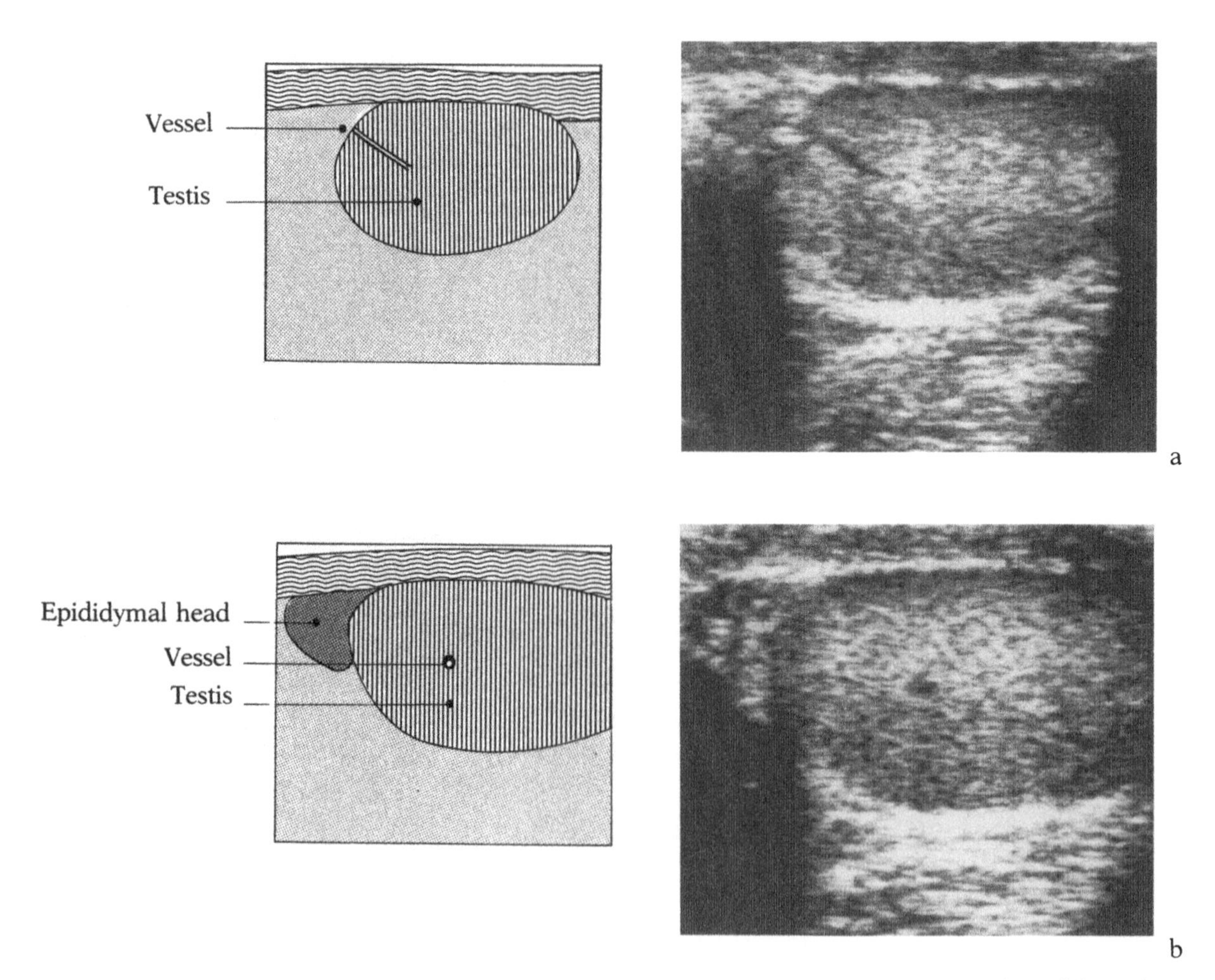

Fig. 17a, b. *Vessels of the testis.* **a** Sagittal section. Transonic tubular vessel over the antero-superior surface of the testis. **b** Transverse section. The vessel is seen as a transonic circular structure without acoustic enhancement posteriorly. In the absence of a varicocele, it corresponds to a normal branch of the testicular artery. A typical Doppler arterial signal can be obtained using pulsed Doppler

The acute scrotum

It is a group of conditions with similar clinical features :

- Sudden onset of signs;
- severe scrotal pain;
- a rapid increase in the size of the scrotal sac;
- the appearance of signs of local inflammation, concomitant or secondary.

There are four major causes for this condition and it may be a difficult diagnostic problem to differentiate them. These are:

- Inflammation of the scrotal contents;
- torsion of the spermatic cord;
- testicular tumours;
- scrotal trauma.

Scrotal ultrasound may be of value in two different clinical contexts (Table 1):

- the commonest is when a firm diagnosis has already been made clinically. The role of ultrasound in this context is to further evaluate the lesion and to assess its severity to guide treatment;
- less commonly, the clinician is uncertain of the diagnosis due to an atypical presentation. Ultrasound is then the examination of choice and should be performed without delay. Its role is diagnostic. In no circumstances must the performance of the ultrasound delay an exploratory orchidotomy when indicated.

Inflammatory conditions of the scrotal contents

For a long time these have been the commonest cause of scrotal pathology. They are almost always of bacterial origin due to sexually transmitted organisms (gonococcus, chlamydia etc.) reaching the scrotum by haematogeneous, lymphatic or direct (urinary reflux) spread. Therefore, there is classically an associated inflammation of the prostate, seminal vesicles or kidneys.

Tuberculosis, although rarely presenting acutely, should always be excluded, particularly in patients with severe periorchitis or in the presence of a septated hydrocele.

Other non-bacterial causes (viral, parasitic, systemic illnesses) are rare and can be suspected by consideration of any relevant previous medial history, ethnic background and clinical context.

Mumps orchitis should also always be considered. This is seen more frequently than bacterial orchitis in atrophic testes but fortunately it is rarely bilateral. The introduction of routine mumps vaccination should lead to its eventual disappearance.

The inflammation can present as epidiymitis, epididymo-orchitis or orchitis with associated funiculitis (of the spermatic cord). The commonest form is epididymo-orchitis.

Ultrasound appearances

- An increase in the volume of either part or all of the epididymis and testis.
- Changes in echo pattern, usually hypo-echoic but sometimes echogenic areas are seen in the subacute phase (corresponding to fibrosis) or in cases of previous epididymitis.

On the other hand the changes in the testis are exclusively a global or localised hypo echogenicity which most often affects the hilum (the most vascular region). In cases of isolated orchitis an analysis of the periphery of the hypo echoic zone is essential; the junction with the healthy parenchyma is indistinct

Table 1. ***Acute testicular enlargement due to inflammation. Diagnostic and therapeutic strategy***

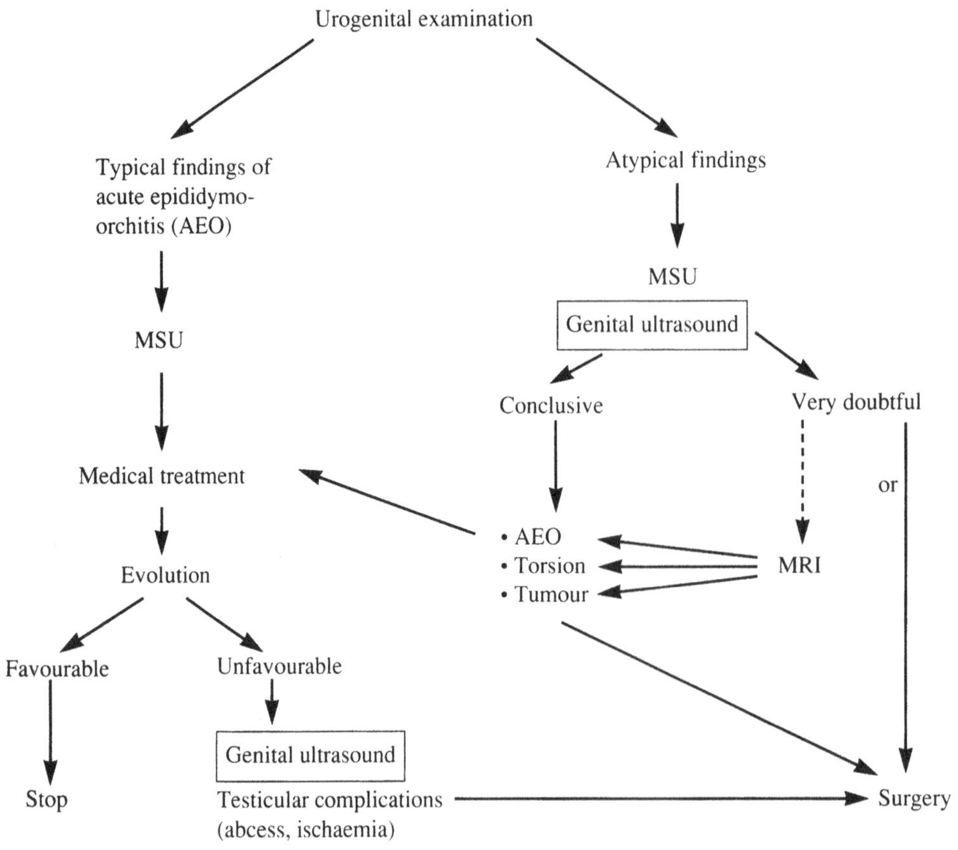

Urogenital examination

Typical findings of acute epididymo-orchitis (AEO)

MSU

Medical treatment

Evolution

Favourable

Stop

Unfavourable

Genital ultrasound

Testicular complications (abcess, ischaemia)

Atypical findings

MSU

Genital ultrasound

Conclusive

Very doubtful

or

• AEO
• Torsion
• Tumour

MRI

Surgery

without any nodularity or specific shape which excludes the possibility of a neoplastic or vascular aetiology.

The presence of echogenic areas in an inflamed testis is rare and should make on question the diagnosis of inflammation. Only a histopathological examination can make the diagnosis of subacute granulomatous orchitis, a rare condition, which gives a pseudo tumour appearance.

- A diffuse thickening of the investing layers of the testis.

- Occasionally there is an associated hydrocele which is always small. If it appears very septated, tuberculosis should be suspected.

Ultrasound can help to monitor treatment, a repeat scan being indicated in the absence of any clinical improvement or if there is a persistent pyrexia.

The scan can assess:

- the *signs of severity* (Table 2) :

•The whole of the epididymis is affected and grossly enlarged with risk of testicular ischaemia due to compression of the vascular pedicle necessitating urgent epididymotomy.

• Marked hypo echogenicity of the testis or small subcapsular, almost anechoic areas indicating necrosis.

• Severe orchitis.

- *Abscess formation.* As a rule this is suspected clinically, but ultrasound can confirm the diagnosis and indicate the location and extent. An abscess appears as a very hypo echoic or anechoic zone sometimes containing a fluid level (layering of necrotic sediment) within the epididymis or less frequently within the testis.

- A *variation of these abnormalities.* If not present, one should reconsider the validity of the initial diagnosis and suspect the presence of a tumour presenting acutely.

In these three circumstances, surgery is indicated, aided by the ultrasound findings. Fortunately, the vast majority of inflammatory conditions affecting the scrotal contents are self limiting requiring medical treatment only.

Table 2. ***Features indicating severe acute epididymo-orchitis***

Diagnostic	
Clinical	Ultrasonic
- Pyrexia, sometimes swinging - Specific area of softening, sometimes painful on palpation - Persistent pain and fever despite medical treatment	- Very enlarged tense epididymis - Very hypoechoic and enlarged testis (presuppurative areas) - Marked periorchitis

Torsions of the spermatic cord

These have several features in common :

- affect adolescents or young adults,

- the most severe presenting symptom is pain,

- they are a surgical emergency due to the risk of ischaemic necrosis and/or haemorrhagic infarction of the testicle resulting in atrophy in the long term.

The only treatment is untwisting of the torsion and bilateral orchidopexy. Delays in diagnosis may result in orchidectomy.

They can also differ in several aspects:

- their type : intra- or extra- vaginal torsion;

- especially in their degree of severity which is related to the number of turns and the tightness of the strangulation. This explains the variable severity of lesions resulting from torsions and is not solely dependent on the time elapsed since the onset of symptoms. Therefore, in cases of a very tight torsion, irreversible testicular damage can occur in a few hours, whereas if the torsion is loose, initial delays in the diagnosis may produce only very mild parenchymal changes and surgical correction can still be of benefit.

Diagnosis by ultrasound is difficult because only atypical cases of torsion, often seen after some delay and simulating suppurative epididymo-orchitis, are referred for an ultrasonic examination.

The ultrasound appearances are varied due to the different forms and the variable delay between the onset of torsion and the performance of the scan (acute to subacute stages up to the tenth day).

Only the unambiguous ultrasound findings which are *helpful in making the diagnosis* will be described :

- Abnormalities of the position of the epididymis and cord, only present if there has been a rotation of 180 degrees along a cranio-caudal or transverse axis; the epididymis or cord passes anteriorly or the epididymal head is rotated beneath the testis.

- Enlargement of spermatic cord greater than 1 cm, usually echogenic (vascular stasis, haemorrhage effusion). The use of pulsed Doppler can be helpful and may demonstrate the absence of an arterial signal from the spermatic artery. However, it must be emphasised that this sign is only seen in cases of a very tight torsion and a persistent Doppler signal does not exclude the diagnosis.

- Hydrohaematocele appearing in the first few hours, sometimes difficult to recognize due to its echogenicity.

- Absence of/or only mild thickening of the investing layers which contrasts with the severity of the other changes seen.

- Normal contra-lateral side.

It is unusual for all these signs to be present in a single case, but the presence of at least two of the first three signs is necessary before a diagnosis of torsion can be made with certainty ultrasonically. Finally, if there is any doubt, an exploratory orchidotomy is justified.

Testicular tumours

Ten per cent of germinal tumours of the testis present acutely, simulating an epididymo- orchitis or torsion. The commonest histological type involved is the embryonic carcinoma which is complicated early on by necrosis and/or haemorrhage resulting in an acute presentation. In fact, these non-seminomatous germinal tumours can be small in size.

On the other hand, seminomas rarely present acutely and when they do, it is usually a large lesion causing testicular enlargement which has been ignored by the patient.

Finally, the spread of the AIDS epidemic has resulted in an increased incidence of testicular lymphoma presenting acutely, occasionally bilaterally, particularly in patients suffering from Kaposi's syndrome.

Ultrasound findings

-Non-seminomatous germinal tumours are seen as a mass lesion, often small and heterogenous within the testicular parenchyma. The ultrasound diagnosis is obvious.

- It is more difficult in the rare acute cases of diffuse seminoma. The negative signs are the most important to differentiate it from epididymo- orchitis; namely, a normal epididymis and absence of thickening of the investing layers.

- In cases of lymphoma, the appearances can be deceptive, especially if bilateral. The key finding is the nodular appearance of the clearly hypo echoic areas within the testis.

In these three circumstances, the results of the ultrasound examination are vital since they confirm the presence of a testicular tumour and lead to surgical exploration by the inguinal approach.

Table 3. ***Principal traumatic lesions of the testis in order of decreasing severity***

Multifragmented and shattered
Fracture - complete - partial width of the breach through the tunica albuginea ± evisceration of the pulp
± Haematoma - subcapsular - perihilar
Contusion

Traumatisms

Only closed trauma of the scrotum, which poses diagnostic and therapeutic problems, will be considered (Table 4).

The majority of authors agree that early surgical intervention in severe trauma (rupture of the tunica albuginea, large haematocele) reduces the risk of testicular necrosis, abscess formation and hence the number of secondary orchidectomies.

Ultrasound has a vital role and may detect severe lesions in the acute situation which were not suspected clinically.

Ultrasound findings

These depend on the severity of the trauma (Table 3).

The shattered testis

Multiple fractures with loss of its normal morphology. In this situation, ultrasound is of little value as the diagnosis is made clinically. Orchidectomy is necessary.

Fracture of the testis

This requires some form of surgical intervention which aims to conserve the whole or part of the testis.

- Either there is a large tear of several centimetres with a disruption of the tunica albuginea and associated evisceration of the parenchyma which is easily recognisable,

- or there is only a limited rupture of the tunica albuginea and it is in these cases where ultrasound may be of value. It may be difficult to recognize and the diagnosis is made with few signs; namely, localised interruption of the echogenic line of the tunica albuginea and loss of the regular contour of the testis.

Haematoceles

These are defined as a blood collection between the two layers of the tunica vaginalis. The ultrasound appearances depend on the age of the haematoma and the degree of liquefaction. When large, they are rarely an isolated finding. Progressive enlargement may be an indication for surgery. In the subacute phase, clots can mask a small testicular fracture. This is why ultrasound should always be performed as early as possible following trauma.

Testicular haematomas

These are usually associated with a fracture. They are rarely an isolated finding and a careful detailed examination of the whole of the testis should be performed. They are seen as hypoechoic zones, often rounded and subcapsular. When present as an isolated finding, no treatment is necessary but a follow-up ultrasound examination three weeks later is indicated in order to exclude an underlying testicular tumour.

Table 4. ***Acute trauma of the scrotum. Diagnostic algorithm***

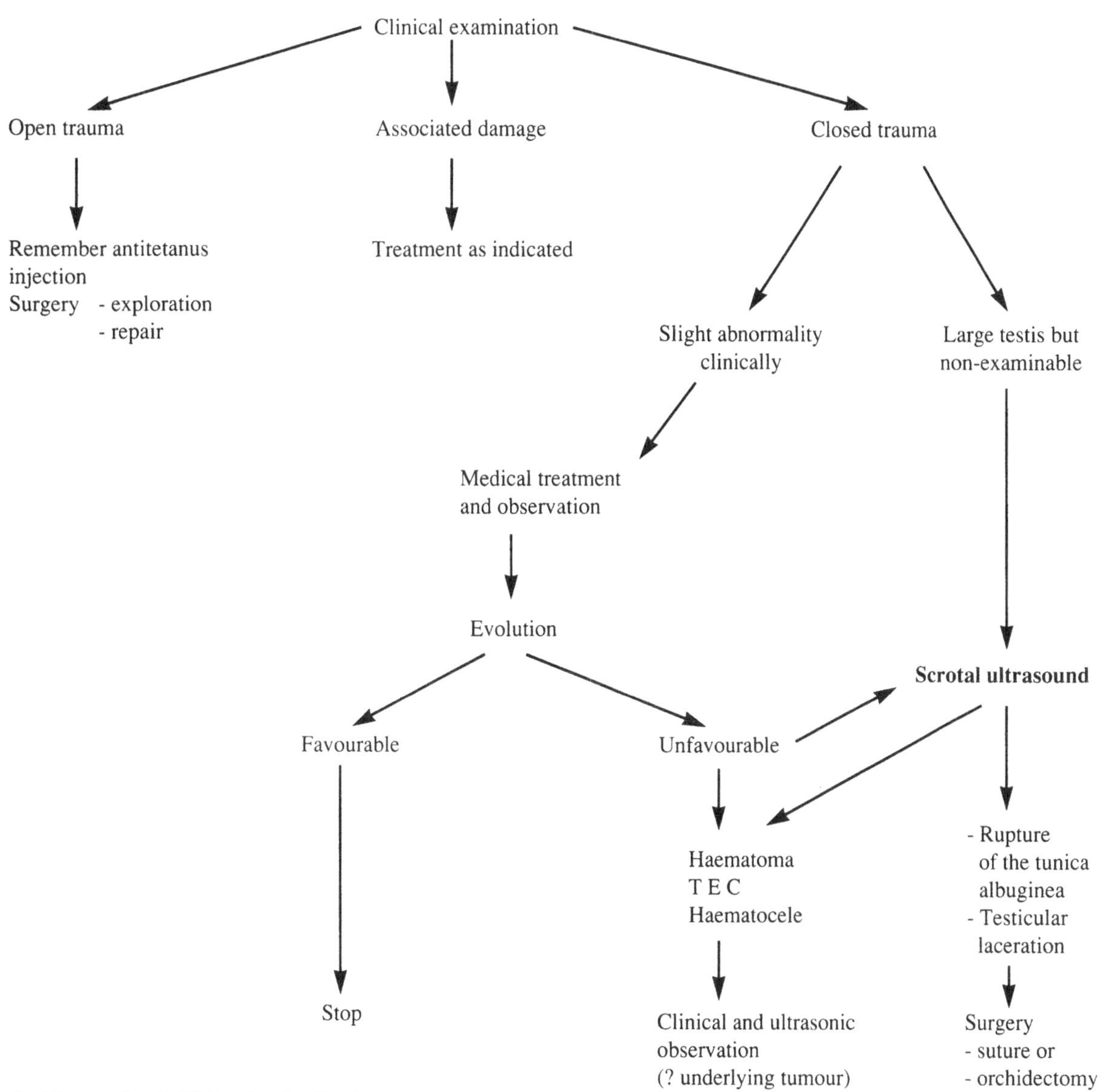

T = Testis ; E = Epididymis ; C = Cord

The acute scrotum

Epididymo- orchitis

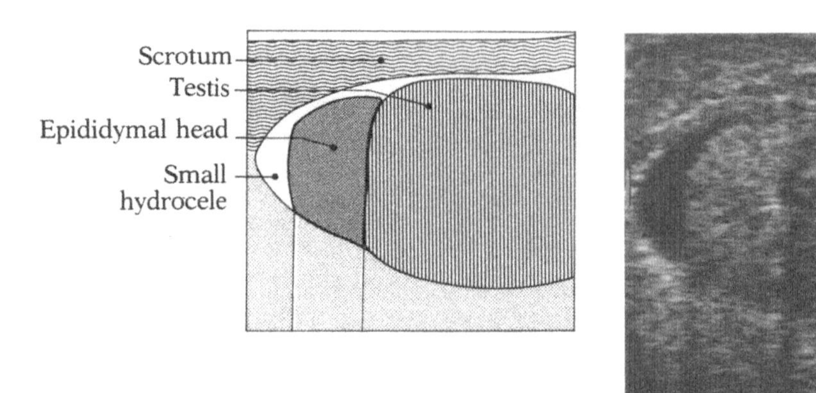

Fig. 1. ***Acute epididymo-orchitis predominantly involving the cephalic portion.*** Sagittal section. Thickened investing layers. Enlarged hyperechoic epididymal head. Markedly swollen testis of uniform hypo echogenicity. Small reactive hydrocele at both poles

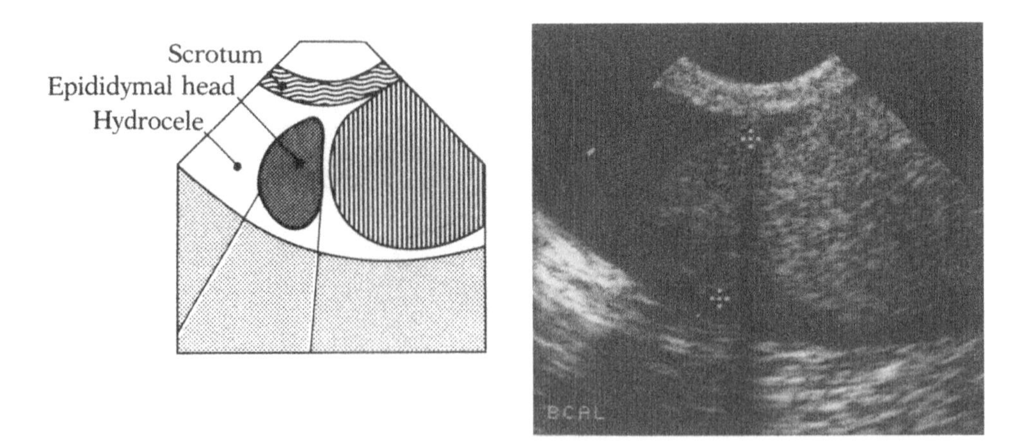

Fig. 2. ***Acute epididymitis of the cephalic portion. Oedematous form.*** Sagittal section of the superior pole. Scrotum virtually normal apart from a large hydrocele. Enlarged epididymal head, parodoxically hypo echoic relative to the testis which is slightly enlarged but retains a normal echo pattern

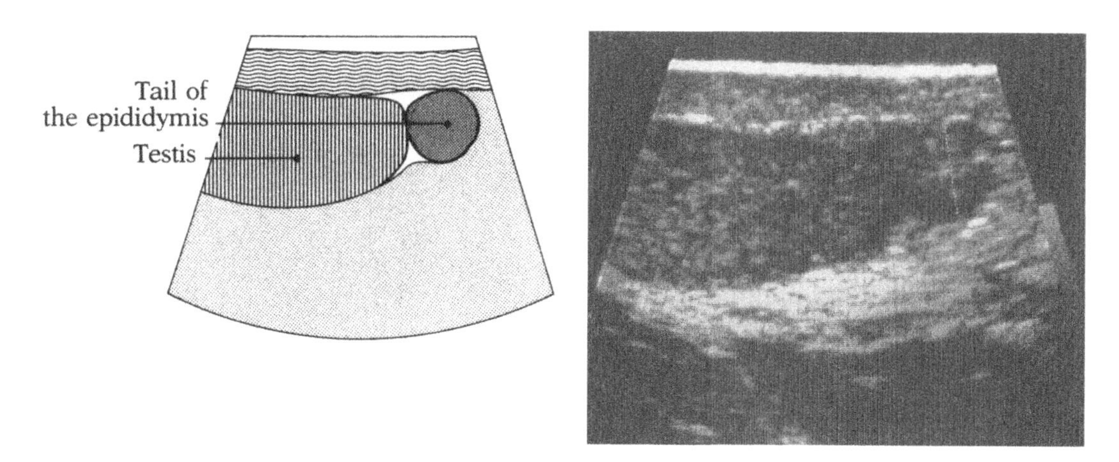

Fig. 3. ***Acute epididymo-orchitis predominantly involving the caudal portion.*** Sagittal section of the inferior pole. Epididymal tail abnormally prominent due to enlargement to almost 1 cm; hypoechoic like the testis

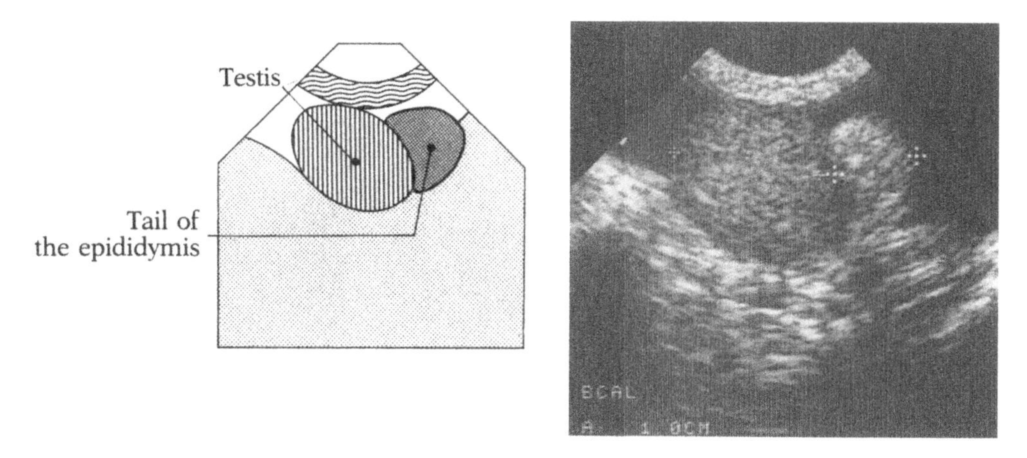

Fig. 4. ***Acute on chronic epididymitis of the caudal portion.*** Transverse section. Enlarged (about 1 cm) hyper echoic (fibrosis) epididymal tail. Normal testis although hypotrophic

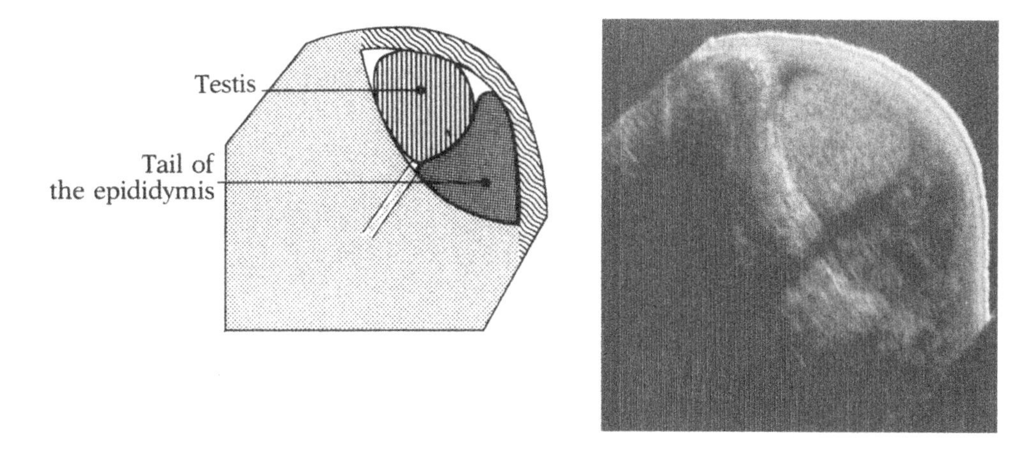

Fig. 5. ***Acute epididymitis affecting the caudal portion.*** Sagittal section. Grossly enlarged epididymal tail. Heterogeneous with areas of hypoechogenicity but no evidence of liquefaction to suggest abscess formation

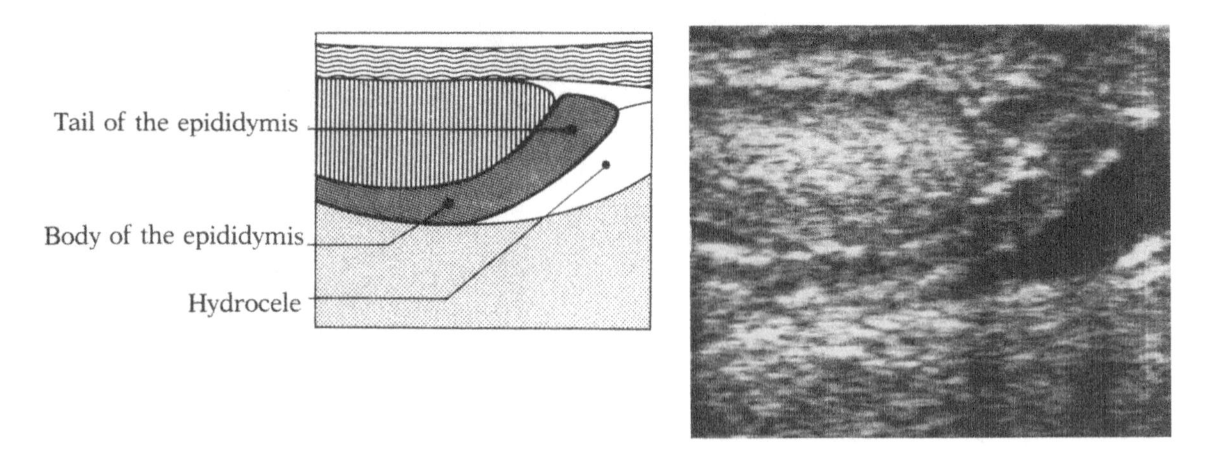

Fig. 6. ***Acute Global epididymitis.*** Sagittal section. Body and tail of epididymis visible due to enlargement, hypoechoic, limited by the echogenic line of the tunica albuginea which outlines a narrow hydrocele at the inferior pole of the testis and fills the postero-inferior interepididymo- testicular recess

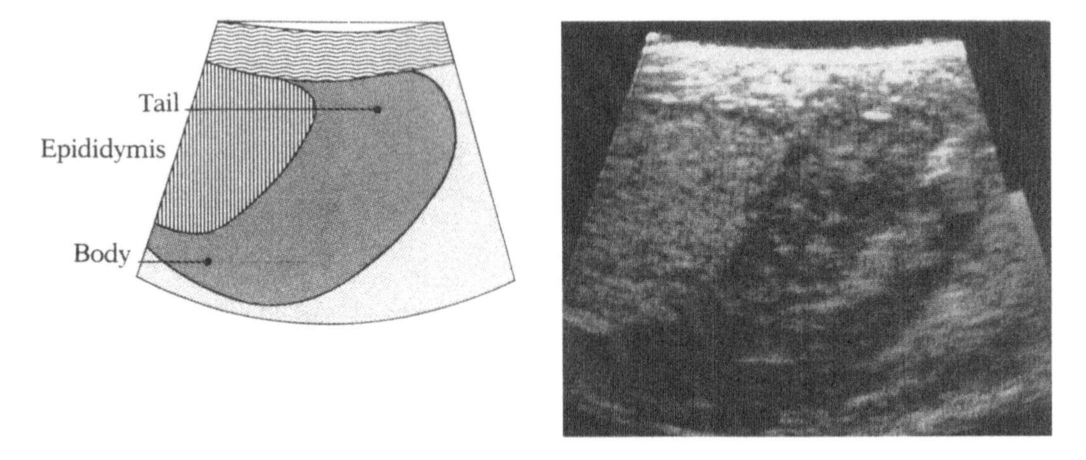

Fig. 7. ***Acute epididymitis affecting the body and tail.*** Oblique section of the inferior pole. Marked enlargement of the body and tail of the epididymis, predominantly hypoechoic and enveloping the testis posteriorly

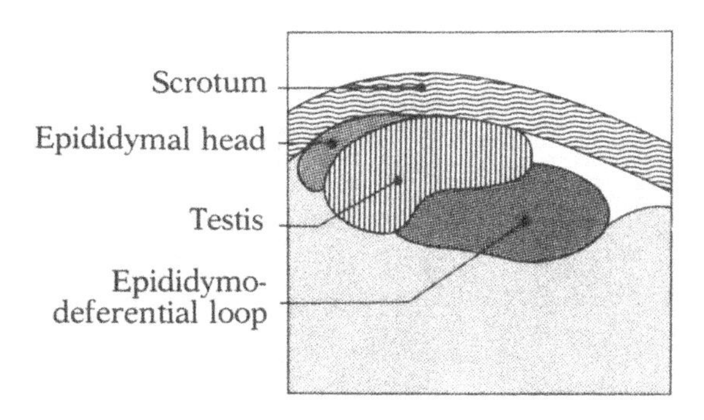

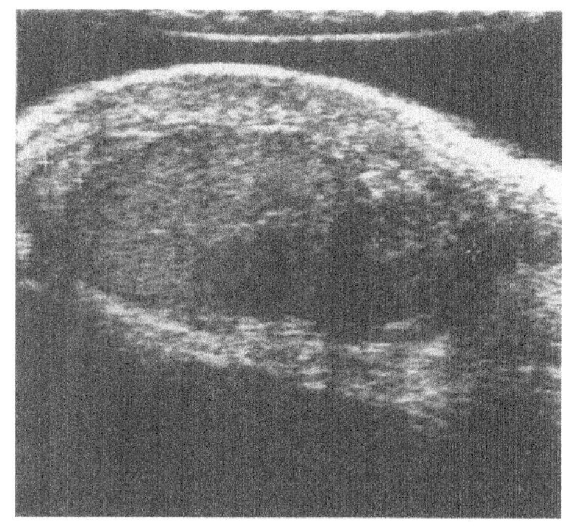

Fig. 8. ***Acute pan-epididymitis.*** Sagittal section. Thickened investing layers. Abnormal epididymis; slight enlargement of the head, appearing abnormally echogenic. Marked tumefaction of the hypo echoic epididymo-deferential loop causing deformity of the testis which has a slightly altered echo pattern

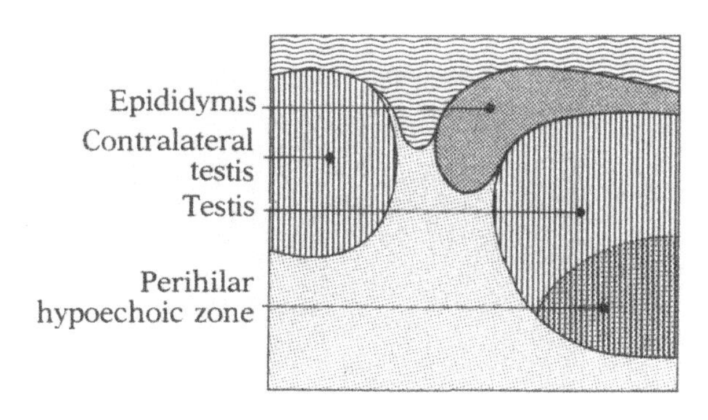

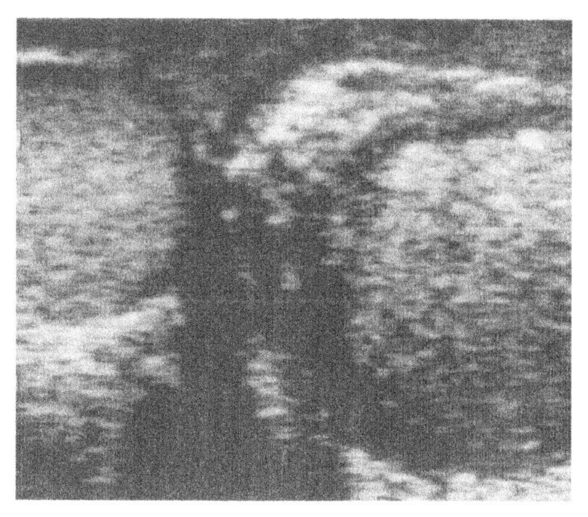

Fig. 9. ***Acute epididymo-orchitis; transverse scan of both testes.*** Abnormalities are evident in the testis compared to the normal contra lateral side; marked enlargement, especially the thickness. Diffuse hypoechogenicity, more pronounced in the perihilar region. Enlarged, fairly echogenic epididymis lying anteriorly (10% of cases)

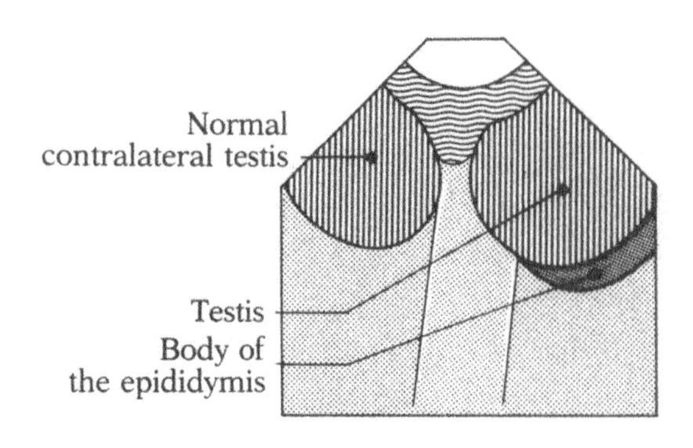

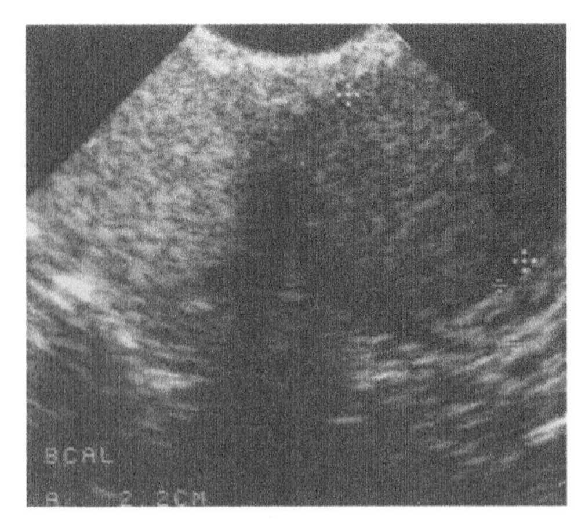

Fig. 10. ***Acute epididymo-orchitis; transverse scan of both testes.*** Testis relatively slightly enlarged but very hypoechoic relative to the normal contra lateral side. Abnormally clear visualisation of the body of the epididymis which appears hyperechoic. Overall, the inflammation has affected primarily the testis and this justifies a careful follow-up clinically and ultrasonically to detect signs of necrosis

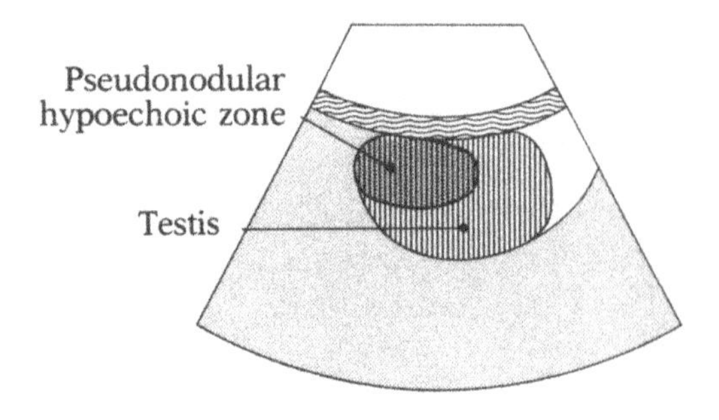

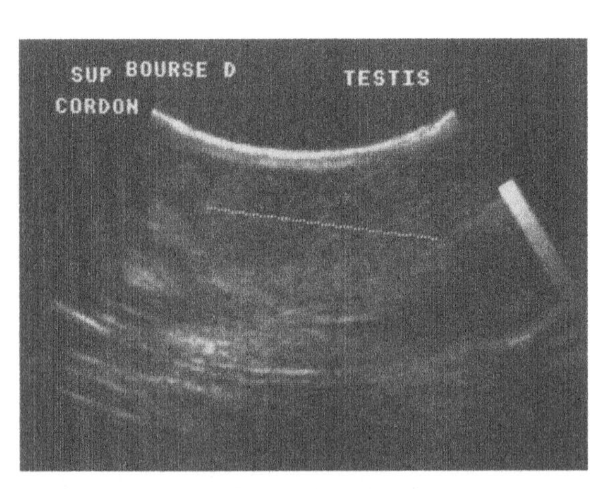

Fig.11. ***Mumps orchitis.*** Sagittal section. No epididymal enlargement. Normal size testis but a poorly defined area of hypoechogenicity is seen anteriorly. Only the clinical context can give the diagnosis of mumps orchitis; a patient of less than 25 years old presenting with a painful testis, slightly enlarged, with associated bilateral parotid swelling and gastro-intestinal problems. The ultrasound finding alone is non-specific, a pseudo tumour

The spermatic cord

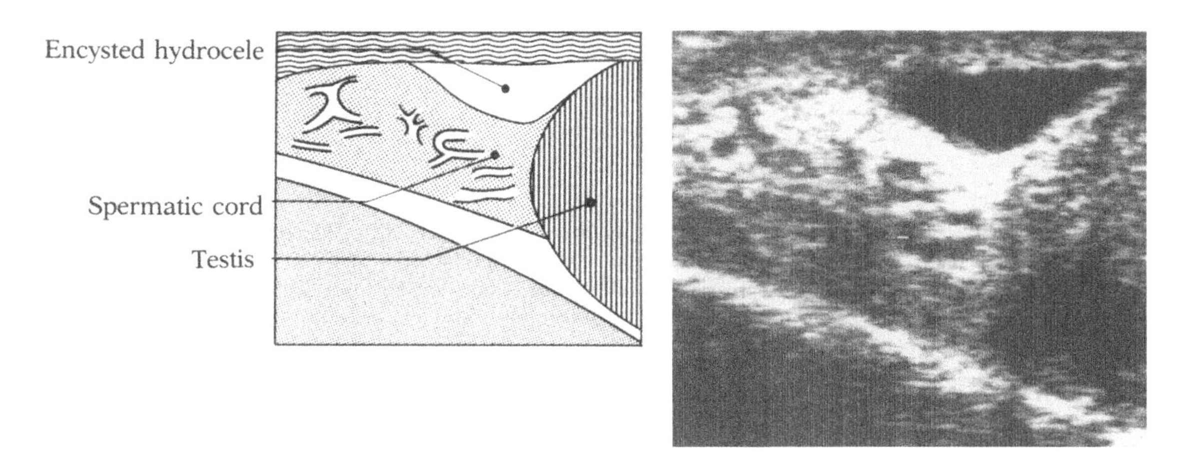

Fig. 12. ***Epididymo-testicular inflammation; associated changes in the spermatic cord.*** Sagittal section through the cord and superior part of the testis; apparent increase in the echogenicity of the fibrous connective tissue in the cord, through which run numerous small dilated vascular structures indicating localised hyperaemia. Small encysted hydrocele

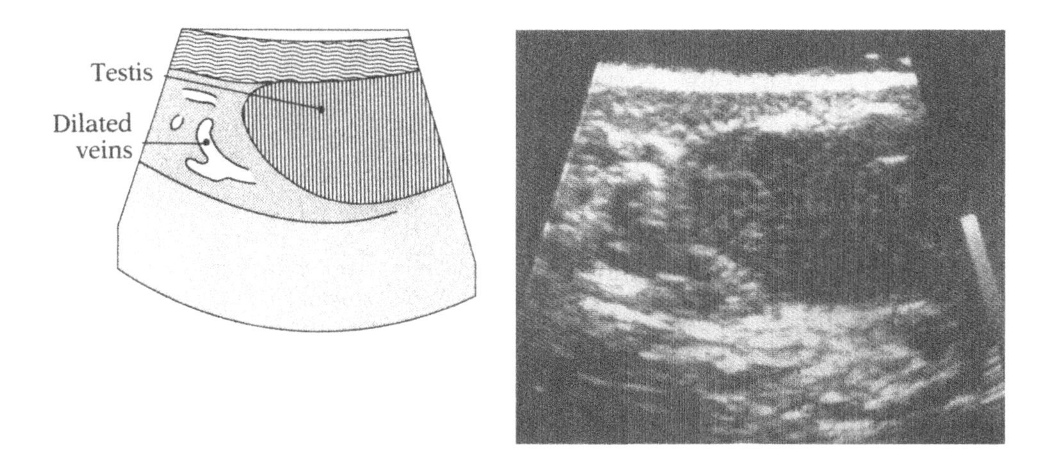

Fig. 13. ***Acute inflammation of scrotal contents abnormalities of the spermatic cord.*** Sagittal section of the superior half of the testis. Severe orchitis (frankly hypoechoic testis) associated with dilated vessels in the cord giving the appearances of varicosities; the appearances are more suggestive of a varicocele enlarged by local inflammation than simply a dilatation of the veins secondary to hyperaemia. However,only the persistence of a varicocele some time after the acute episode can confirm the diagnosis. In any case, the real size of the varicocele cannot be determined in the acute phase due to enlargement as a result of the local inflammation

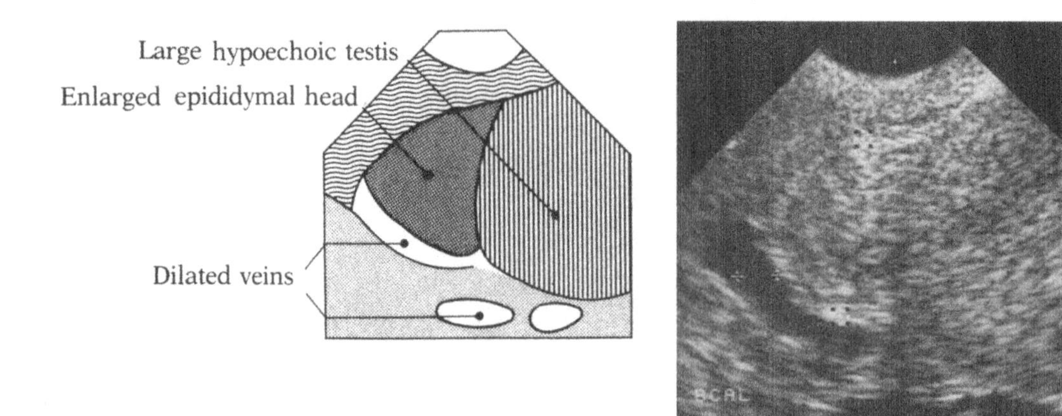

Fig. 14. ***Acute inflammation of the scrotal contents; associated varicocele.*** Section at the same level. Marked acute epididymo-orchitis associated with clear dilatation (greater than 5 mm) of the veins of the anterior spermatic plexus; this degree of dilatation indicates a definite associated varicocele in this case. However, the appearances may be aggravated by the associated hyperaemia

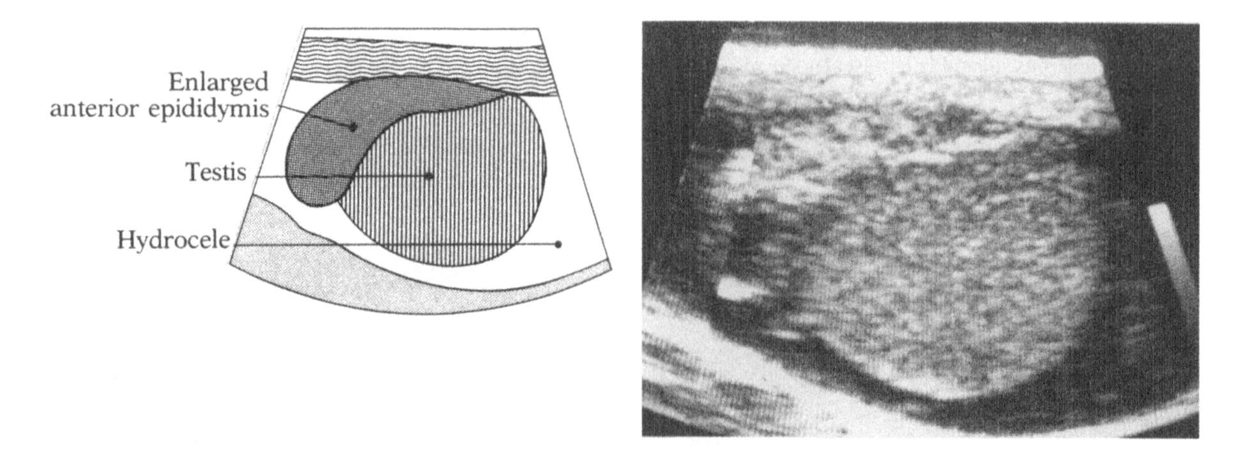

Fig. 15. ***Acute inflammation of the scrotal contents; differential diagnosis with torsion of the spermatic cord.*** Sagittal section. Anterior position of the epididymis which is enlarged and echogenic, especially in the head. It can be differentiated from a torsion along the cranio-caudal axis by: thickening of the investing layers, a hydrocele which is not septated and above all, the absence of an enlarged echogenic cord situated in an abnormally anterior position. However, sometimes a firm diagnosis is not possible and in these cases an exploratory scrototomy is indicated

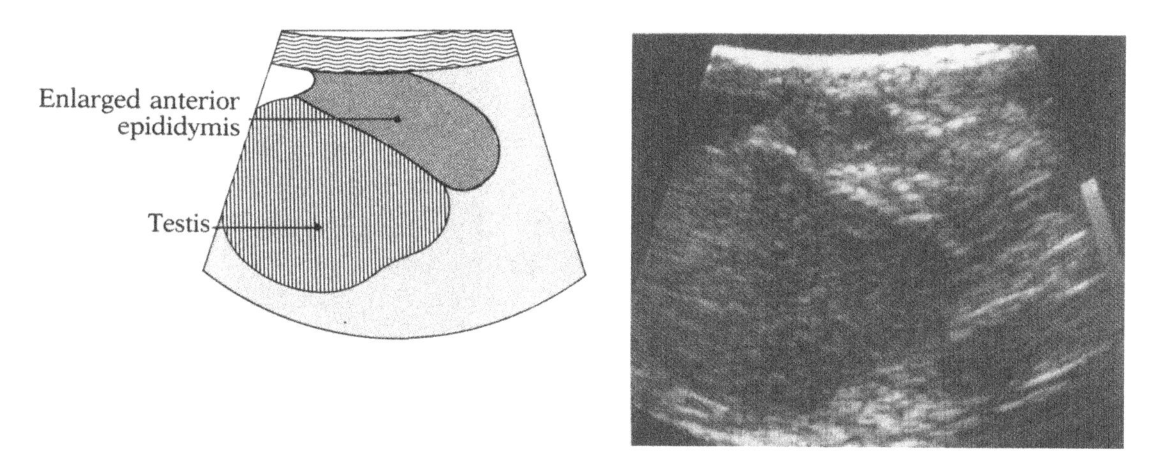

Fig. 16. ***Acute inflammation of scrotal contents; differential diagnosis with torsion of the spermatic cord.*** Sagittal section of the inferior pole. Anterior position of the epididymis which is echogenic and enlarged, particularly in the region of the tail. The diagnostic criteria are the same with, in addition, visualisation of an homogenous hypoechoic testis and enlargement of its width

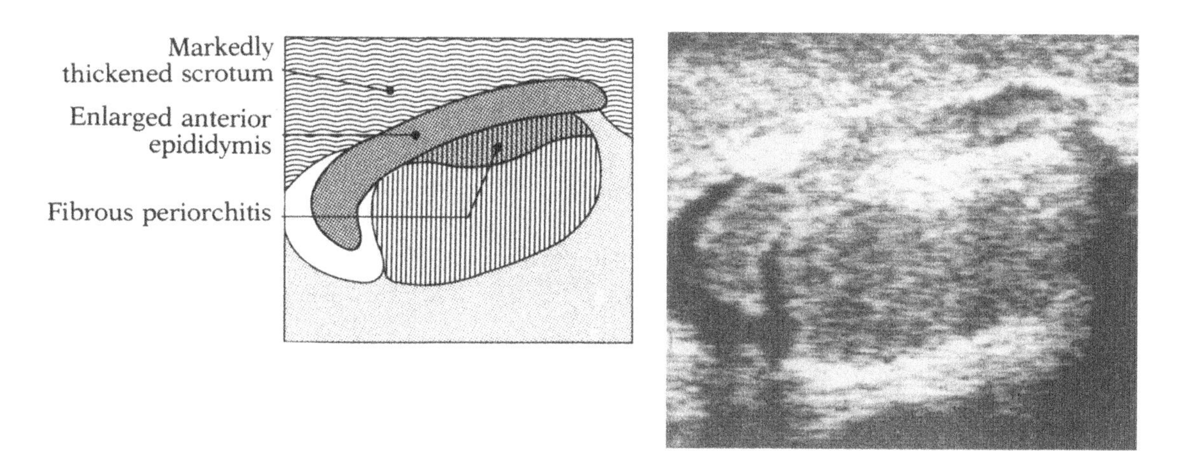

Fig. 17. ***Acute inflammation of the scrotal contents; differential diagnosis with torsion of the spermatic cord.*** Sagittal section. Anterior position of the epididymis which is enlarged in all three segments and appears heterogeneous. In this case the differentiating feature is a marked thickening of the investing layers which are attached to the body of the epididymis. This is only seen in inflammatory conditions

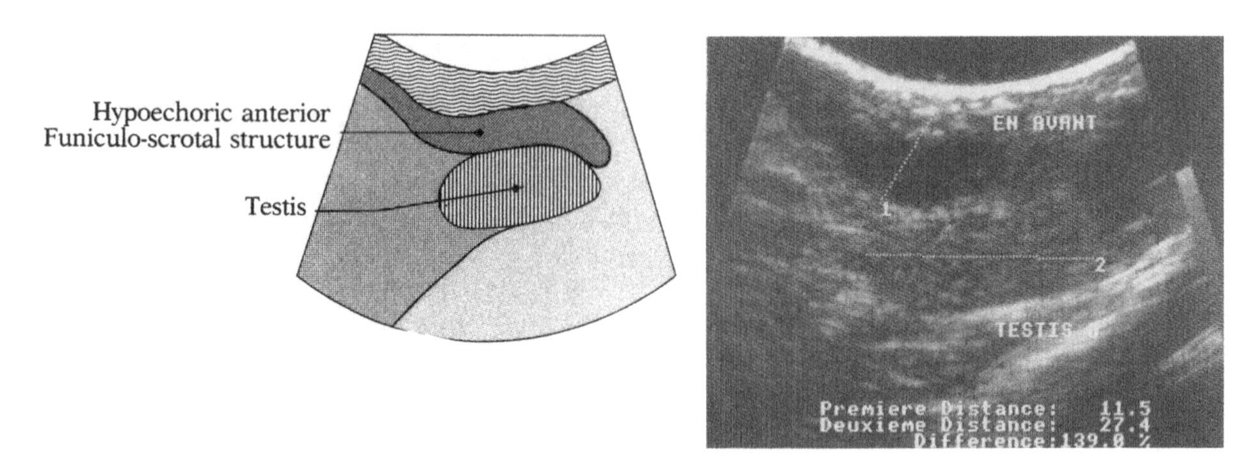

Fig. 18. ***Acute inflammation of the scrotal contents; differential diagnosis with other pathology of the spermatic cord.*** Previous history of orchidopexy for ectopic testis. Finger shaped anterior hypoechoic structure leading towards the inguinal canal. The testis is displaced posteriorly, has a normal echo pattern but appears atrophic (reduced thickness). Abnormal position of the junction of the epididymis and cord as a result of the orchidopexy. The features against this being a torsion (which is not excluded but excessively rare after orchidopexy) are: the hypoechogenicity of the structure and the small testis with a normal echo pattern. Conclusion: Oedematous funiculo-epididymitis with pseudo tumour formation (surgically proven)

The investing layers

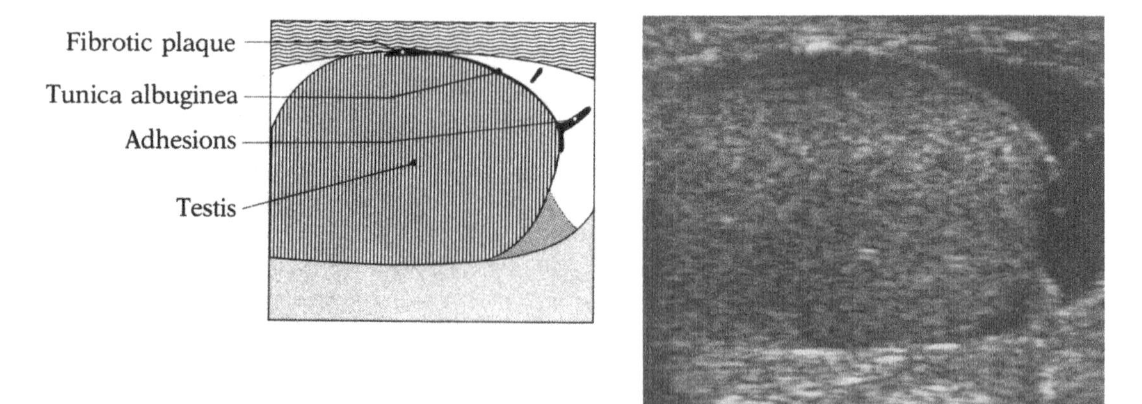

Fig. 19. ***Acute inflammation of the scrotal contents;investing layers.*** Sagittal section of the inferior pole. Enlarged hypoechoic testis. Tunica albuginea is well seen with some echogenic fibrotic plaques. Small reactive hydrocele. The parietal layer of the tunica vaginalis is adherent to the inferior pole of the testis

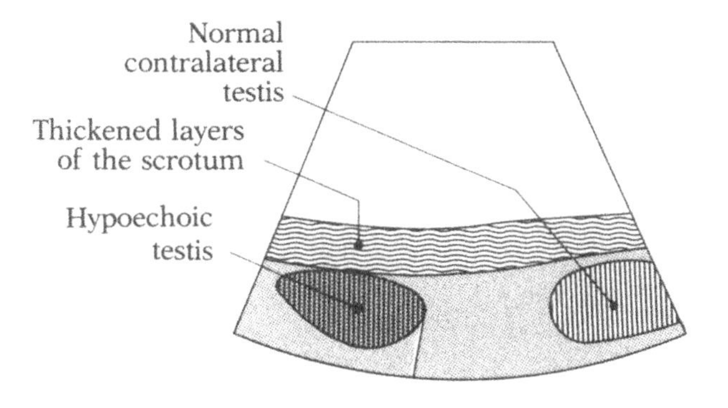

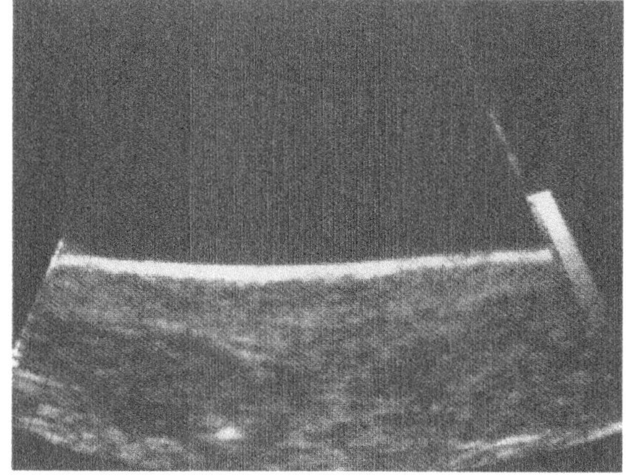

Fig. 20. ***Acute inflammation of the scrotal contents; investing layers.*** Transverse section of both testes. The testes are high in position, small and are held in a small capacity scrotum. Orchitis of the hypotrophic testis (hypoechoic relative to the opposite side). The slight thickening of the investing layers is made more prominent by the plane of the section through the cremasteric fasciculi and the high position of the testes

Severe forms and complications

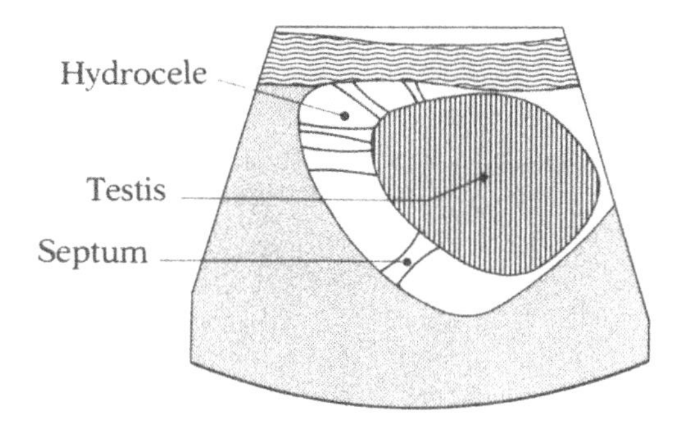

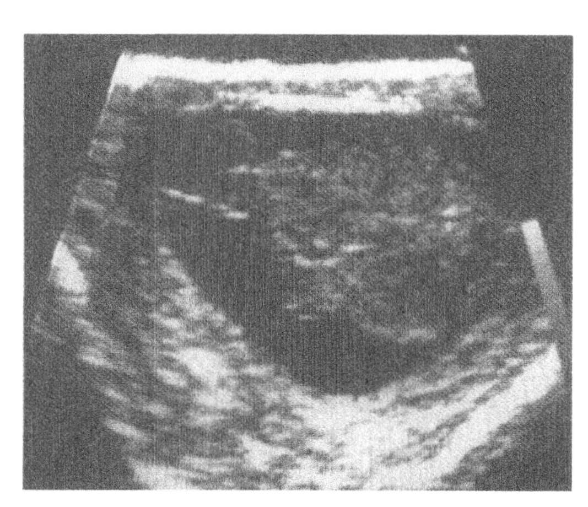

Fig. 21. ***Acute inflammation of the scrotal contents; investing layers; signs of severity.*** Transverse section. Orchitis associated with a small septated hydrocele; the severity of this periorchitis raises the possibility of tuberculosis which should be excluded

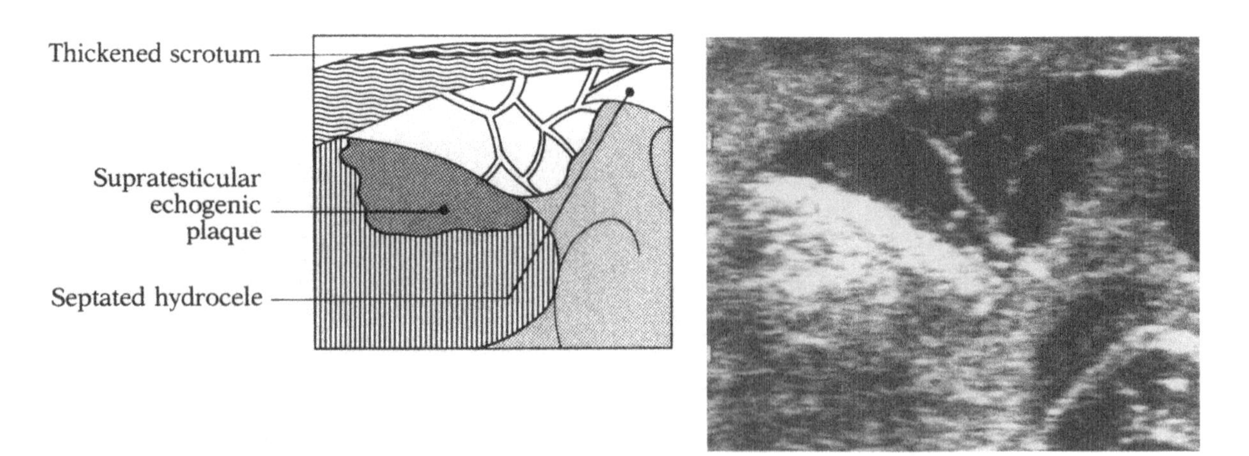

Fig. 22. ***Acute inflammation of scrotal contents; investing layers; signs of severity.*** Oblique section of the inferior pole. The severity of the epididymo- orchitis is indicated by the intense periorchitis: hyperechogenic areas covering the inferior pole of the testis; very thickened investing layers; septated hydrocele

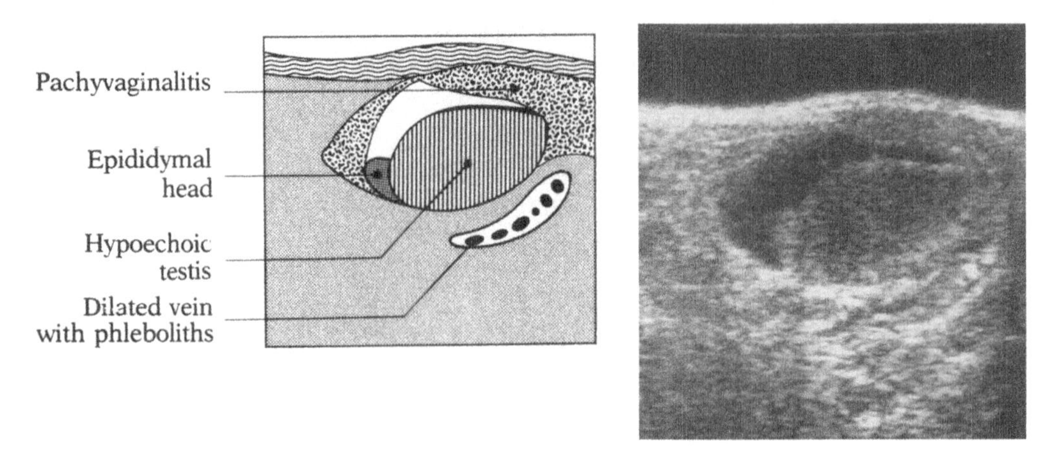

Fig. 23. ***Acute inflammation of the scrotal contents; investing layers; signs of severity.*** Sagittal section. Severe orchitis is shown by the definite hypoechogenicity of the parenchyma (tunica albuginea abnormally prominent), thickening of the investing layers, particularly of the parietal layer of the tunica vaginalis, a pseudo tumour appearance. Note the phleboliths, hyperechoic flecks in the cremasteric plexus of this elderly diabetic

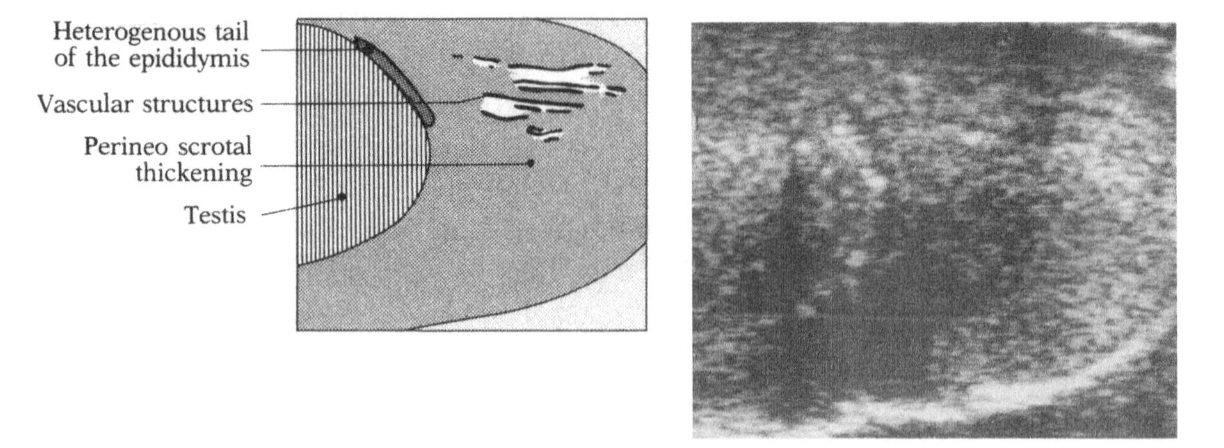

Fig. 24. ***Acute inflammation scrotal contents; investing layers; signs of severity.*** Oblique section of the perineo-scrotal junction. Very severe epididymo-orchitis: heterogenous epididymal tail (barely distinguishable from the testis), punctuated by areas of hyperechogenicity. Heterogenous thickening by several centimetres of the base of the scrotum extending into the anterior perineum with small veins running through. Major risk of fistula formation

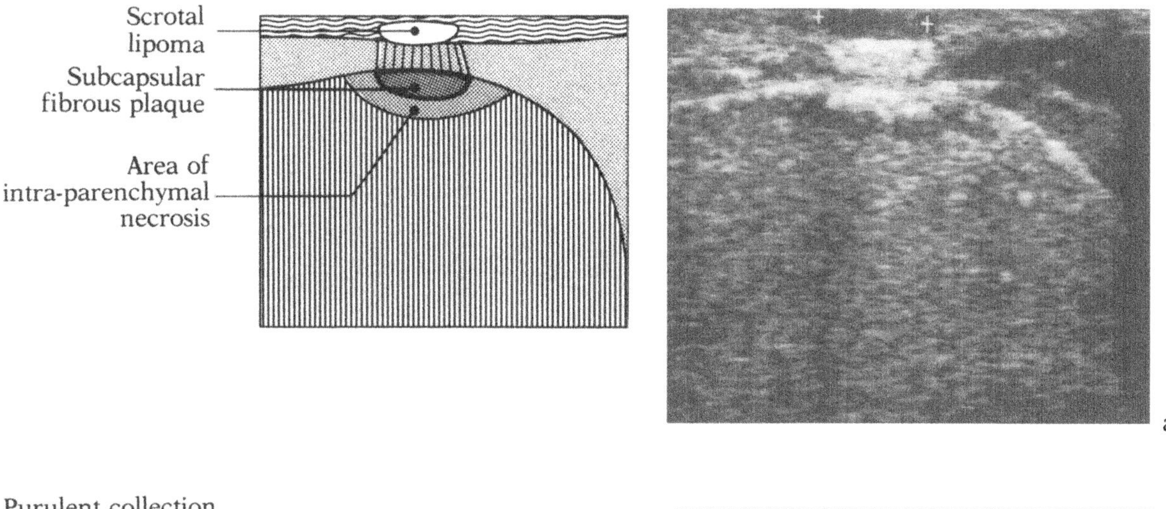

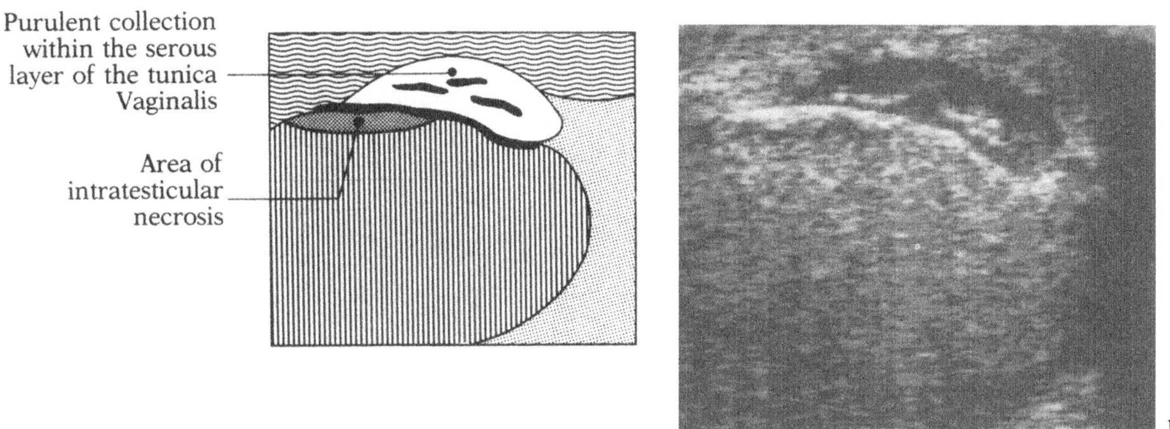

Fig. 25a, b. ***Acute epididymo-orchitis. Complications. Testicular necrosis.*** No improvement clinically with medical treatment. Palpable area of softening within the testis. **a** Sagittal section. Enlargement of the antero- medial portion of the scrotum. Two abnormalities are evident: a scrotal lipoma of about 1 cm (regular hypoechoic nodule) whose acoustic posterior enhancement must not hide the changes in the underlying testis; localised fibrotic thickening of the tunica albuginea surrounding a well circumscribed hypoechoic halo within the testis: necrosis confirmed surgically. **b** Enlargement of the inferior pole of the testis. A small purulent collection with a fluid level is shown anterior to the necrotic area in the testis

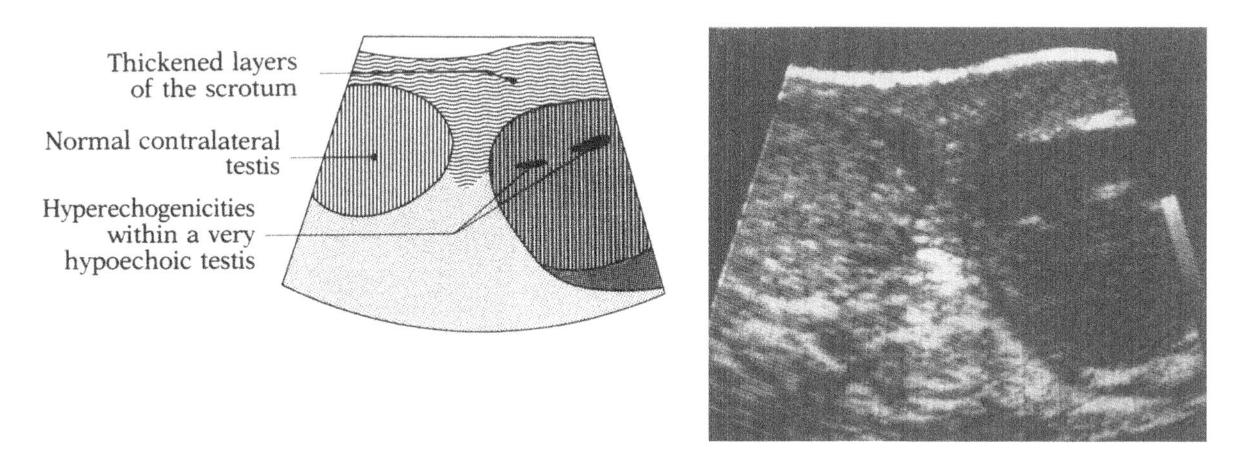

Fig. 26. ***Acute epididymo-orchitis. Cutaneous complications.*** Transverse section through both testes. Severe orchitis (marked hypoechogenicity) with thickening of the investing layers, including the median raphe, mainly hypoechoic punctuated with several small hyperechoic areas. These findings would suggest possible fistula formation and is an indication for parenteral antibiotic treatment

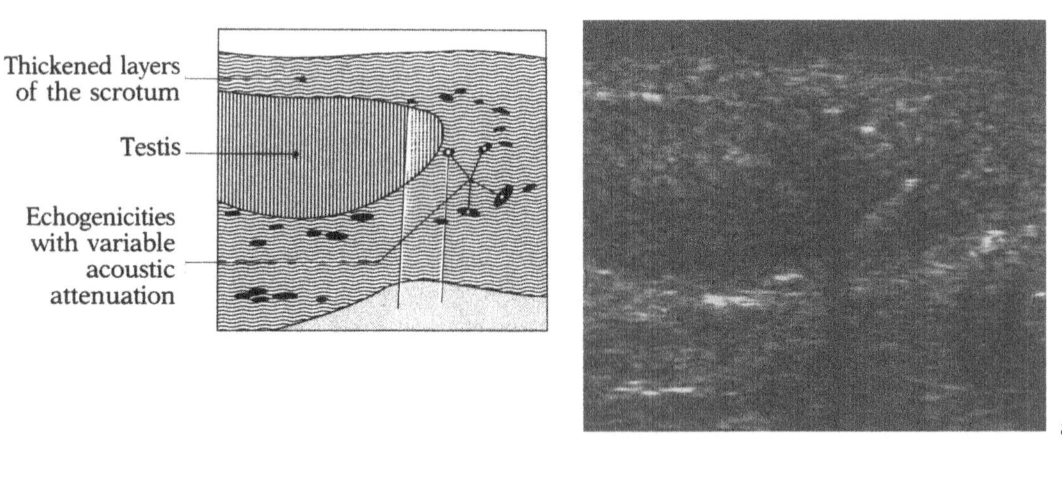

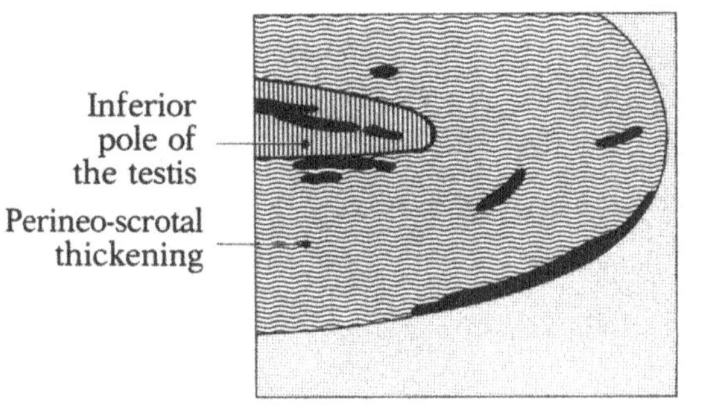

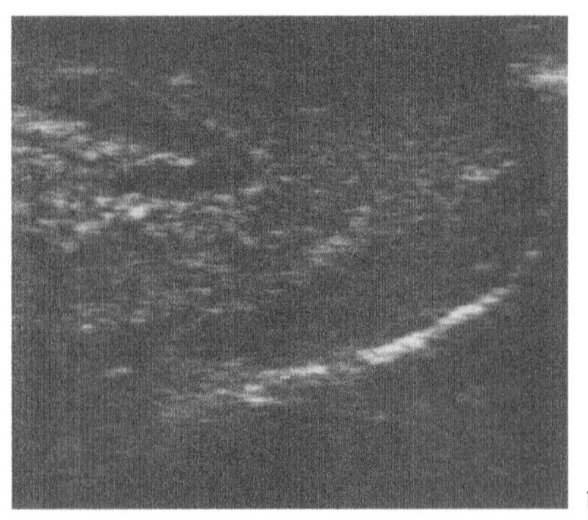

Fig. 27a, b. ***Hyperacute pseudo- gangrenous perineo- scrotal candidiasis.*** Patient on chemotherapy. Pancytopenia. Presented with a pyrexia and severe tumefaction, pain and inflammation of the scrotum and perineum. **a** Sagittal section of inferior pole. Healthy testis but surrounded, particularly at the inferior pole by a massive hypoechoic infiltration of the investing layers with attenuating echogenicities giving the appearance of pseudogangrene. **b** Section through the perineoscrotal area.The cutaneous and subcutaneous infiltration extends to the perineum anteriorly. Conclusion: The picture suggests Fournier gangrene; it was, in fact, a hyperacute candidiasis confirmed by the isolation of Candida Albicans and the rapid response to parenteral antifungal treatment

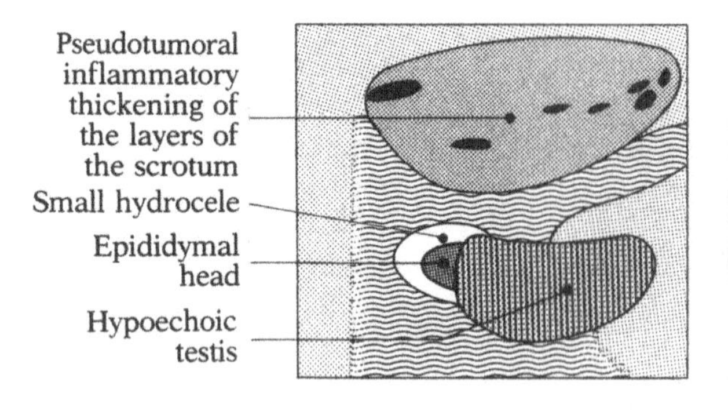

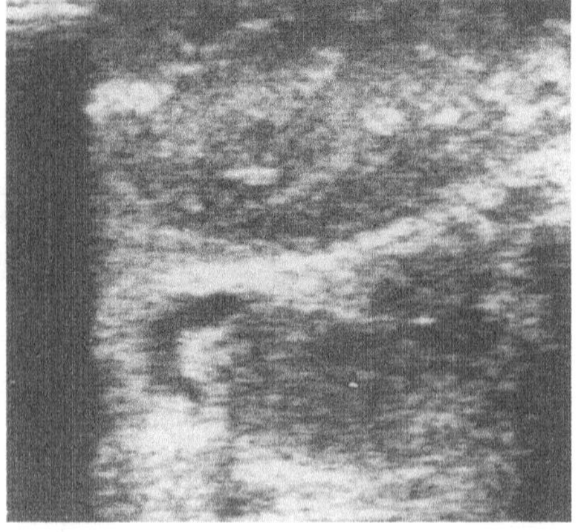

Fig. 28. ***Acute inflammation of the investing layers of the testis; pseudo tumour appearance.*** Sagittal section (slightly magnified). Epididymo- orchitis (hypoechoic testis, echogenic epididymal head surrounded by a hydrocele) adjacent to an inflammatory, heterogeneous and presuppurative mass involving the investing layers, a true pseudo tumour. Risk of cutaneous fistula formation

Torsions of the spermatic cord

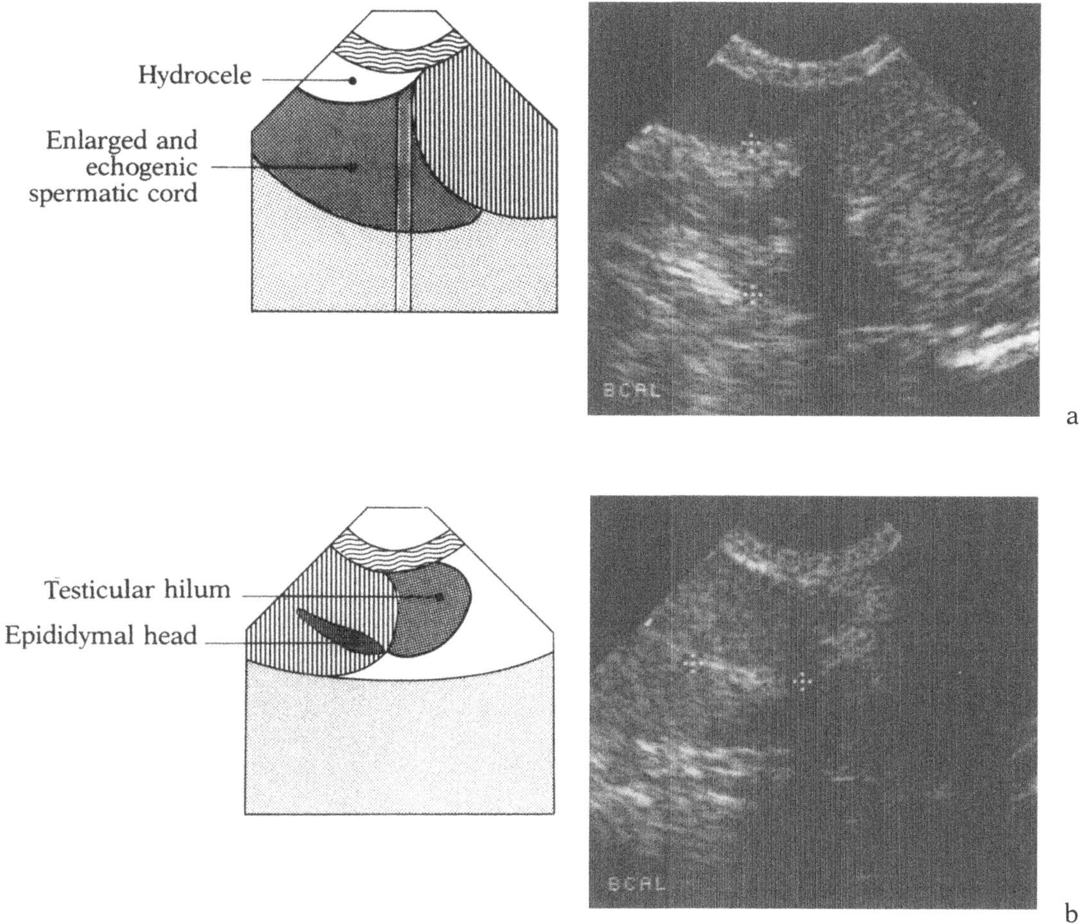

Fig. 29a, b. ***Acute 180 degree torsion of the spermatic cord.*** Ultrasound performed six hours after onset of pain. **a** Sagittal section of the superior pole of testis. Spermatic cord clearly enlarged, greater than 1.5 cm and abnormally hyperechoic. Small reactive hydrocele. Non-visualisation of the epididymal head. **b** Sagittal section of the inferior pole of testis. Abnormal position of the epididymal head (slightly enlarged and echogenic) and the hilum of the testis. Cranio-caudal rotation of 180 degrees of the epididymis and testis due to torsion of the cord. Surgical confirmation. Surgical untwisting and orchidopexy

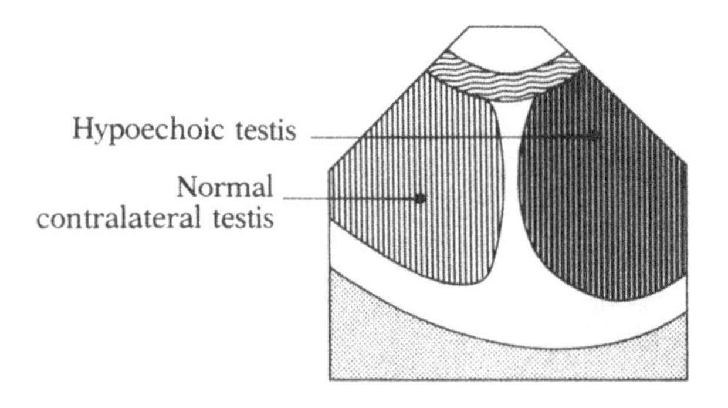

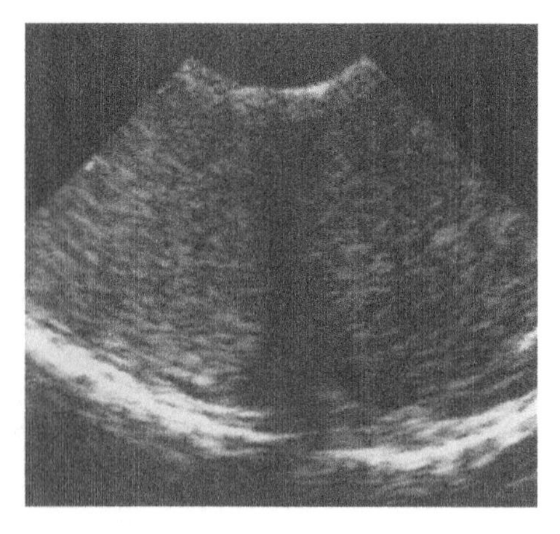

Fig. 30. ***Acute torsion of the spermatic cord; transverse sections of both testes.*** On the side of the torsion, the left, the testis is hypoechoic and enlarged compared to the normal side. The changes are due to venous stasis caused by torsion of the vascular pedicle

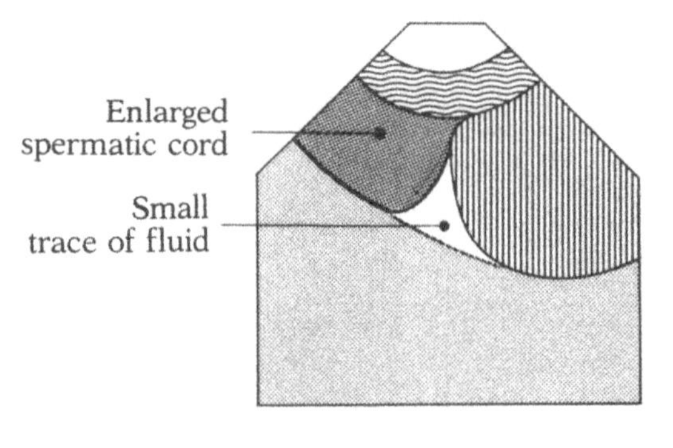

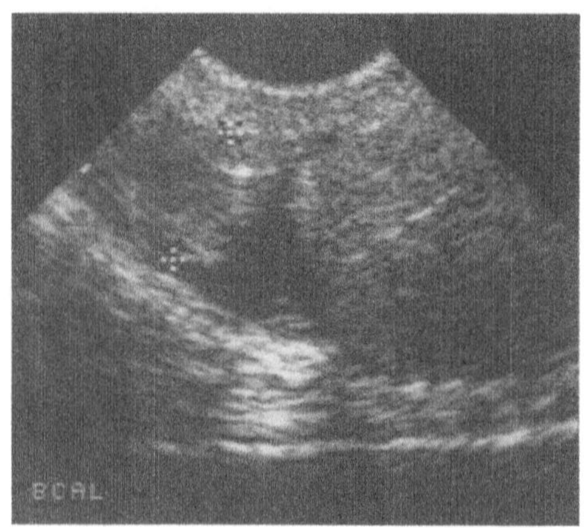

a

Spermatic cord

Epididymal head

Testis

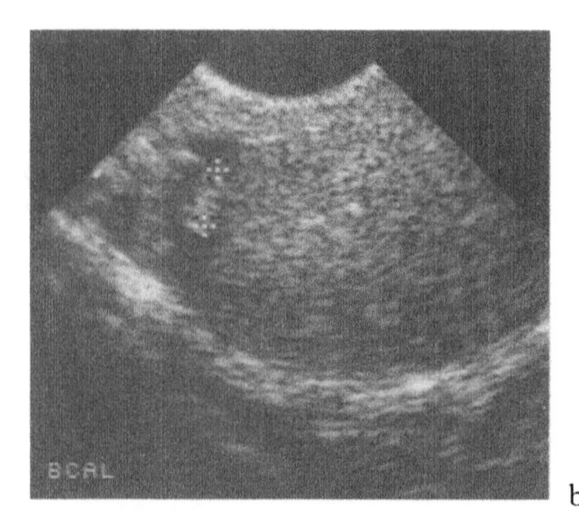

b

Fig. 31a, b. ***Subacute loose torsion of the spermatic cord.*** Ultrasound after eight hours. **a** Sagittal section of the superior pole. Cord abnormally visible due to enlargement, hypoechogenic (loose torsion), persistent Doppler arterial signal. **b** Sagittal section. Small epididymal head remains in place. Testis slightly tumefied, almost normal echo pattern. Conclusion: Loose torsion of a single turn, surgically proven

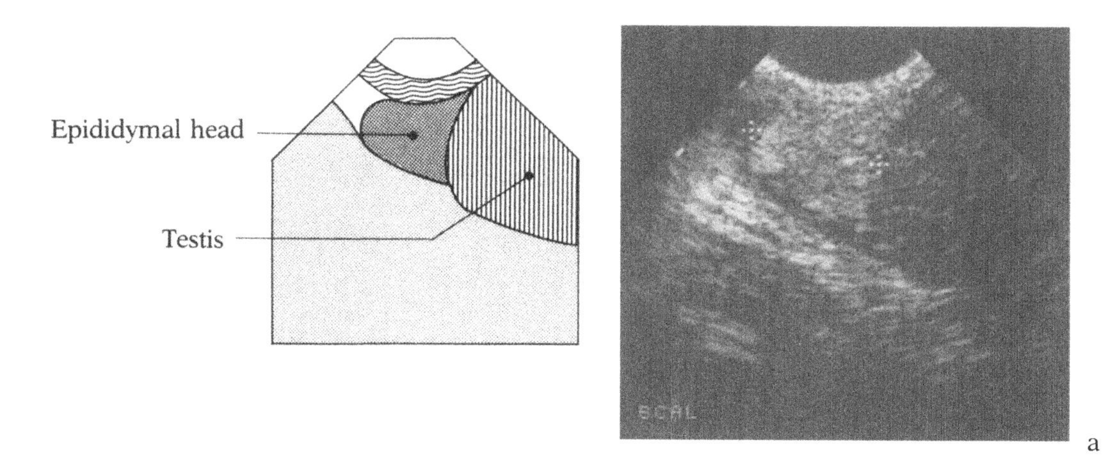

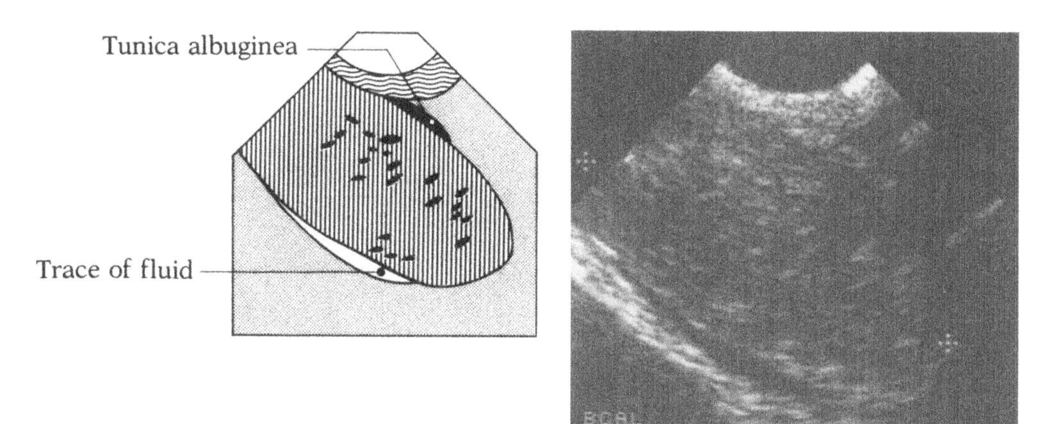

Fig. 32a, b. ***Tight torsion of spermatic cord in the subacute stage.*** Ultrasound performed twelve days following the onset of pain in one testis in a forty five year old man, initially treated as epididymo- orchitis with antibiotics and anti-inflammatory drugs. **a** Sagittal section of the superior pole. Epididymal head in place, but slightly enlarged and hyperechoic (congestion). **b** Sagittal section of the inferior pole. Almost normal size of testis but very abnormal echo pattern: diffuse hypoechogenicity but heterogeneous, punctuated by small scattered hyperechoic areas. Tunica albuginea abnormally visible: testicular infarction. Note a small fluid collection in the postero- inferior interepididymo- testicular recess. Conclusion: Tight torsion of cord in the subacute stage with necrosis of the testis. Surgical confirmation: tight torsion of two turns. Epididymo- orchidectomy

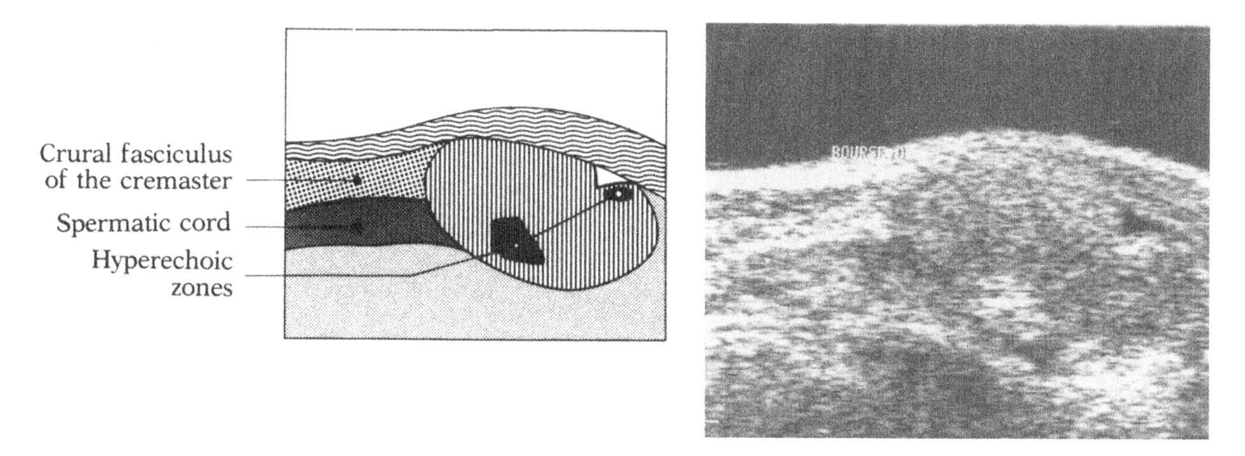

Fig. 33. ***Tight torsion of the spermatic cord in the subacute stage.*** Ultrasound on the second day since onset of an illness followed by scrotal pain in a fifteen year old adolescent. Sagittal section. Thickened investing layers. Several testicular abnormalities: its position: retraction to the inguinal ring from where the crural fasciculus of the cremaster muscle arises; its size is reduced with poorly defined contours; its echo pattern: very heterogeneous/ hypoechoic with hyperechoic sub-capsular plaques. The cord is enlarged and hypoechoic. Conclusion: Ischaemic testicular necrosis due to a tight torsion, surgically proven. Orchidectomy necessary

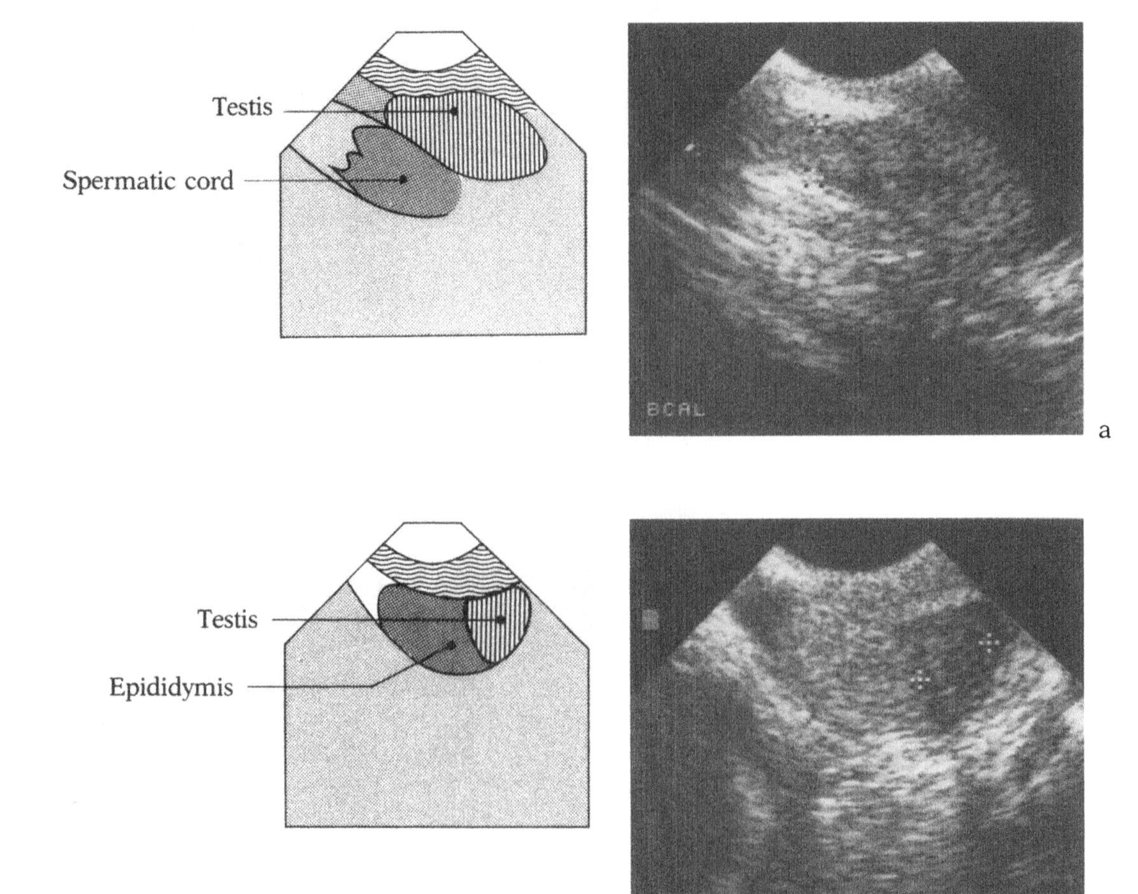

Fig. 34a, b. ***Subacute torsion of the cord in crypt-orchidism corrected surgically during childhood.*** Ultrasound in a fifteen year old adolescent on the second day since onset of pain in the testis which had been surgically fixed in childhood. **a** Sagittal section. Small atrophic testis, hypoechoic. Posteriorly is an echogenic band corresponding to the cord. **b** Transverse section. The very echogenic epididymis is larger than the hypotrophied testis. Conclusion: The appearances are not those of an epididymo-orchitis but are suggestive of a torsion (despite the previous history of orchidopexy). Surgically confirmed

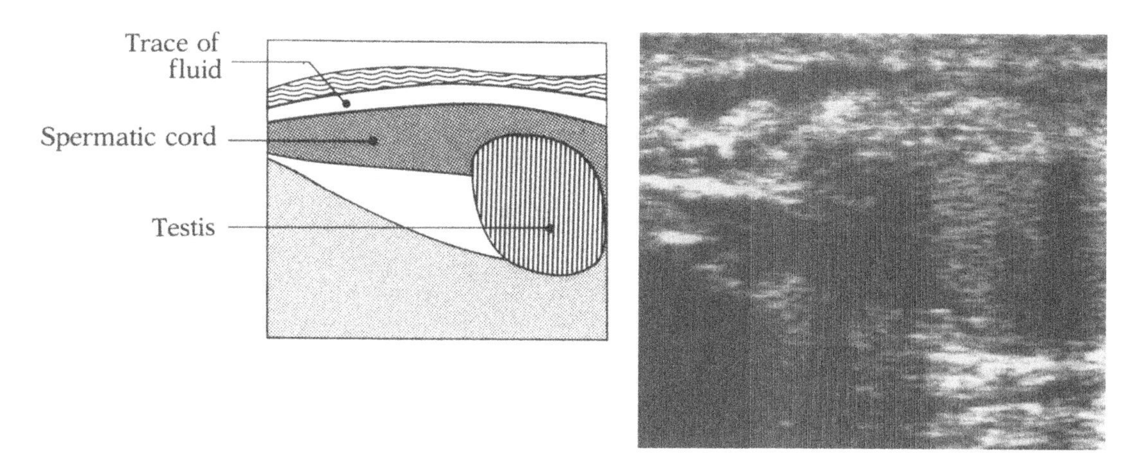

Fig. 35. ***Incomplete torsion of the spermatic cord in the subacute stage.*** Ultrasound on the second day following onset of severe pain in the testis in a twenty-eight year old man. High sagittal section: enlarged echogenic cord passing anterior to a minimally enlarged and slightly hypoechoic testis. Small amount of fluid outlining the abnormal cord anteriorly: torsion of half a turn, not tight at operation. Bilateral orchidopexy

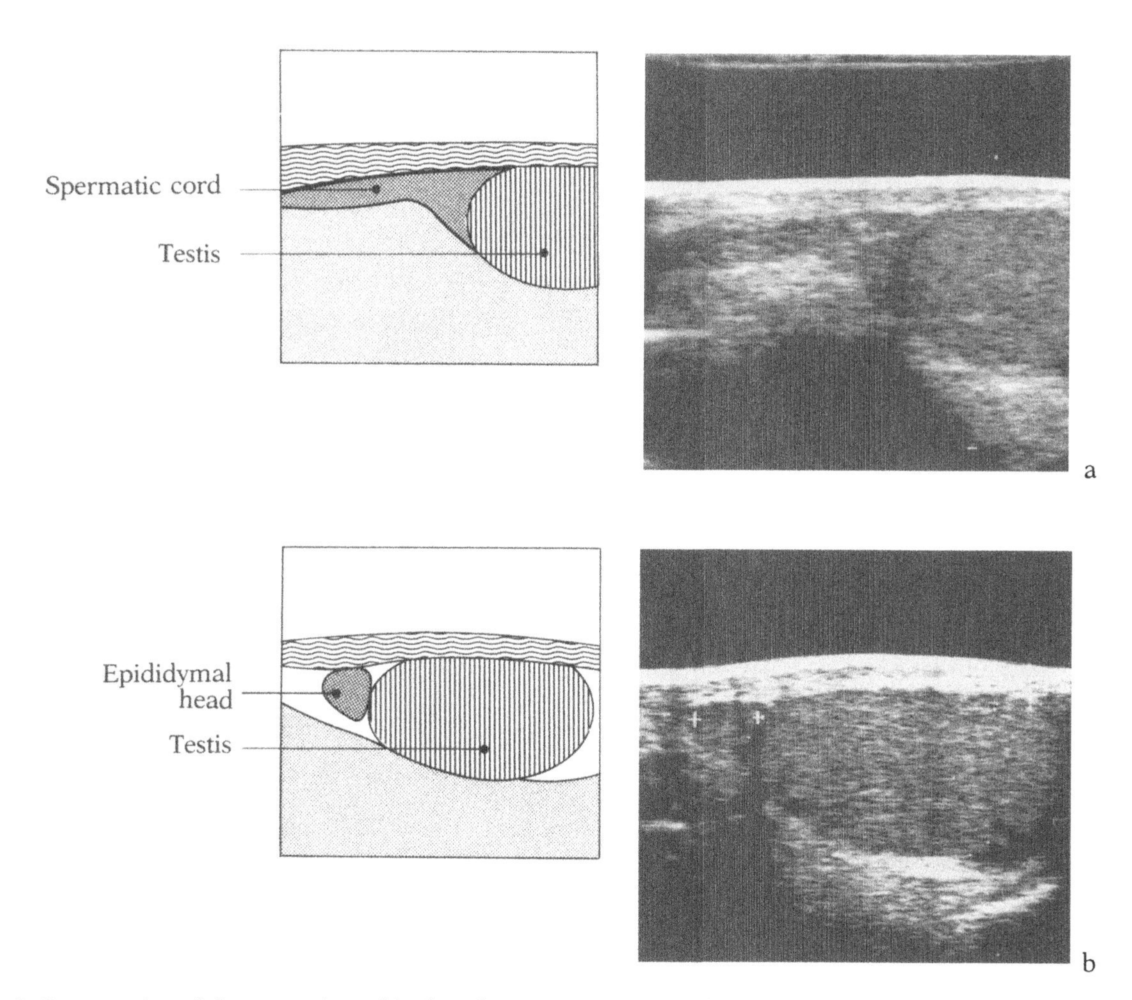

Fig. 36a, b. ***Loose torsion of the spermatic cord in the subacute stage.*** Ultrasound on the third day since onset of scrotal pain in a twenty year old man. **a** High sagittal section. Normal testis. By contrast the cord is abnormally visible and hyperechoic. **b** Paramedian section: Visualisation of epididymal head in a normal position and not enlarged. Conclusion: No features to suggest inflammation, but signs suggesting a loose torsion having little effect on the epididymis or testis. Surgical confirmation

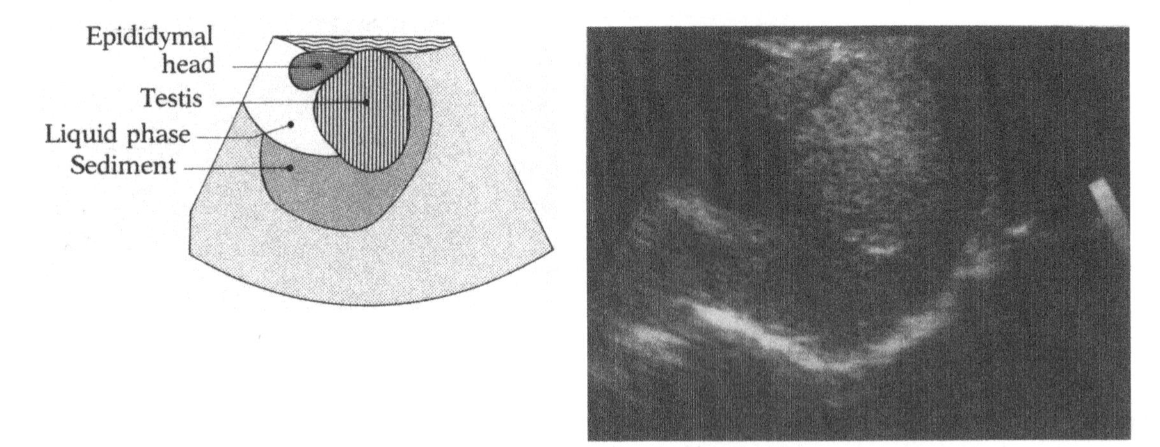

Fig. 37. ***Subacute torsion of spermatic cord. Differential diagnosis with scrotal trauma.*** Ultrasound performed on a foreign patient who was confused and unintelligible. Definite testicular pain with slight enlargement. Transverse section. Epididymal head is slightly less echogenic than the testis, itself virtually normal. By contrast, there is a large effusion between the two layers of the tunica vaginalis in two phases: a moderately echogenic sediment above which lies an echofree fluid phase. Appearances could suggest a post traumatic haematocele undergoing liquefaction but the presence of an enlarged cord indicates torsion. Surgically proven torsion with a serosanguinous exudate. This amount of fluid is most commonly seen following trauma (pseudo- traumatic appearance)

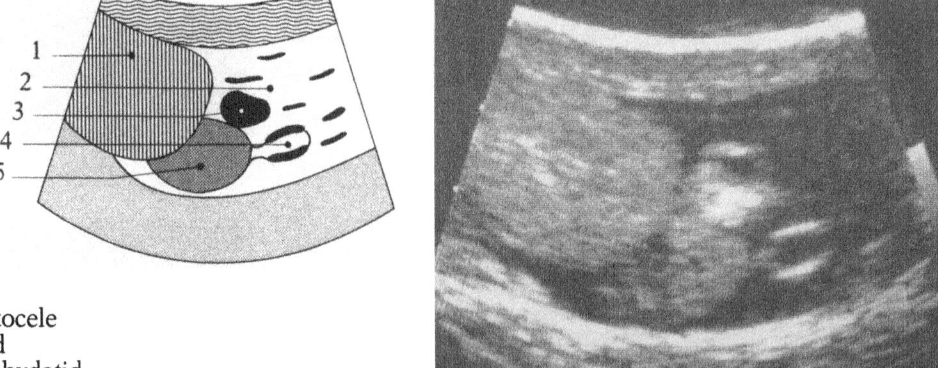

Fig. 38. ***Loose torsion of the spermatic cord.*** Ultrasound on fourth day following onset of scrotal pain. Sagittal section inferior pole. Below the inferior pole of the testis is seen an oblong structure which is the cephalic portion of the epididymis, confirmed by the proximity of two small rounded structures, one solid and the other vesicular. These are the two hydatids - the sessile above and the pedunculated below. Loose torsion through 180 degrees of the cord as indicated by the minimally altered echo pattern of the epididymis and testis even after four days

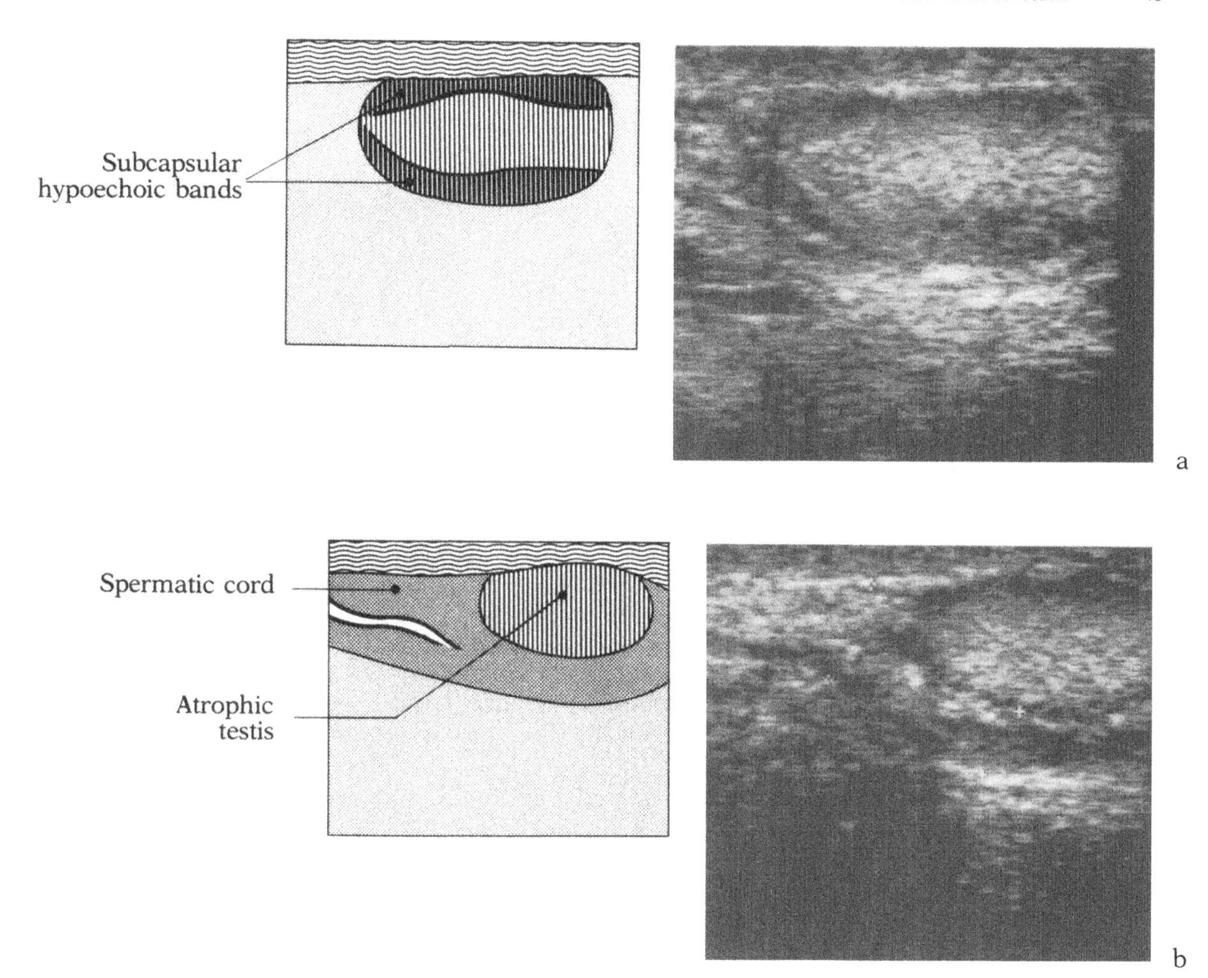

Fig. 39a, b. ***Missed torsion of the spermatic cord.*** Ultrasound one month following onset of pain in the testis, then inflamed in a thirty seven year old man. No improvement on medical treatment. **a** Sagittal section. Slightly small testis with markedly altered echo pattern: peripheral hypoechoic band. **b** Sagittal section superior pole. Testicular atrophy is apparent. The cord remained abnormally visible and echogenic. Conclusion: Ischaemic necrosis of the testis secondary to an undiagnosed torsion. Orchidectomy

Tumours of the testis

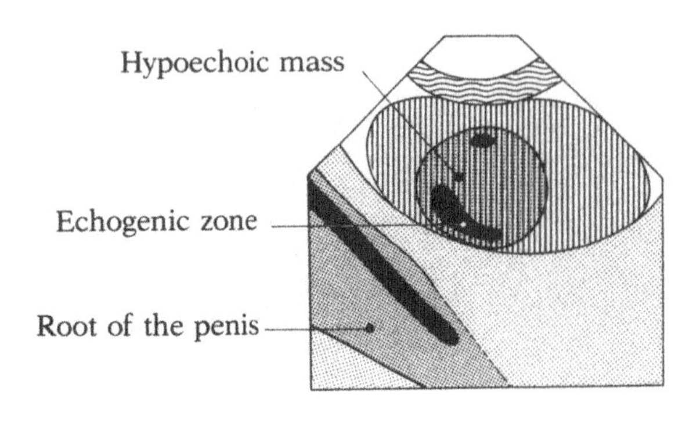

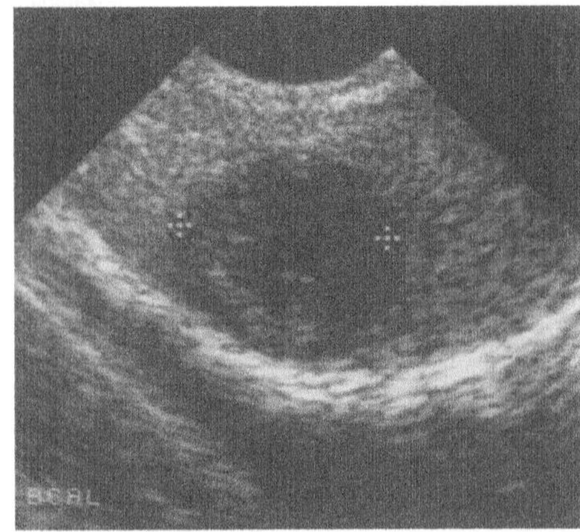

Fig. 40. ***Germinal tumour of the testis - haemorrhagic embryonic carcinoma*** . Severe pain one evening in a young man of twenty. No urinary symptoms or ascended testes. Sagittal section: Rounded 1.8 cm solid and hypoechoic tumour within the testicular substance in the perihilar region; some echogenic areas within the lesion. Haemorrhagic embryonal carcinoma found at operation. Histological sections of the cord revealed tumour emboli within the veins which are likely to be related to the situation of the lesion at the hilum

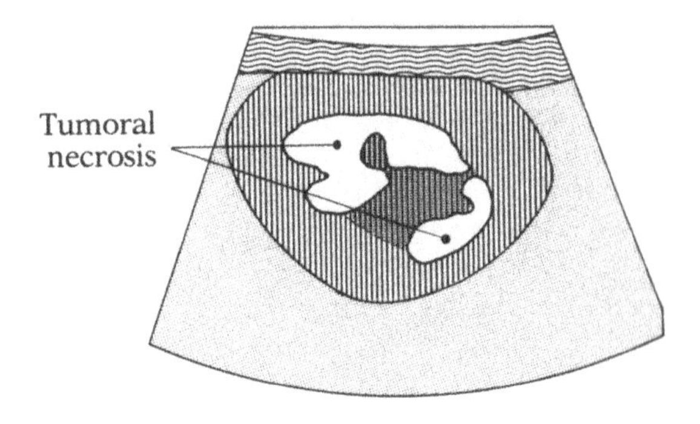

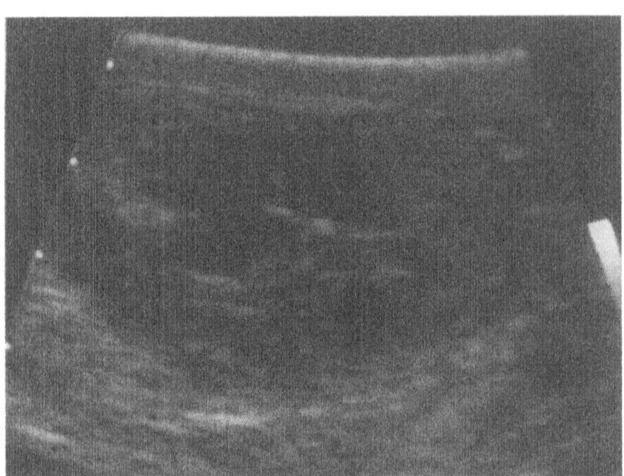

Fig. 41. ***Germinal tumour of testis: necrotic seminoma.*** Resolving episode of unilateral pain in the lumbar and inguinal regions in a forty two year old man. Two weeks later, large painful and inflamed testis on the ipsilateral side. Sagittal section. Large heterogeneous testis with small, very hypoechoic areas without posterior enhancement, central and confluent. Almost complete necrosis of tumour mass confirmed at orchidectomy

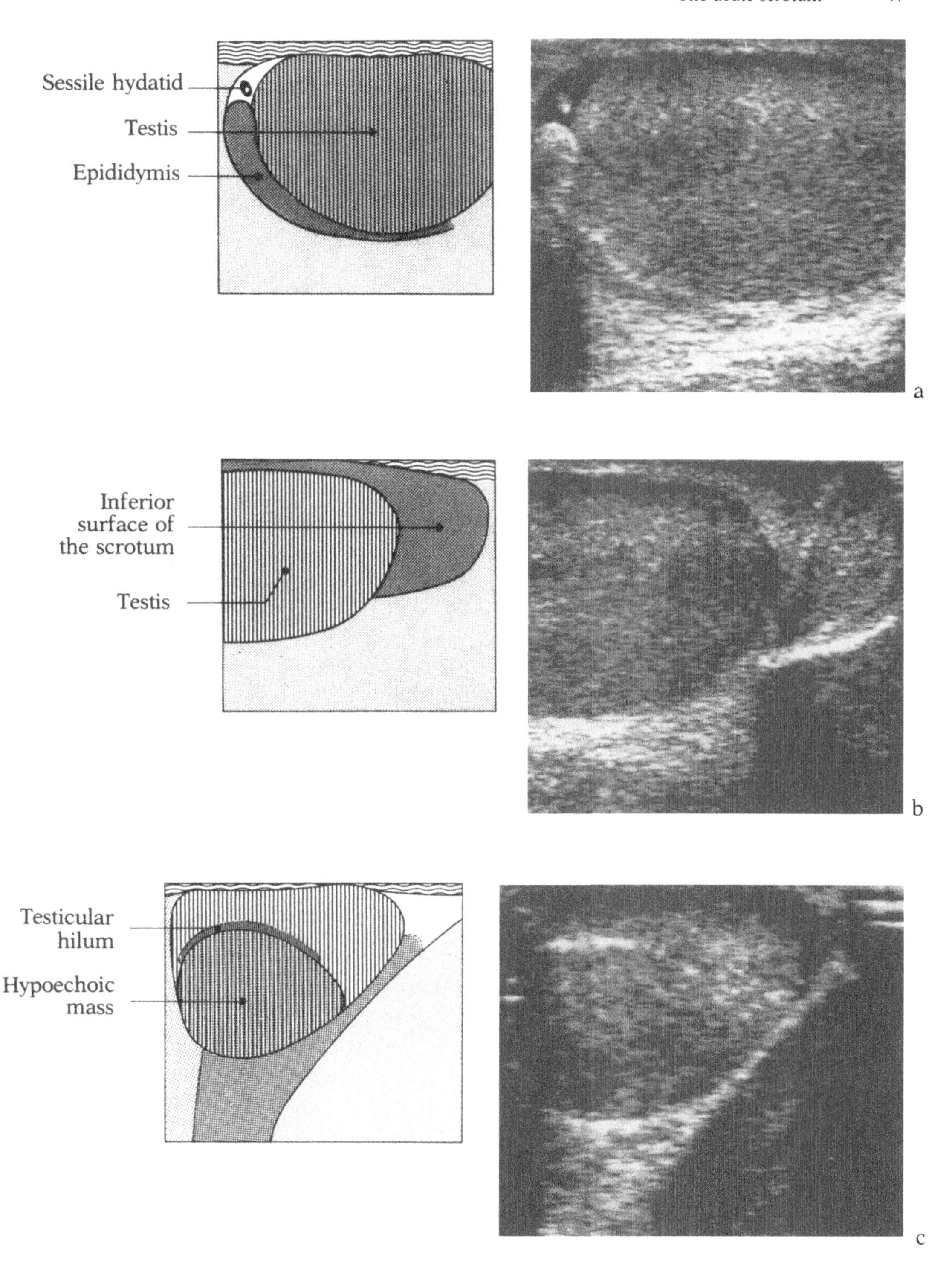

Fig. 42a-c. ***Bilateral testicular lymphoma.*** Patient of forty years with AIDS and Kaposi syndrome. Onset of inflamed, very painful left testis with pyrexia. **a** Sagittal section of the left testis: very large diffusely hypoechoic testis with no evidence of nodularity. Enlargement of the whole of the epididymis, heterogeneous, poorly distinguished from the testis particularly in the region of the body. Note a sessile hydatid. **b** Sagittal section inferior pole. Beneath the lower pole of the testis there is a significant inflammatory infiltration of the investing layers. **c** Transverse section of the asymptomatic right testis: showing anterior displacement of the hilum by a large nodular hypoechoic mass within the testis. Diagnosis: Testicular tumour, in this clinical context-lymphoma. Conclusion: Bilateral non-Hodgkin lymphoma of high grade malignancy infiltrating the tunica albuginea and left epididymis. Bilateral orchidectomy

Traumatisms

Major trauma

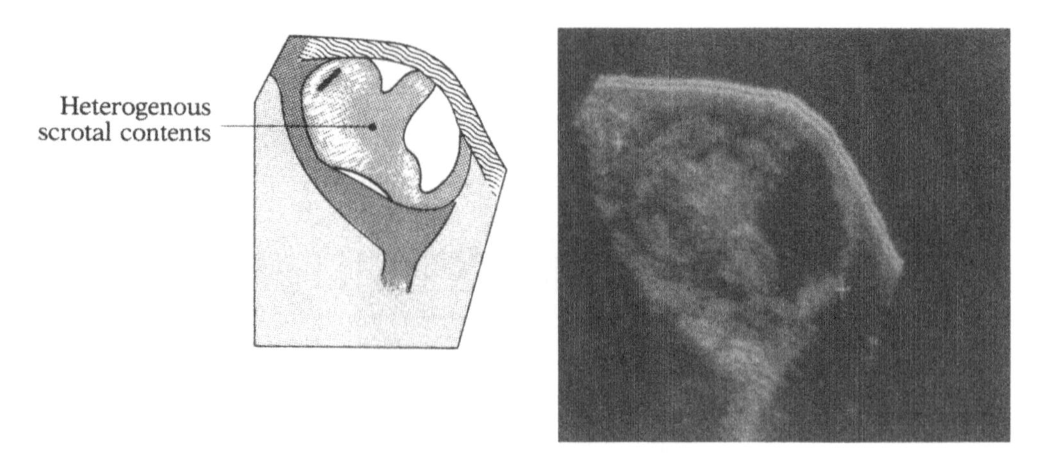

Fig. 43. ***Shattered testis.*** Ultrasound on the *fifth day*. Sagittal section: No recognisable testis can be seen within the scrotum, not even part of the testis. Orchidectomy necessary

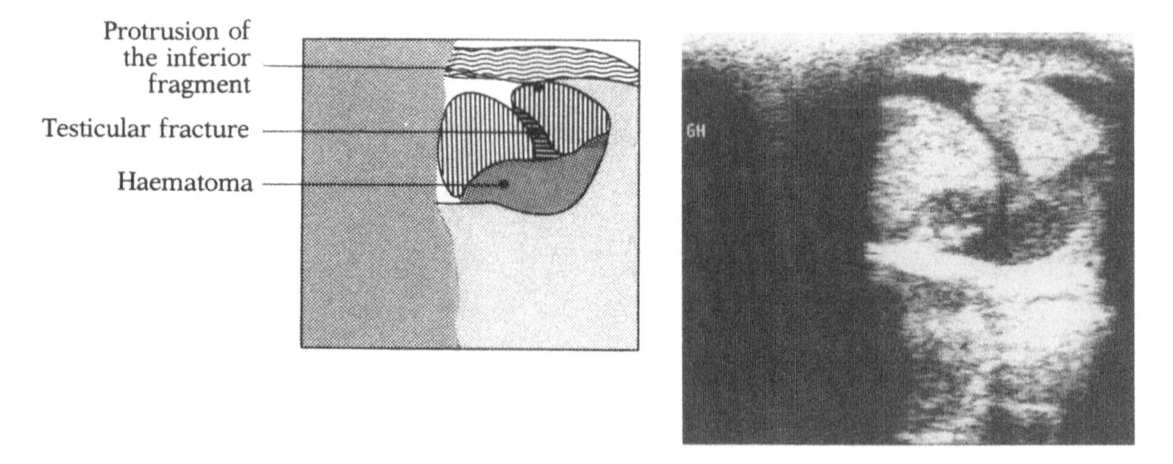

Fig. 44. ***Fractured testis with evisceration of the parenchyma.*** Ultrasound *six hours* following direct trauma (kicked). Sagittal section: thickened investing layers. Testis fractured in two by a tear which extends to the abnormal border of the inferior portion indicating an evisceration of the parenchyma into the tunica vaginalis. Posterior to the fracture is an oblong hypoechoic haematoma. Operation: subcapsular orchidectomy with conservation of the epididymis

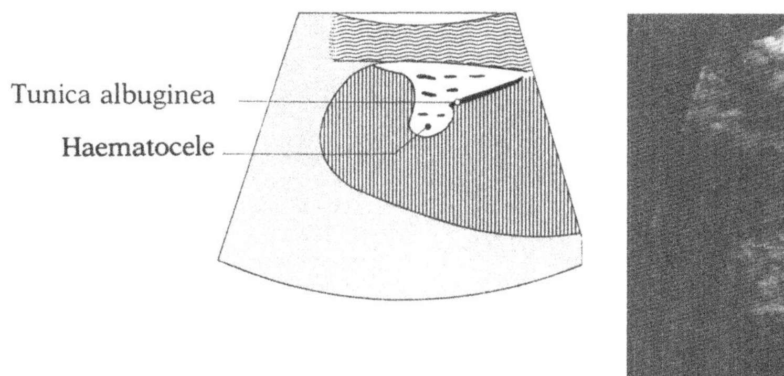

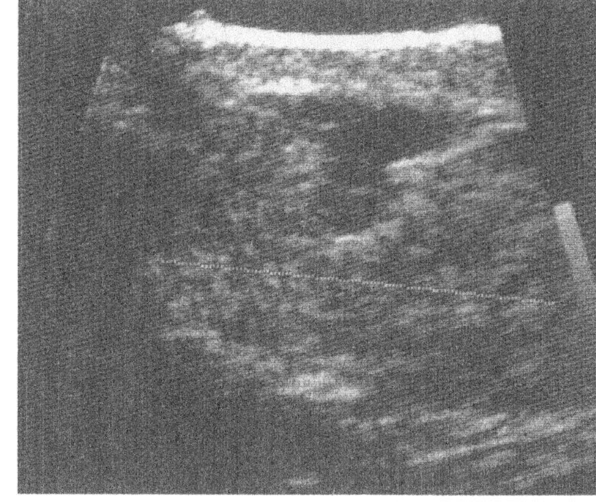

Fig. 45. ***Fractured testis.*** Ultrasound *three hours* following trauma. Sagittal section: rupture of the tunica albuginea anteriorly indicated by a less than 1 cm. interruption of its echogenic line with a parenchyma tear filled with a small haematocele. The rest of the testis has a grossly abnormal echo pattern, the relatively small size of the tear makes conservative surgical repair possible

Trauma of moderate and minor severity

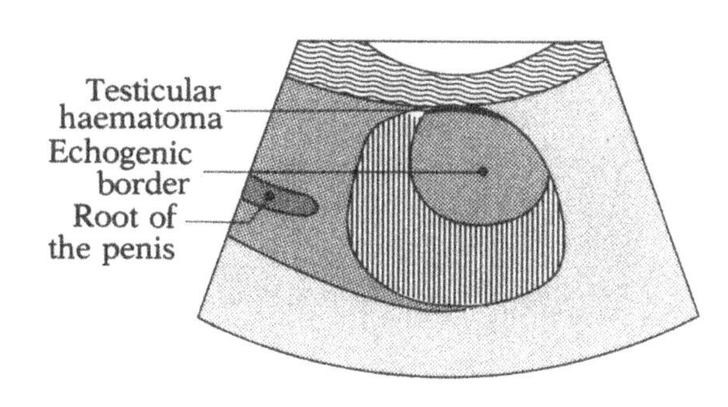

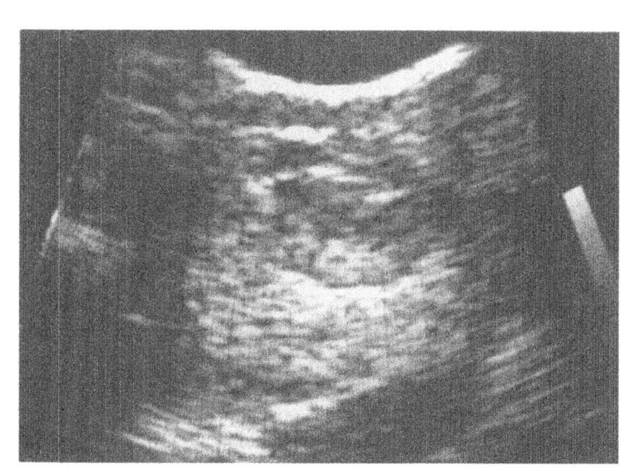

Fig. 46. ***Testicular haematoma.*** Ultrasound the day following trauma (hit by a ball). Transverse section: rounded structure of 1 cm essentially hypoechoic in the anterior half of the testis (whose morphology is conserved) due to a haematoma. An associated rupture of the tunica albuginea should be excluded, although unlikely in this case as the echogenic line adjacent to the contusion is intact

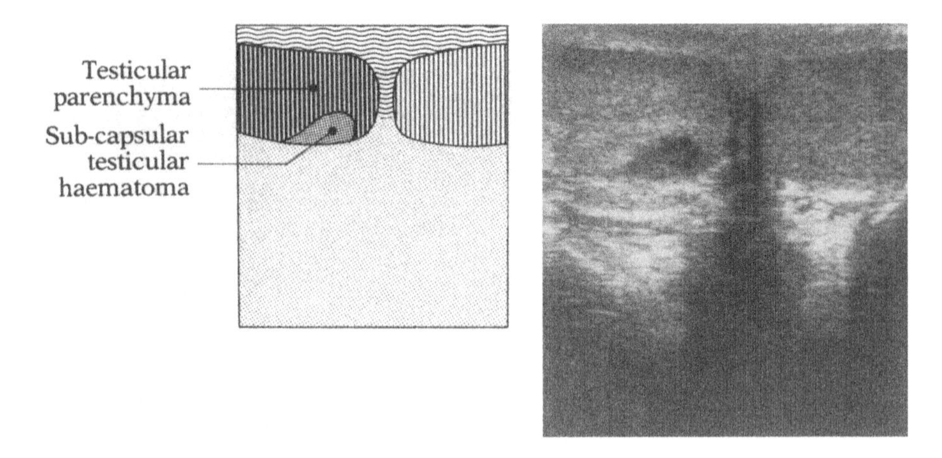

Fig. 47. ***Testicular haematoma.*** Ultrasound on the *third day*. Transverse section both testes: subcapsular haematoma causing some compression of the testis which appears slightly echogenic, relative to the contralateral normal side (Image courtesy of Dr. Tordjmann). Conservative treatment

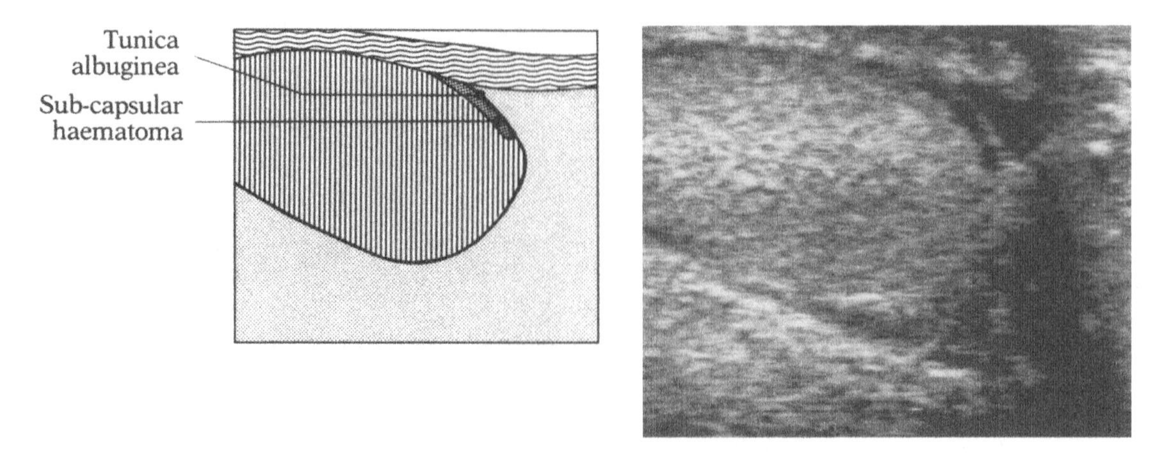

Fig. 48. ***Subcapsular haematoma.*** Ultrasound on *fifth day* due to persistent pain in the inferior pole of the testis. Sagittal section: discrete hypoechogenic subcapsular band with preservation of the echogenic line of the tunica albuginea. Conservative treatment

Haematoceles

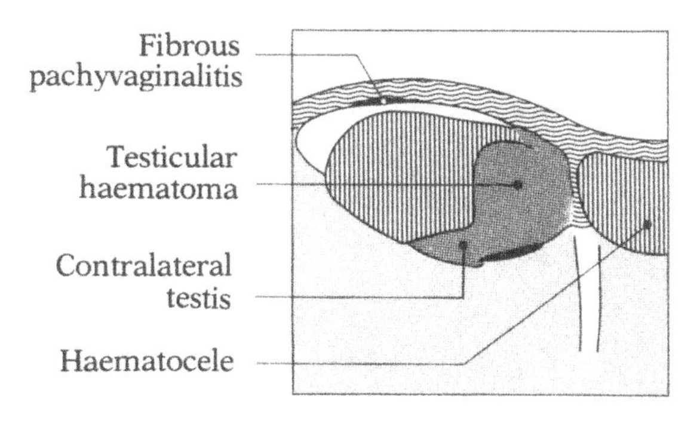

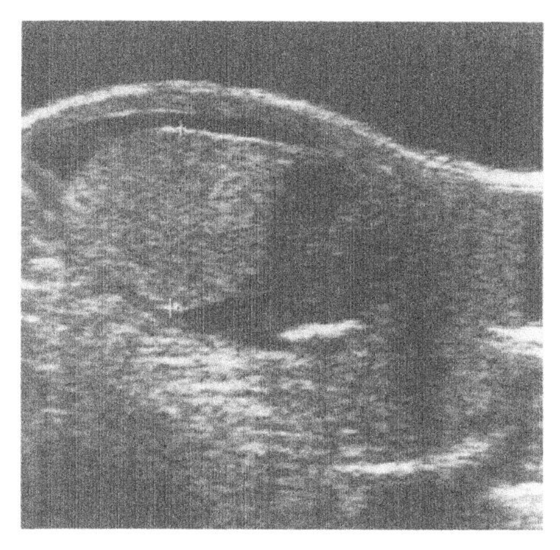

Fig. 49. ***Contusion of the epididymis and testis with haematocele.*** Ultrasound performed *three weeks* following violent trauma. Persistently enlarged and painful testis. Sagittal section: recognisable morphology of the testis but there is effacement of the inferior pole by a hypoechogenic area extending into the tunica vaginalis and particularly into the posterior interepididymotesticular recess as a tongue-like process. The epididymal tail is also swollen. Note the thickening of the investing layers by echogenic fibrous tissue

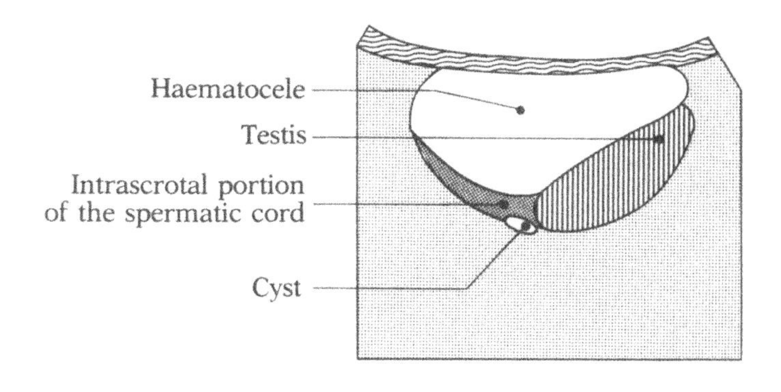

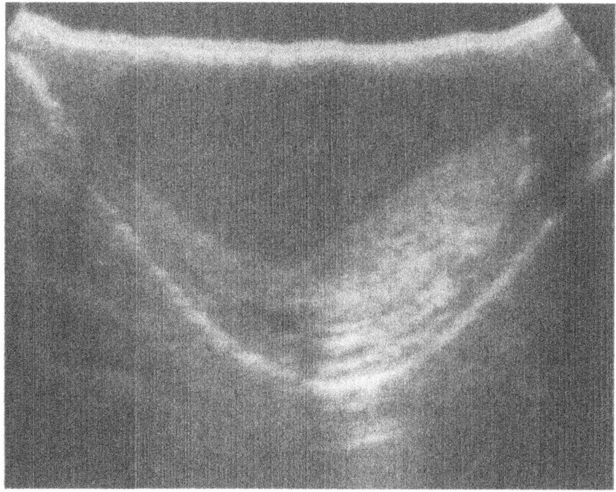

Fig. 50. ***Acute haematocele.*** Ultrasound *three hours* after direct blow to scrotum. Transverse section: Large collection of blood in the tunica vaginalis, recent in view of the fine homogenous echoes. It extends towards the intact base of the testis and is stretching the spermatic cord. Note a small incidental dystrophic cyst

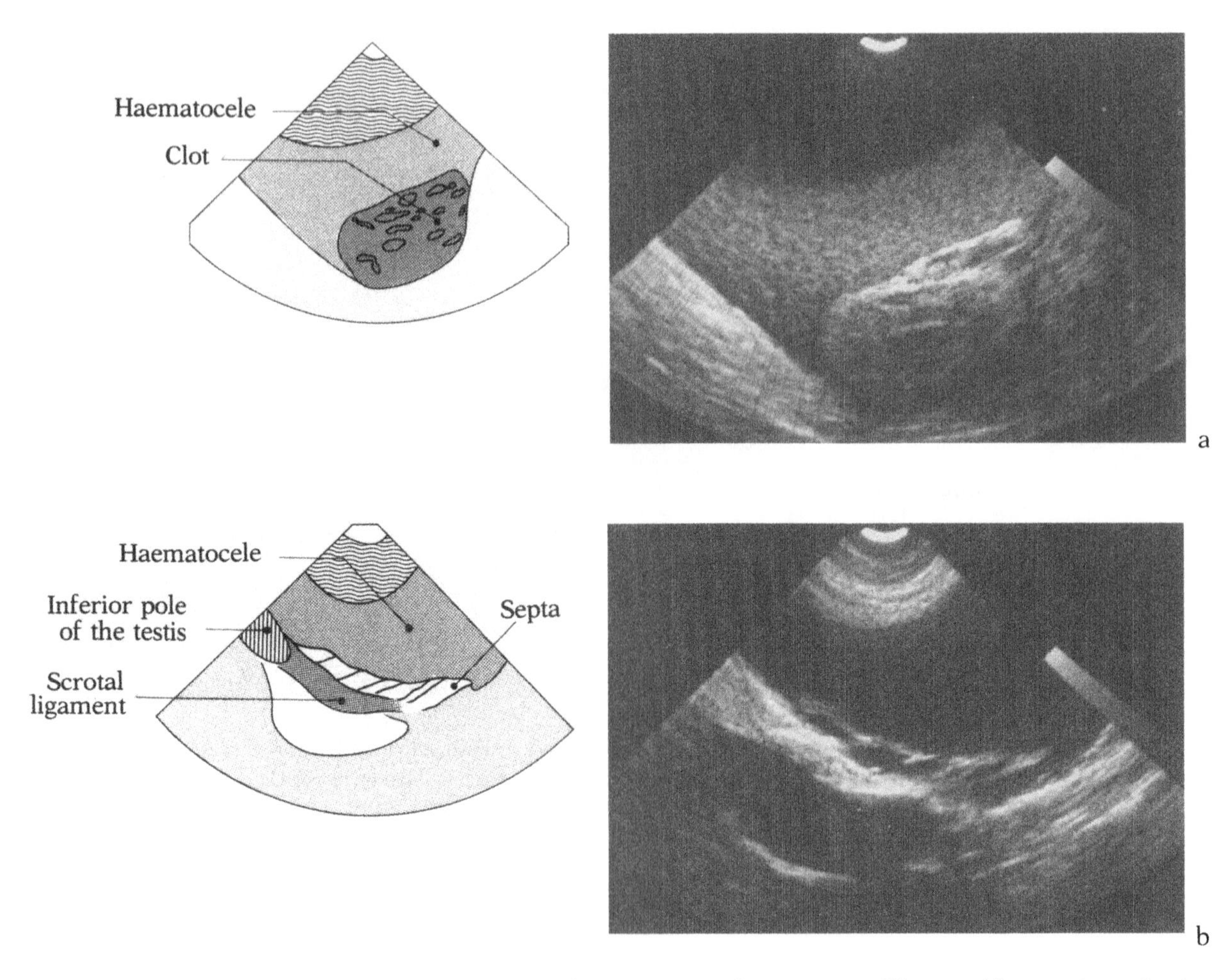

Fig. 51a, b. ***Spontaneous bilateral haematocele secondary to anticoagulant treatment.*** Ultrasound in an anticoagulated man with polyarteritis presenting with progressive painless scrotal swelling. **a** Transverse section of left testis (slightly enlarged): large collection of blood in the tunica vaginalis in two phases: One is an organised echogenic sedimented clot, the other is superficial, homogeneous and slightly echogenic due to more recent haemorrhage. **b** Sagittal section inferior pole of right testis. Mainly liquid collection, layered with projections around the scrotal ligaments. Old, almost completely liquefied haematocele

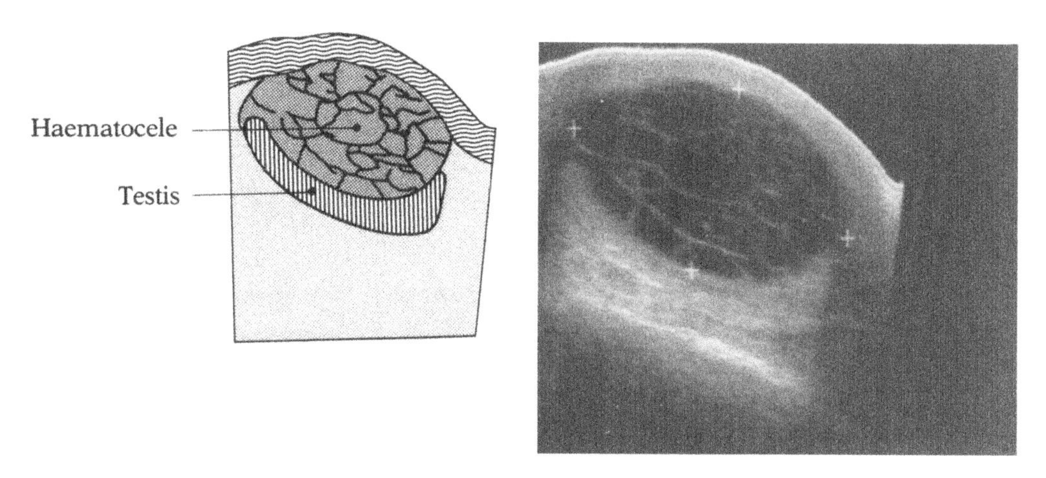

Fig. 52. ***Old haematocele.*** Sagittal section: Intrascrotal rugby ball shaped mass, organised in a regular fashion with alternating areas of liquid and clot characteristic of an old haematoma. Marked compression and deformity of the normal testis

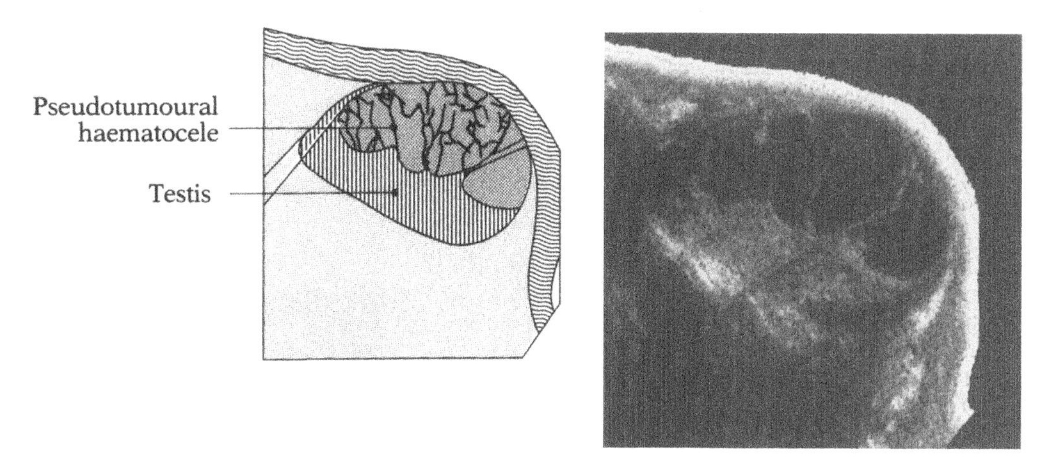

Fig. 53. ***Pseudo tumour appearance of an haematocele.*** Sagittal section: Echogenic clots running through the anterior blood collection causing retraction of the very deformed testis by adhesions. In the absence of trauma, these appearances could be due to a large necrotic tumour in the anterior half of the testis

Spermatic cord and investing layers

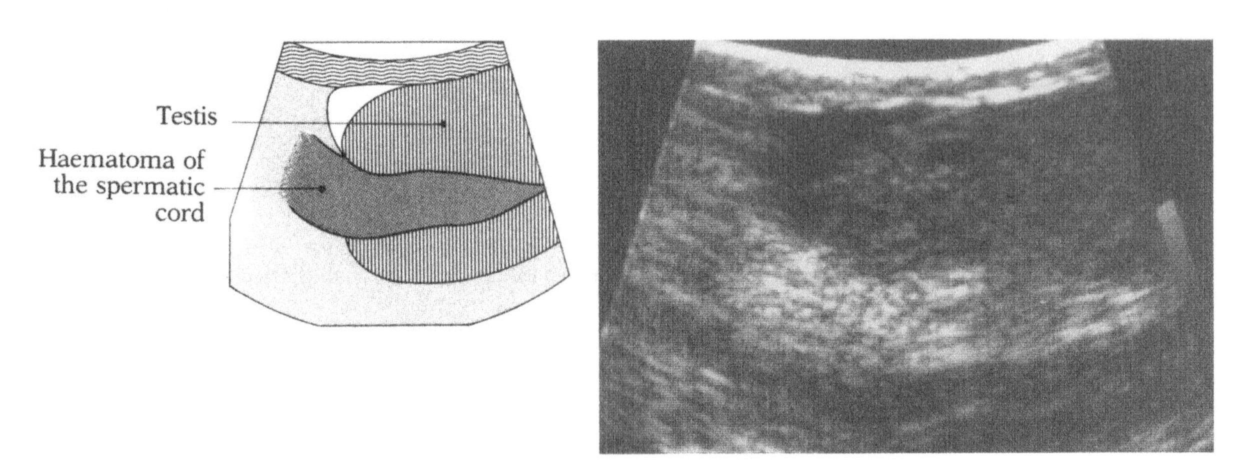

Fig. 54. ***Haematoma of the cord.*** Pain in the right testis following minimal trauma in a man on anticoagulants. Transverse scan: Echogenic enlargement (greater than 1 cm) of the cord as far as the hilar region. Normal testicular parenchyma. Haematoma of spermatic cord predisposed to by anticoagulant therapy

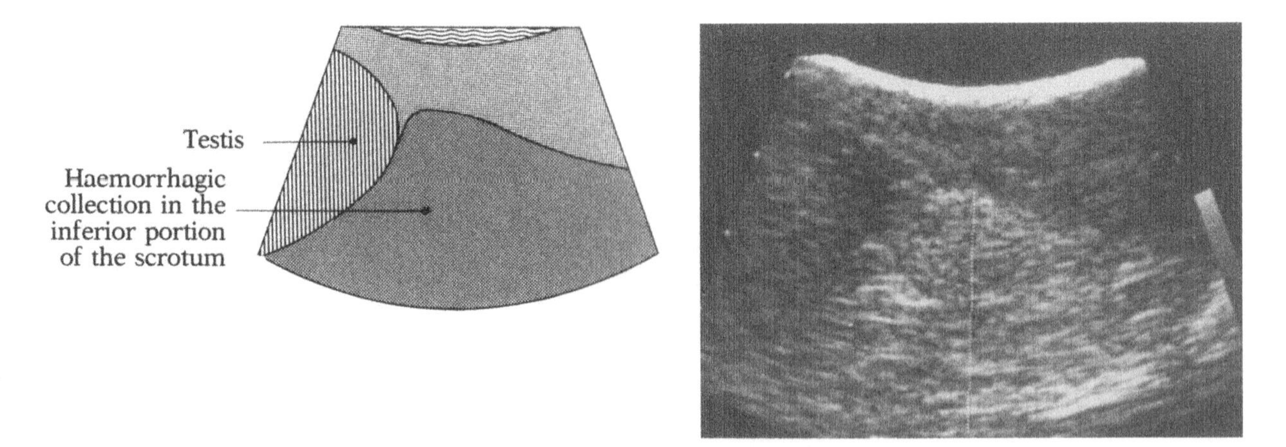

Fig. 55. ***Scrotal contusion.*** Pains in the penis and scrotum following a straddle injury on a ladder. Oblique section inferior pole: thickening of several centimetres of the inferior scrotal area infiltrated by a very echogenic serosanguinous effusion: haematoma of insufficient size to justify drainage

Complications and sequellae

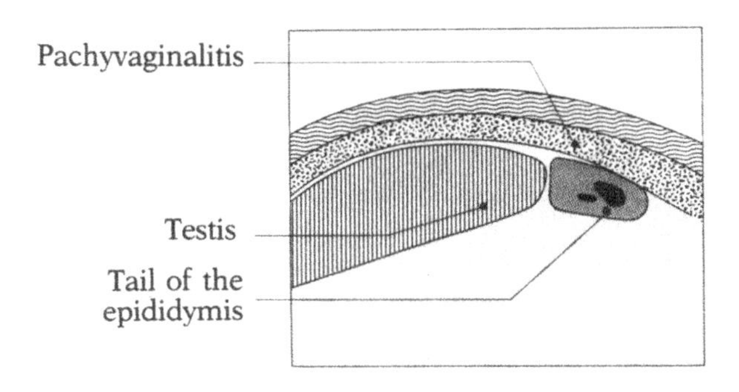

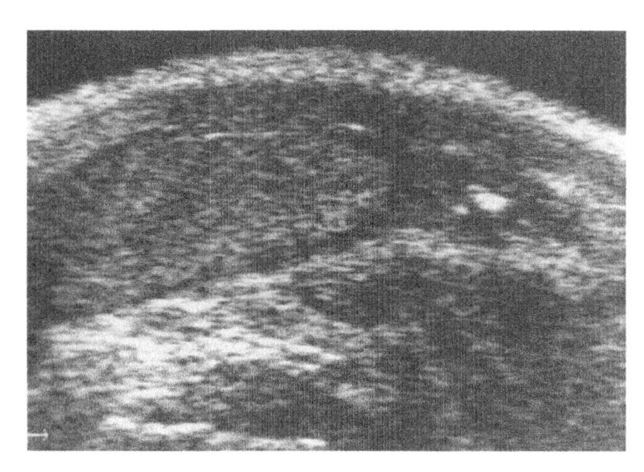

Fig. 56. ***Abscess.*** Same patient as in Fig.49, presenting *two months* later with fever and pain in the previously traumatised testis. Sagittal section: testis with normal echo pattern including the inferior pole but slightly hypotrophic (thickness less than 20 mm). Inferiorly the tail of the epididymis appears enlarged, heterogeneous, hypoechoic, punctuated with echogenic areas. Note also the thickened investing layers. Abscess at the tail of the epididymis requiring a segmental epididymectomy

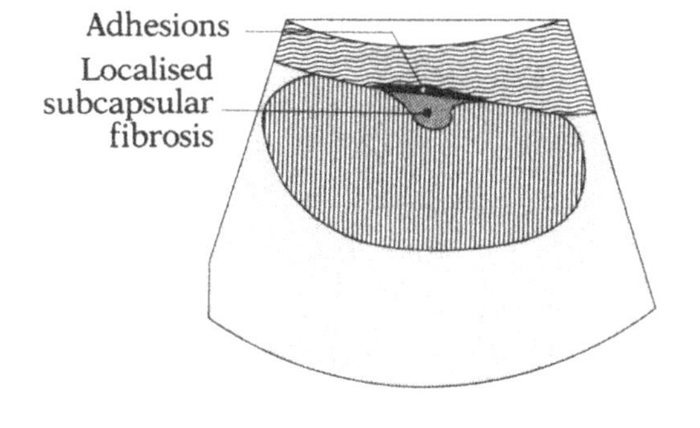

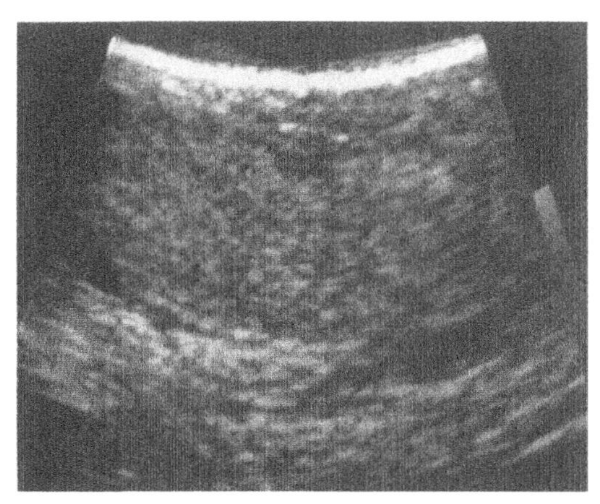

Fig. 57. ***Fibrosis.*** *Four months* after subcapsular haematoma of the testis. Sagittal section: fibrosis of the residual cavity appearing as a small echogenic band deep to the anterior part of the tunica albuginea in the mid part of the testis. The rest appears normal. Note the poorly visualised investing layers over the anterior testicular surface, definitely due to adhesions

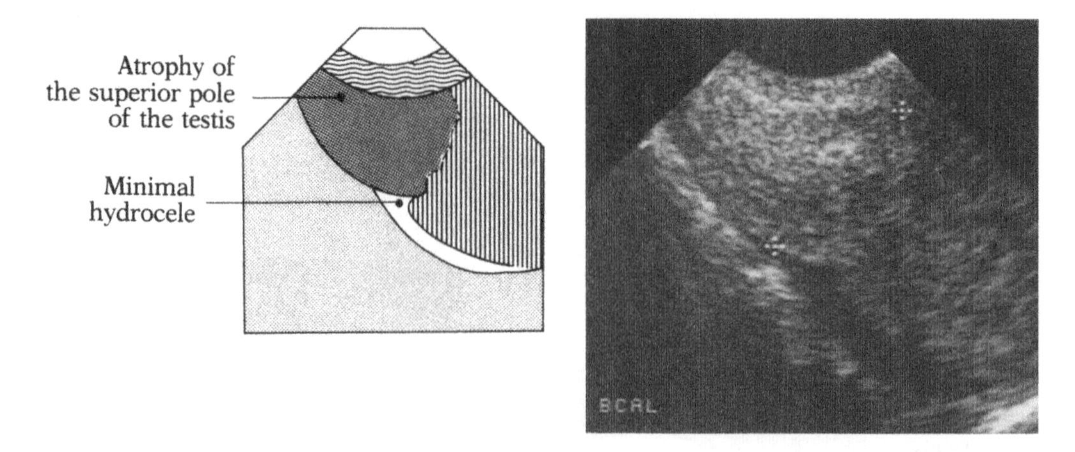

Fig. 58. ***Testicular atrophy.*** Persistent pain in the testis *three months after* trauma which was ignored. Sagittal sections superior pole. Deformity of the testis appearing as a notch on the posterior surface outlined by thin layer of fluid in the tunica vaginalis. There is a reduction in the size of the superior part which appears abnormally echogenic relative to the rest of the testis. Atrophic fibrosis of the superior pole without doubt secondary to an injury of the testicular branch of the spermatic artery

The chronically enlarged scrotum

A set of conditions characterised by a common clinical picture:

- progressive scrotal enlargement over several weeks, months or years;
- paucity of symptoms, often limited to a vague feeling of heaviness.

The conditions fall roughly into two pathological groups:

- inflammatory and benign conditions, represented by hydroceles with pachy-vaginalitis;
- neoplastic and malignant conditions, essentially testicular tumours.

Tumours and pseudo tumours of the testicular appendages are very rare and seldom encountered ultrasonically.

Due to the extreme contrast of these two diametrically opposed groups of conditions, it is imperative for the Clinician to make a definitive diagnosis in the presence of a chronically enlarged scrotum. Therefore, when the diagnosis remains uncertain on clinical grounds (scrotum indurated and testis not palpable, transillumination unhelpful, obese or extremely anxious patient), ultrasound can be of great diagnostic value (Table 1).

Hydroceles

Definition

A hydrocele is an effusion of fluid between the two layers of the tunica vaginalis. It consists of a clear, light yellow coloured fluid which is quite rich in protein. The mechanism of formation is due to an obstruction of the lymphatic reabsorption of the normally secreted fluid by the parietal layer of the tunica vaginalis which is itself always thickened, sometimes markedly so. The condition is, in general, benign and tends to occur in elderly subjects.

Ultrasound findings and characteristics of a hydrocele

The diagnosis of a hydrocele is usually very easy: a transonic collection of free fluid which surrounds the testis and epididymis. Associated thickening of the parietal layer of the tunica vaginalis is seen as a fairly regular hypoechoic line, occasionally with echogenic plaques due to localised areas of fibrosis, sometimes calcified.

Three features should be defined ultrasonically:

The site of the hydrocele

Determine whether the hydrocele is:

- *free* (commonest);
- or *encysted*, usually at the inferior or superior pole of the testis;
- or *funiculo-vaginal* (least frequently), that is to say extending along the spermatic cord due to non-obliteration of the distal part of the peritoneo- vaginal canal;
- or *communicating* with the main peritoneal cavity (complete failure of closure of the canal).

The size of the hydrocele and whether or not bilateral

Hydroceles are bilateral in 10% of cases, often asymmetrical, being large on one side and small on the other.

Table 1. ***Testicular enlargement due to tumours. Diagnostic algorithm***

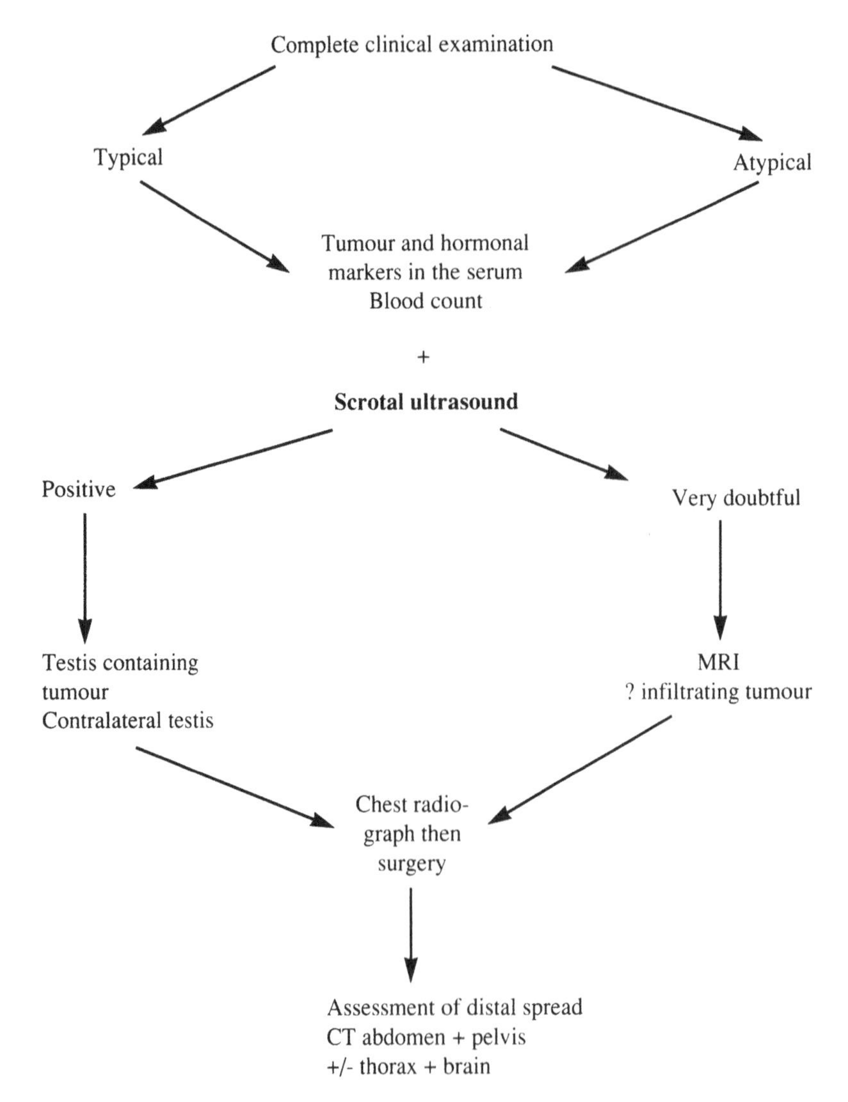

The type of the hydrocele on ultrasound

This can give some indication of the aetiology. It may be:

- a *simple* hydrocele, the commonest, completely anechoic;

- a *septated hydrocele* with echogenic septa which connect the testis and epididymis to the parietal layer of the tunica vaginalis. These appearances raise the possibility of Tuberculosis or infection of a previously simple hydrocele;

- a *"cholesterol"* hydrocele recognized by its "snowstorm" effect due to multiple small echoes throughout the collection indicating an abnormally high level of cholesterol crystals. This type is most frequently seen in obesity, diabetes or hyperlipidemia and indicates that the hydrocele is old;

-*"lithiasis"* within a hydrocele. These are seen as echogenic particles of a few millimetres, highly attenuating, mobile (stand the patient up) and layered out. They are small mixed calcified concretions. This appearance can also be seen in a detached hyatid which has become fibrosed and secondarily calcified, although the particles are larger in this instance.

Associated signs

It is imperative to look for these:

- above all, an underlying testicular tumour must

Table 2. ***OMS classification of the histological types of testicular tumours***

Germinal tumours	Seminoma Embryonic carcinoma Associated forms Polyembryonic Choriocarcinoma Teratoma (dysembryonic)
Tumours of the supporting tissues	Leydig cell tumours Sertoli cell tumours Granulosa tumours
Tumours of the lymphatic and haemopoietic tissues	Acute leukaemia
Secondary tumours	Metastases (prostate ++, lung, kidney, colon, stomach)
Varied tumours	Carcinoid tumour
Primordial gonadal tumours	Gonadoblastoma Other tumours

be excluded by a detailed study of the testicular parenchyma. An associated tumour is a rare but recognised feature;

- fairly commonly, the hydrocele is secondary to an inflammation of the epididymis, indicated by a nodule of variable echogenicity;

- finally, where there is a suspected or pre-existing underlying carcinoma, the presence of ascites should be excluded.

The great majority of hydroceles are primary and benign. Treatment is dependent on the size of the hydrocele and the resultant symptoms caused, varying from no treatment at all to aspiration or operative intervention.

Testicular tumours

Malignant tumours of the testis are rare (1%-3% of malignancies in the male) but, along with lymphomas, are the second most common cause of death in young males.

Primary tumours are the commonest, the majority of which consist of the germinal tumours (90%) which affect mainly young patients. Secondary tumours (metastases, lymphoma) classically occur in elderly patients but the increased frequency of testicular lymphoma in patients with AIDS is altering this age distribution (Table 2).

Ultrasound diagnosis

The question posed by the Clinicians is simple: are the testes normal ultrasonically; or is there an intraparenchymal abnormality necessitating surgical exploration via the inguinal approach?

In this context there are five distinct steps in the ultrasound examination: the first three are essential to determine whether orchidotomy is necessary and assess the spread of the lesion. The last two are really accessory since they will not alter the decision whether to operate or not:

- *Ultrasonic diagnosis of an intratesticular parenchymal mass partially solid and therefore almost certainly a tumour:*
  - obtuse angles at the junction between the lesion and the testicular parenchyma;
  - orthogonal sections, the lesion is intraparenchymal on all sections;
  - echopattern: the appearances of the lesion are not at all characteristic of a simple cyst.
- *Exclude a contralateral testicular tumour; by a*

Table 3. ***TNM classification of the spread of primary testicular tumours***

Stage	
T0	No detectable tumour
T1	Tumour limited to the testis
T2	Tumour extension through the tunica albuginea
T3	Tumour invasion of the rete testis or epididymis
T4a	Invasion of the spermatic cord
T4b	Invasion of the scrotum

detailed analysis and comparison of the parenchymal echopattern.

- *Look for local extension and evidence of lymphadenopathy* ; particularly the lumbo-aortic lymph nodes, which extend from inferiorly to the level of the vascular pedicle of the kidney, on the ipsilateral side to the tumour. Inguinal lymphadenopathy is very rare and is seen mainly in cases of previous anterior testicular surgery (for ectopic testis, orchidopexy etc.).

-*Additional features suggesting tumour type.* The ultrasound findings taken in conjunction with the age and previous medical history of the patient can give further clues to the diagnosis. In no circumstances is the aim to give the histology as this is exclusively the domain of the histopathologist. However, ultrasound can help to plan the extent of the surgery pre-operatively.

- *Look for signs of tumour extension into the testicular appendages* (Table 3). This is, in practice, of little interest for two reasons:

• the surgery anyhow will consist of an orchidectomy with high ligation of the cord,

• microscopic spread, especially into the tunica albuginea and epididymis, will be missed ultrasonically.

Follow-up

- After unilateral orchidectomy, annual ultrasound of the remaining testis is indicated to look for a contra lateral tumour.

- In the very rare cases of tumourectomy (tumours of the stroma of the gonad), ultrasound confirms the absence of any alterations in the testicular parenchyma around the post-operative cavity.

Tumours and pseudotumours of the testicular appendages

Tumours of the testicular appendages

These are extremely rare.The aims of the ultrasound examination are:

- *To make the diagnosis of a solid extra-testicular mass* :
  - by the classical radiological signs:
    - the centre of the mass projects outside the testis,
    - the angles at the junction are acute;
  - the echopattern.

This first stage confirms the extra-testicular position of the lesion and therefore, if surgery is indicated, the testis can be conserved.

- *Additional features for a more precise diagnosis.* In effect, the organ of origin and position of the tumour will determine the surgical approach:

• if the tumour arises in the spermatic cord, the approach will be via the inguinal route;

• if not, depending on the size of the lesion, a simple scrototomy could be considered.

Secondary tumours (metastases, lymphoma) which are not within the testis are extremely rare.

Primary tumours make up the vast majority of tumours of the appendages. They are in general of mesenchymal origin and usually benign. They are almost always asymptomatic apart from the tumours of the cord which are often large and present with a feeling of heaviness in the scrotum.

Despite their rarity, the principal tumours should be recognized by the Ultrasonologist because they have distinct ultrasonic appearances.

Adenomatoid tumour

This is the commonest paratesticular tumour (30 per cent). It is benign, usually affecting middle aged patients and tends to be situated in the tail of the epididymis. A regular hypoechoic nodule in the epididymal tail seen in a subject without any history of previous infection should raise the possibility of this diagnosis. A follow-up ultrasound three months later is reasonable in order to confirm there has been no growth of the lesion and that no further treatment is necessary.

Fibrous pseudotumour

This is otherwise known as: fibromatous or reactive periorchitis, fibroma, inflammatory pseudotumour.

It is also benign, affecting the same age group and is the second most common tumour of the testicular appendages. In 50 percent of cases there is an associated hydrocele. It develops mainly from the tunica vaginalis and generally presents in the form of several solid nodules of variable size around the testis. The ultrasound appearances are fairly typical.

Surgery consists of localised excision of the lesion and conservation of the testis.

Cystadenoma of the head of the epididymis

This is a hamartoma. This benign tumour is characterised by an ectasia of the efferent tubules and is therefore seen either within or adjacent to the epididymal head. It has been described in association with Von Hippel Lindau disease.

Ultrasonically it appears as a mass with mixed solid / cystic elements of variable size within the epididymal head.

Rhabdomyosarcoma

This is a malignant tumour of children, adolescents and very young adults. It arises almost exclusively in the intrascrotal portion of the spermatic cord. Occasionally it is difficult to be certain of its origin and to differentiate it from other tumours of the testicular appendages. As a rule, it is a large tumour. Ultrasonically it appears as a large, solid and heterogeneous inguino-scrotal mass lying above the testis.

Following orchidectomy and clearance of the inguinal lymph nodes recurrence is seen in 10 per cent of cases.

Other mesenchymal tumours of the cord (leiomyosarcoma, liposarcoma) are much rarer, affecting older adults and the histopathological diagnosis is often not suspected.

Mesothelial hyperplasia and mesothelioma of the tunica vaginalis

Mesothelioma of the tunica vaginalis is very rare. Histopathological diagnosis can be difficult.

Ultrasonically, the problem is the interpretation of atypical thickening of the parietal layer of the tunica vaginalis, discovered during the investigation of a hydrocele.

The following characteristics of the thickening should be noted:

- diffuse or localised,
- en plaque or frankly nodular,
- solid, moderately echogenic or vesicular,
- regular or irregular, serrated.

In the vast majority of cases the thickening is localised and regular, occasionally with a small cystic area: the appearances are those of a simple benign hyerplasia.

Exceptionally, the thickening has a worrying appearance (frankly nodular, heterogeneous and irregular) which suggests the possibility of malignant degeneration and is an indication for surgical confirmation.

Pseudotumours

These are basically inguino-scrotal hernias which, in patients who are difficult to examine, cannot be diagnosed clinically and are ultrasonically misleading.

Inguino-scrotal hernias are of two types:

-Either congenital, due to non-obliteration of the peritoneo-vaginal canal passing, therefore, through the spermatic cord (indirect hernias),

-or acquired, commonest in the adult, due to an evagination of the peritoneum which extends either through the large opening of the inguinal canal into the cord (indirect external oblique hernias) or outside the cord (direct hernias).

The ultrasonic appearances are dependent on the anatomical structures within the hernia:

-fat : variable size, echogenic sheet above and behind the testis. This is the commonest type.

-loop of intestine. The appearance varies depending on the bowel contents: faeces, air or fluid. If fluid filled, the appearance is that of a rounded structure with an anechoic centre; air filled loops appear as echogenic highly attenuating arcs. A careful search should be made to detect the presence of peristaltic movement.

The frequently encountered heterogeneous appearance (fat and bowel) must not be misdiagnosed as a tumour of the cord. The inability to clearly define the limits of the mass ultrasonically is a good clue for doingt the right diagnosis of hernia.

The chronically enlarged scrotum

Inflammatory pathology: hydroceles

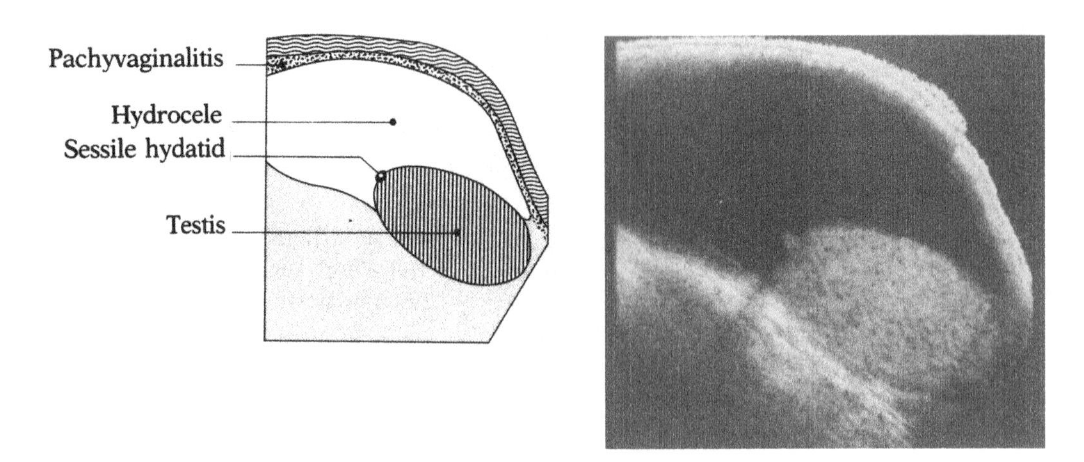

Fig.1. ***Simple hydrocele.*** Sagittal section. A large fluid collection in the tunica vaginalis outlining a sessile hydatid. Thickened parietal layer of the tunica vaginalis. Testis normal

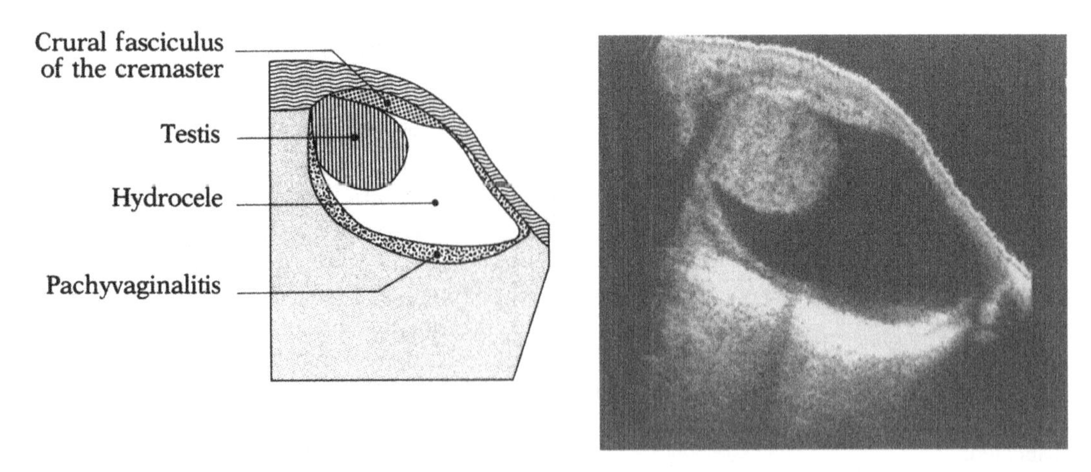

Fig. 2. ***Hydrocele with frank pachyvaginalitis (inflammatory thickening of the tunica vaginalis).*** Sagittal section. Large hydrocele with definite diffuse thickening of the parietal layer of the tunica vaginalis appearing as a band of intermediate echogenicity close to the deep surface of the investing layers. This can be differentiated from the triangular, echogenic and antero-posterior crural fasciculus of the cremaster muscle. The normal testis has a "ringing bell" appearance in the centre of the hydrocele

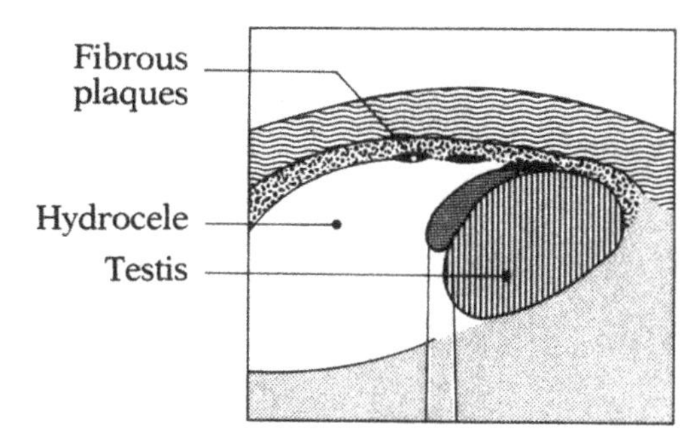

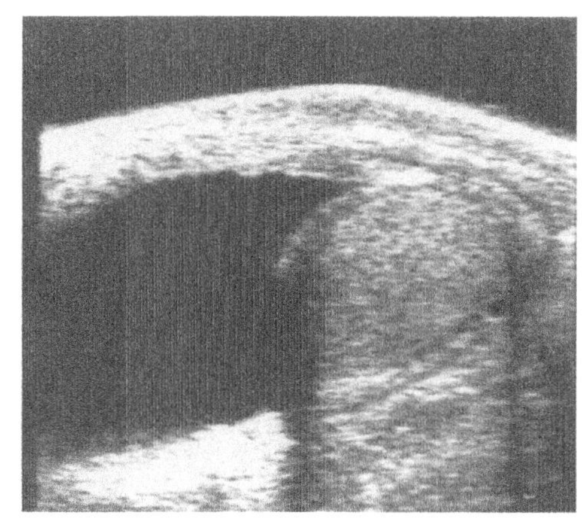

Fig. 3. ***Hydrocele and fibrous cephalic epididymitis.*** Sagittal section. Large hydrocele pushing the testis against the inferior scrotal surface. Pachyvaginalitis with fibrous areas indicated by echogenic lines. The fibrous anterior epididymis appears calcified casting an acoustic shadow behind the head

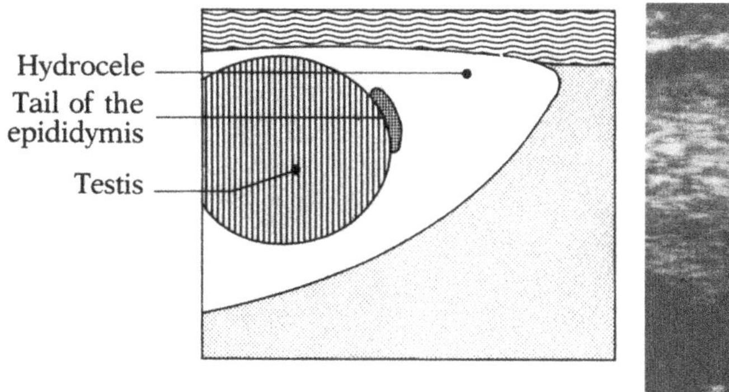

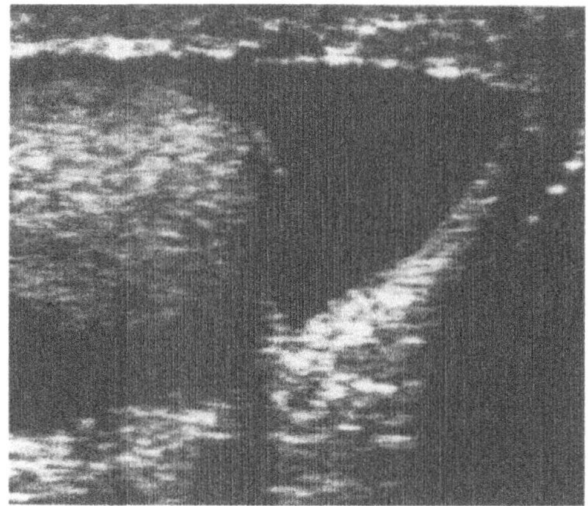

Fig. 4. ***Hydrocele and fibrous caudal epididymitis.*** Sagittal section of the inferior pole. The hydrocele is adjacent to a normal size epididymal tail which appears abnormally visible due to fibrosis

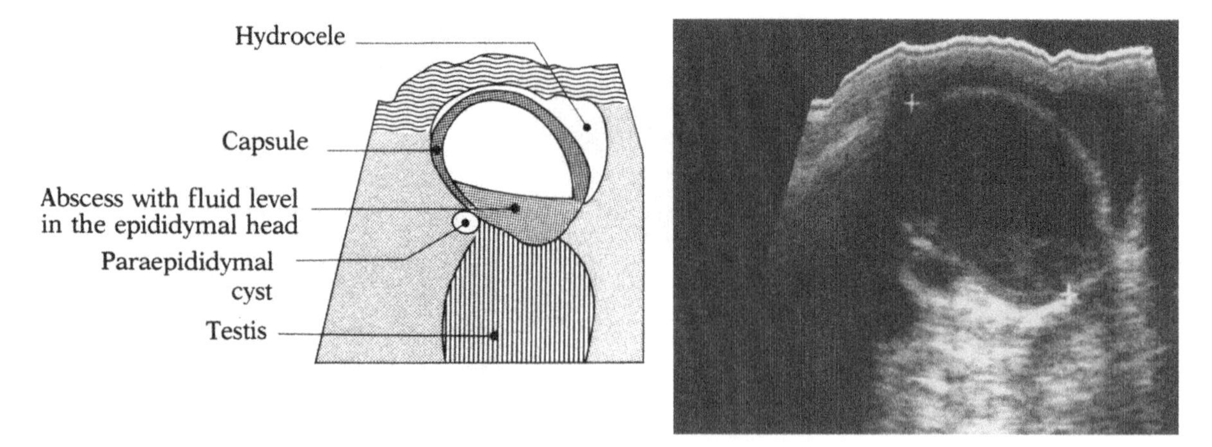

Fig. 5. ***Hydrocele and epididymal abscess.*** Transverse section with magnification of the anterior half of the scrotal sac. A small hydrocele adjacent to a rounded structure of almost 2 cm situated anterior to the testis. The appearances indicate a complex cyst due to superadded infection as shown by its echogenic wall and fluid levels

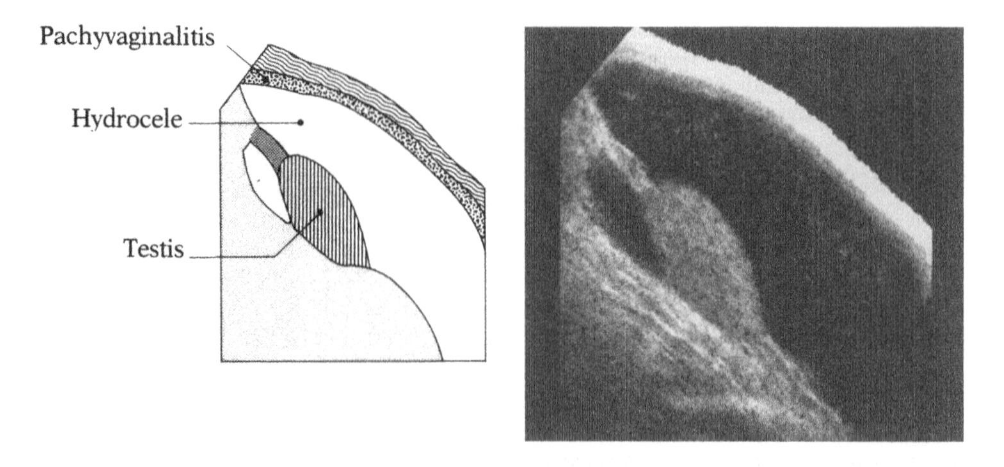

Fig. 6. ***Cholesterol hydrocele.*** Sagittal section. A large hydrocele which does not appear transonic as in a simple hydrocele but contains multiple, very fine and diffuse echoes which are very suggestive of cholesterol crystals within the collection

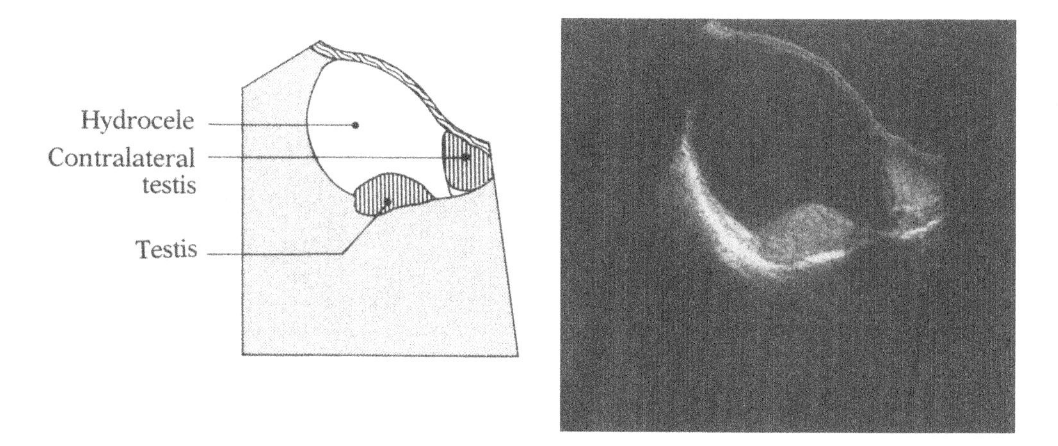

Fig. 7. ***Hydrocele: position of the testis.*** Transverse section of both testes. Large hydrocele developing anteriorly displacing the testis horizontally against the posterior scrotal wall

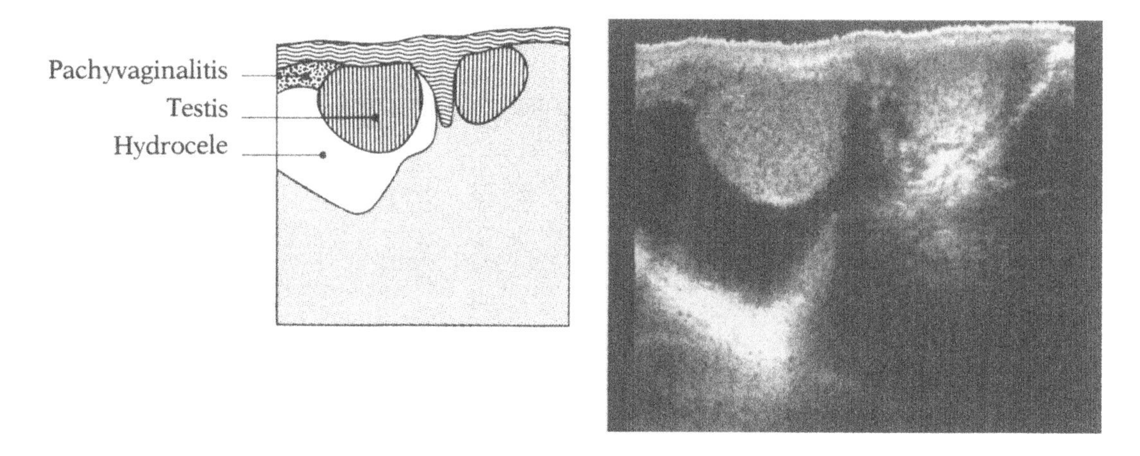

Fig. 8. ***Hydrocele: position of the testis.*** Transverse section of both testes. Medium size hydrocele postero-superiorly pushing the testis anteriorly and medially against the median raphe

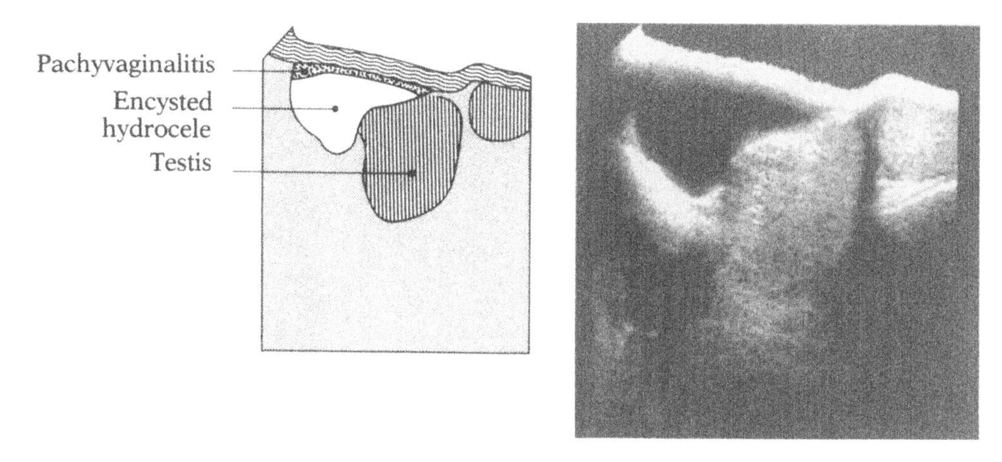

Fig. 9. ***Hydrocele: position of the testis.*** Transverse scan of both testes. Antero-superior hydrocele with pachyvaginalitis displacing both the testes infero-posteriorly and medially

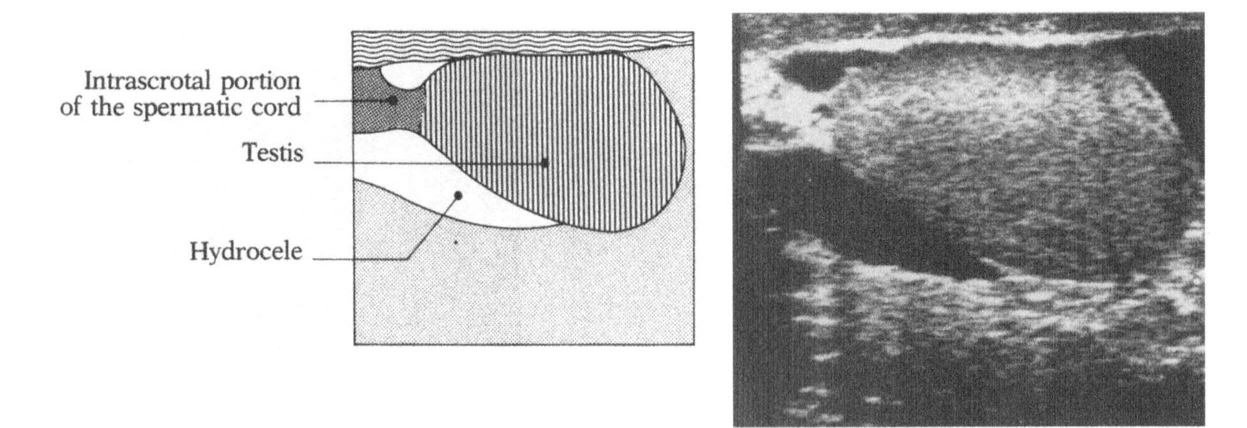

Fig.10. ***Hydrocele: morphology.*** Sagittal section. Free, medium size hydrocele outlining the spermatic pedicle and filling the antero- superior interepididymo-testicular recess

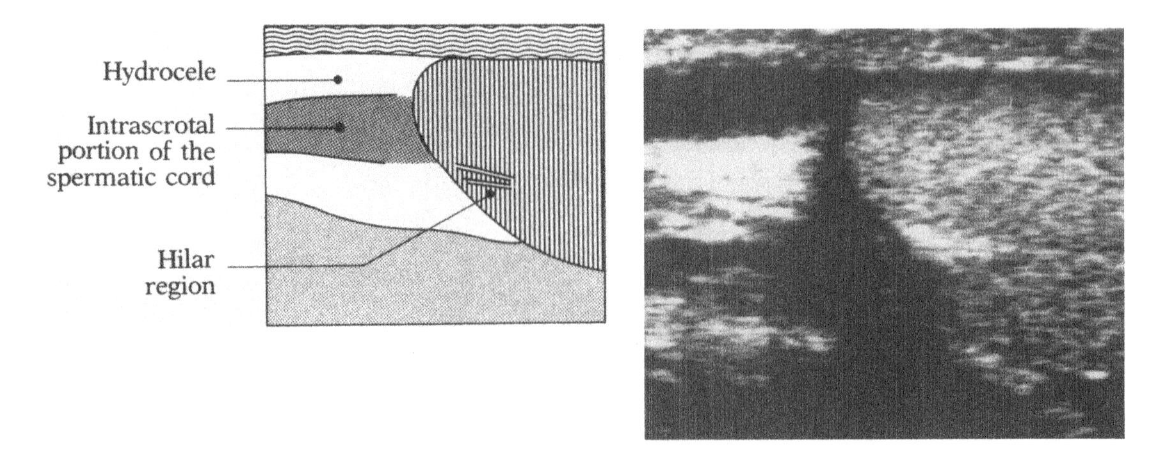

Fig.11. ***Hydrocele: morphology.*** Sagittal section of the superior pole. Small hydrocele surrounding the cord, highly echogenic due to the posterior enhancement from the collection

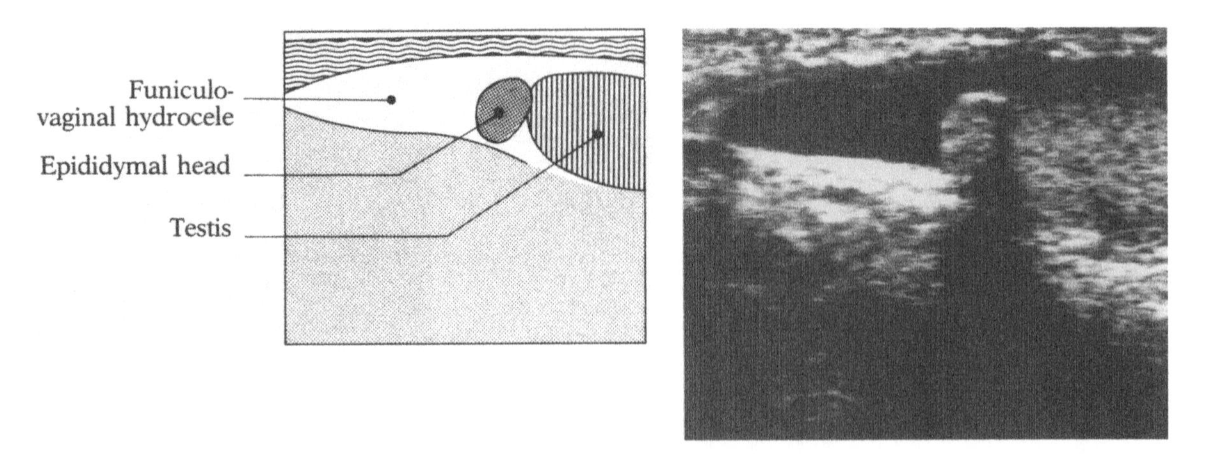

Fig.12. ***Funiculo-vaginal hydrocele.*** Sagittal section of the superior pole. Small tubular hydrocele extending above the head of the epididymis

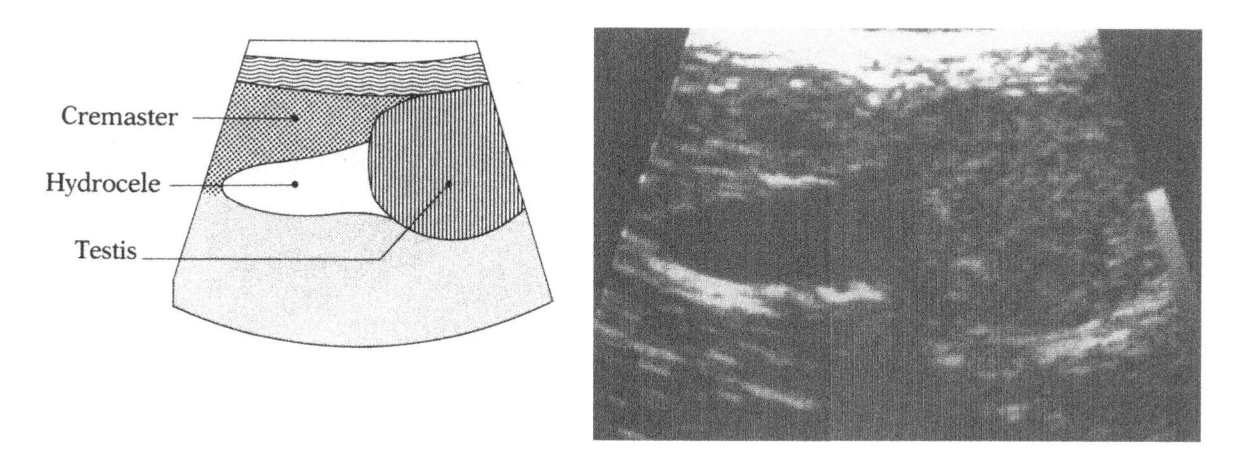

Fig.13. ***Hydrocele with a freely mobile testis.*** Sagittal section of the inguino-scrotal region. A small hydrocele adjacent to a hypertrophied crural fasiculus of the cremaster muscle. The hydrocele is a satellite lesion to an intermittently high lying testis

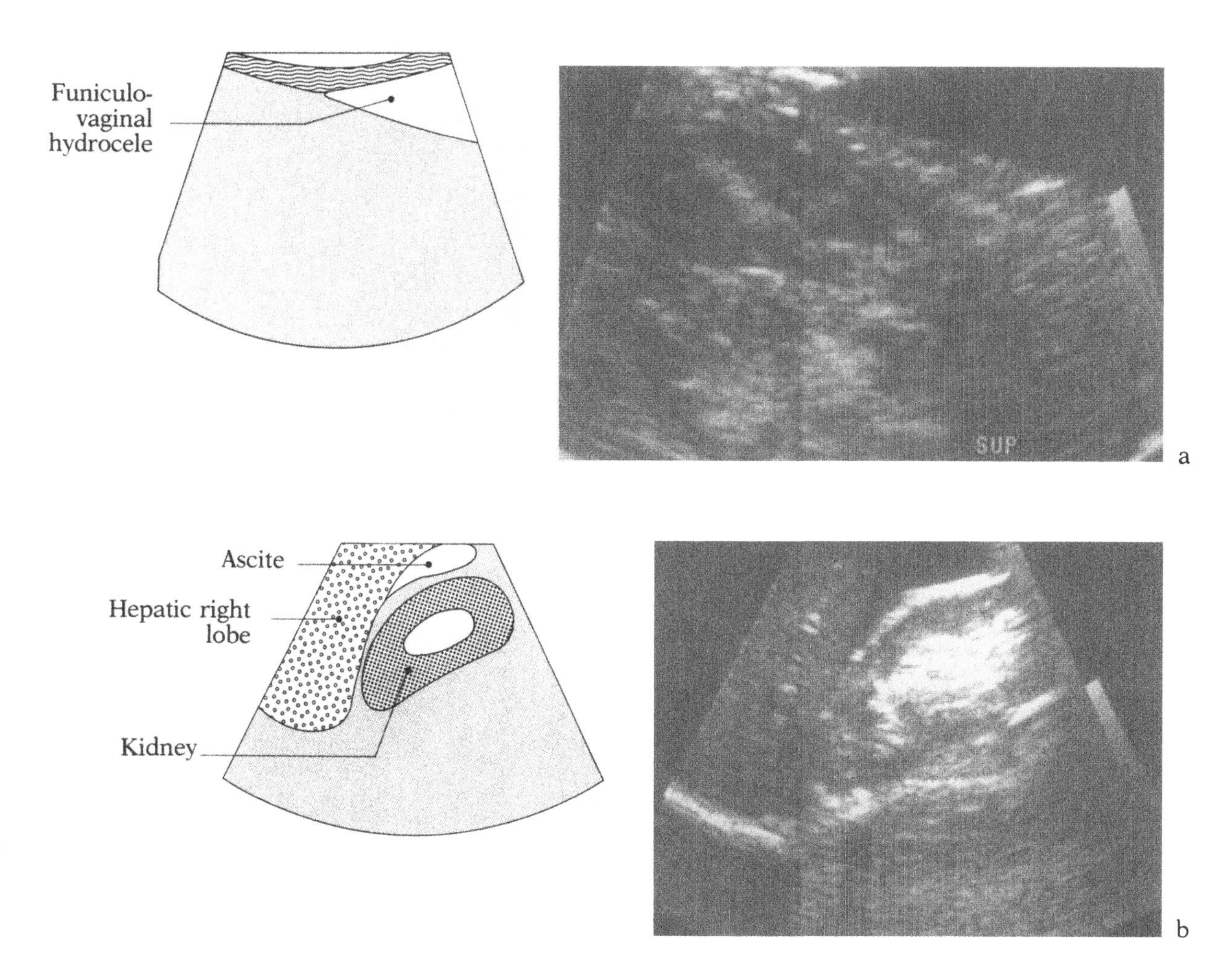

Fig.14a, b. Funiculo-vaginal hydrocele associated with a carcinoma. Recent feeling of heaviness in the testis in a man who had recently undergone a gastrectomy for gastric cancer. **a** Sagittal section of the superior portion of the testis. Small hydrocele filling the lower portion of the non-obliterated peritoneo-vaginal canal. **b** Sagittal section of the right hypochondrium: ascites in the interhepato- renal recess. Conclusion: Given the history of carcinoma, a hydrocele with ascites is probably secondary to peritoneal carcinomatosis

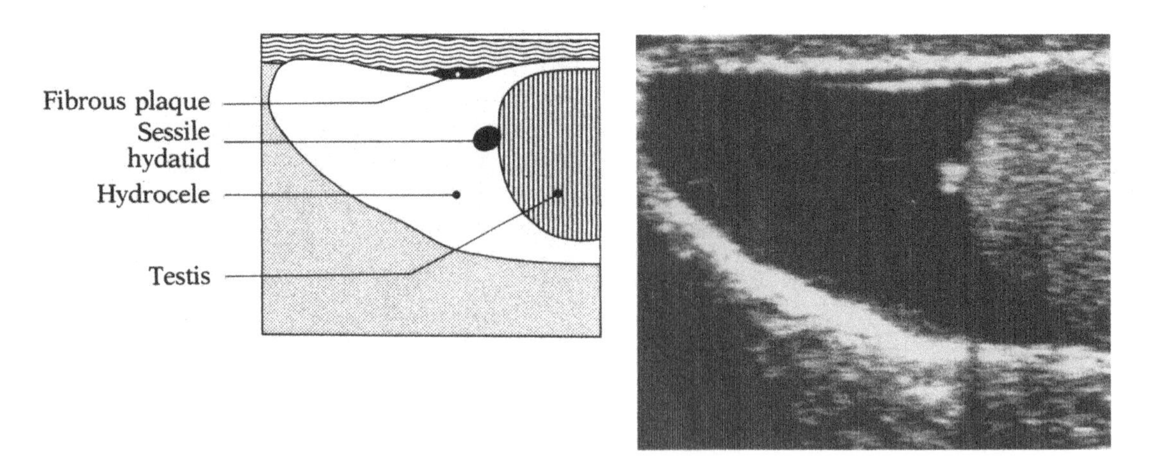

Fig. 15. ***Hydrocele of the superior pole.*** Sagittal section. Completely transonic hydrocele, localised to the superior part of the scrotal sac, surrounding a very echogenic sessile hydatid (due to fibrosis)

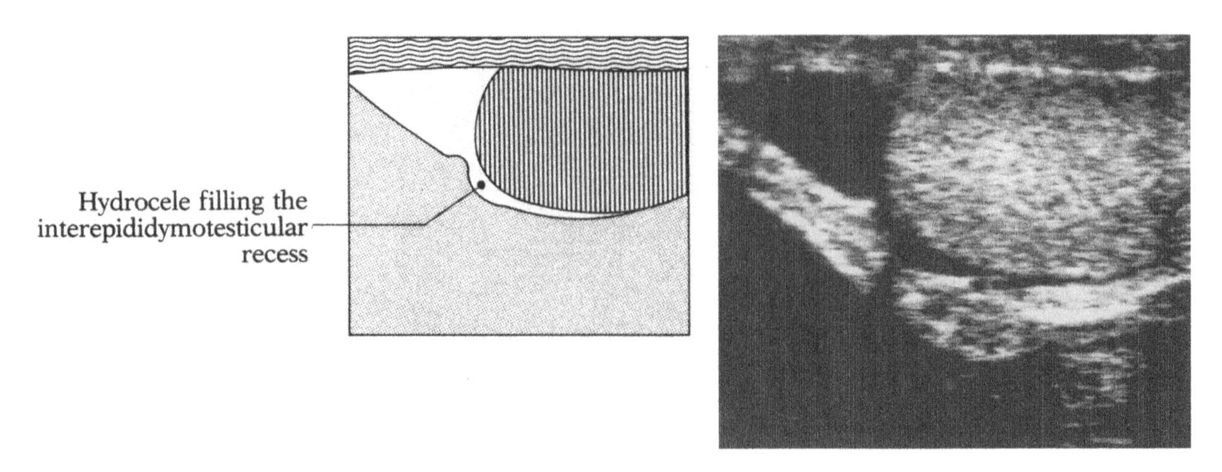

Fig. 16. ***Hydrocele of the superior pole.*** Sagittal section. Small fluid collection filling the postero-superior interepididymo-testicular recess

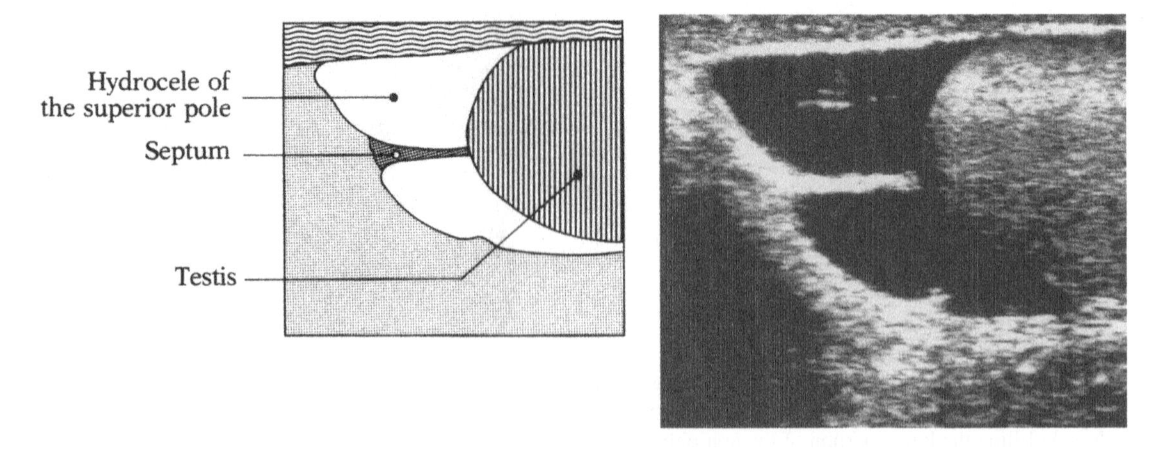

Fig. 17. ***Biloculated hydrocele of the superior pole.*** High sagittal section. The hydrocele is divided by an echogenic fibrous septum extending from the postero-superior surface of the investing layers to the superior pole of the testis

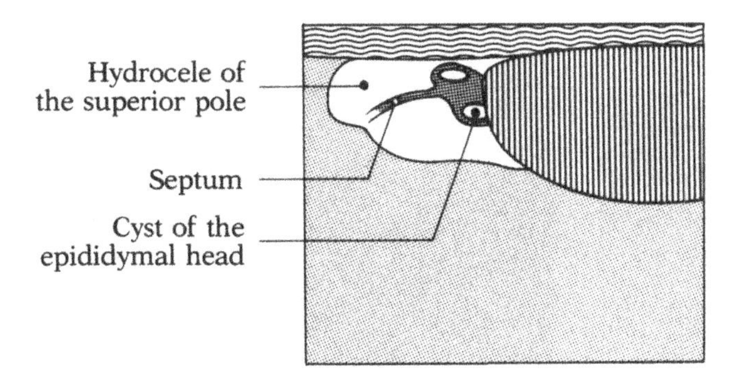

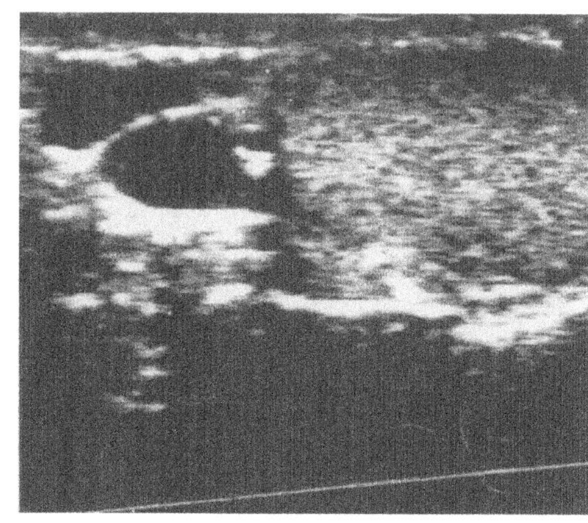

Fig. 18. ***Biloculated hydrocele of the superior pole.*** In view of its small size, it may be suggestive of a dystrophic para-epididymal cyst which has in fact, a more rounded shape and is often situated antero-superiorly. Sometimes, however, it is not possible to be absolutely certain of the diagnosis

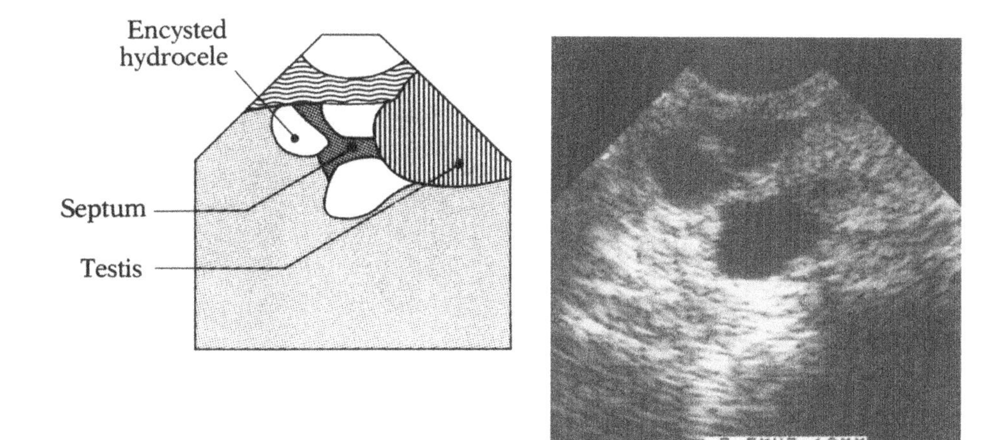

Fig. 19. ***Trifoliate hydrocele of the superior pole.*** There are several adhesions between the two layers of the tunica vaginalis, forming septa within the collection. Same diagnostic problem to differentiate it from a possible dystrophic cyst

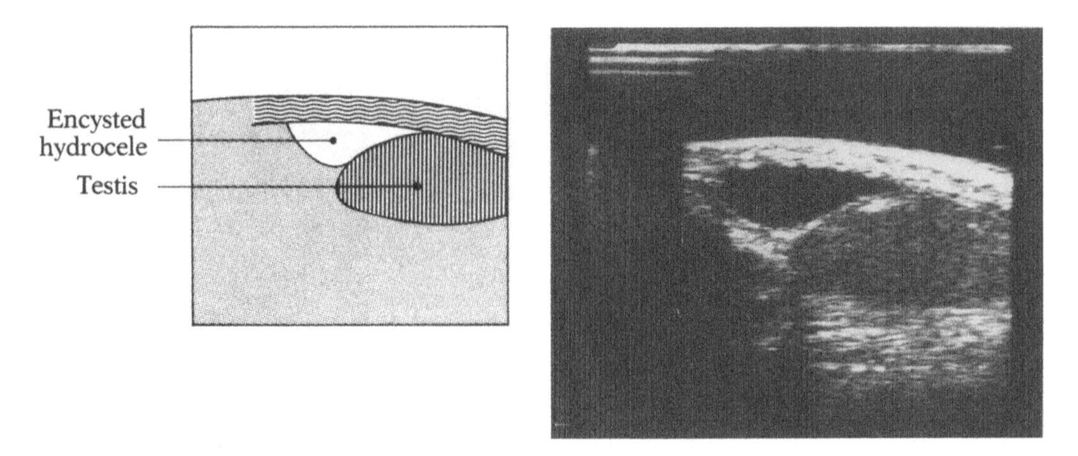

Fig. 20. ***Encysted hydrocele of the superior pole.*** Sagittal section. Truly encysted hydrocele due to adhesions which are surrounding it. The testis is pulled downwards

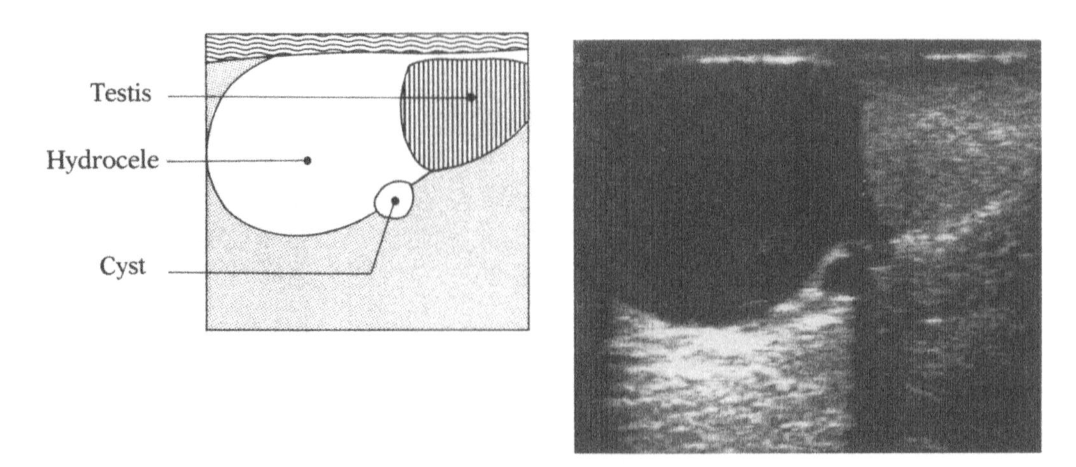

Fig. 21. ***Encysted hydrocele of the superior pole with a parietal cyst.*** Transverse section. Large hydrocele localised to the superior pole of the scrotal sac associated with a small cystic structure of a few millimetres arising from the parietal layer of the tunica vaginalis, encysted by fibrous tissue. Not to be mistaken for a tumour of the tunica vaginalis

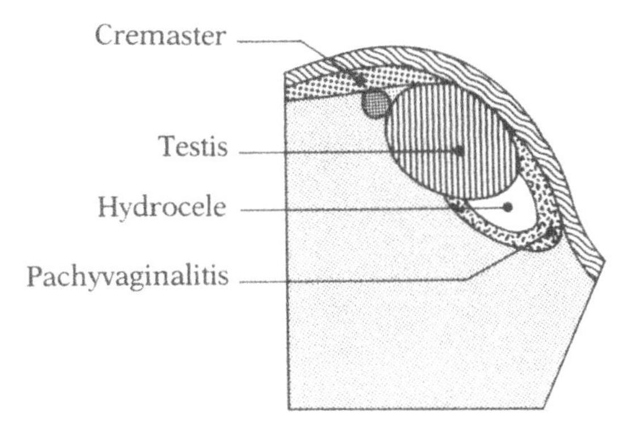

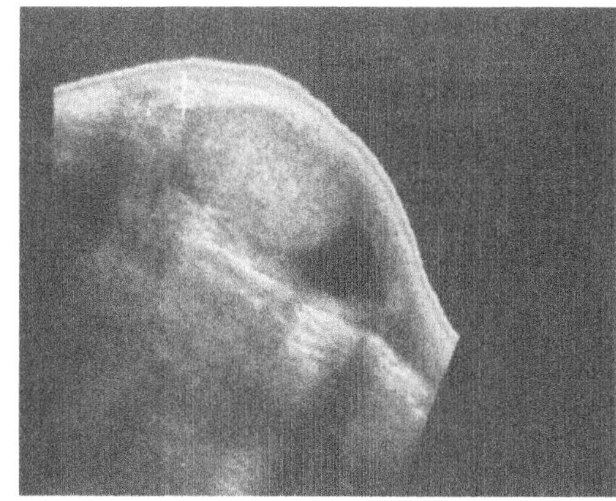

Fig. 22. ***Hydrocele of the inferior pole.*** Sagittal section. The fluid collection under the testis has a fluid level associated with a marked pachyvaginalitis. Note the contracted cremaster muscle recognised by the antero-superior echogenic band over the deep surface of the scrotum

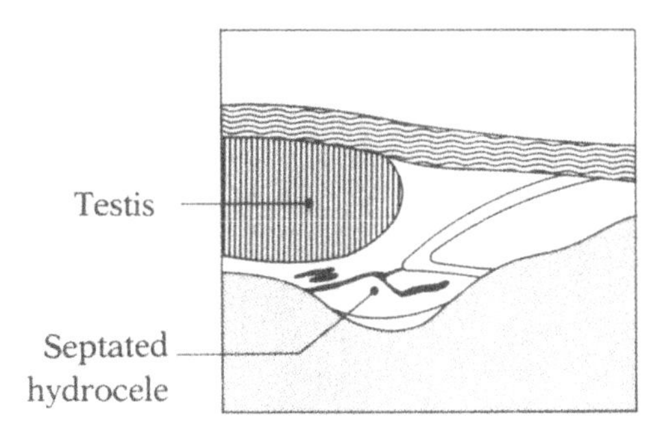

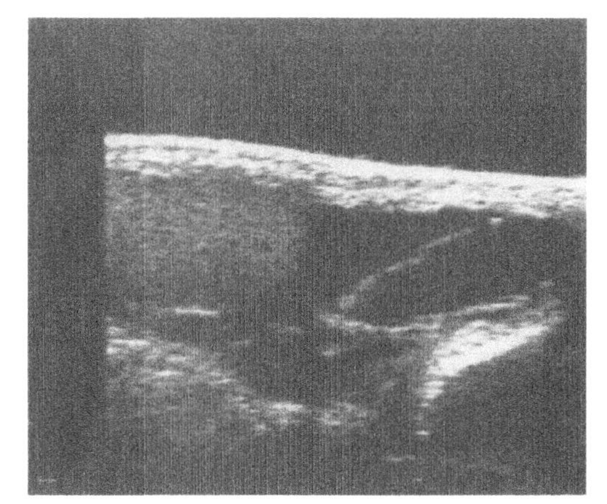

Fig. 23. ***Multi-loculated hydrocele of the inferior pole.*** Sagittal section of the inferior pole. Beneath the testis, the fluid collection is separated by several septa. With these appearances and the absence of any history of trauma, tuberculosis must be excluded

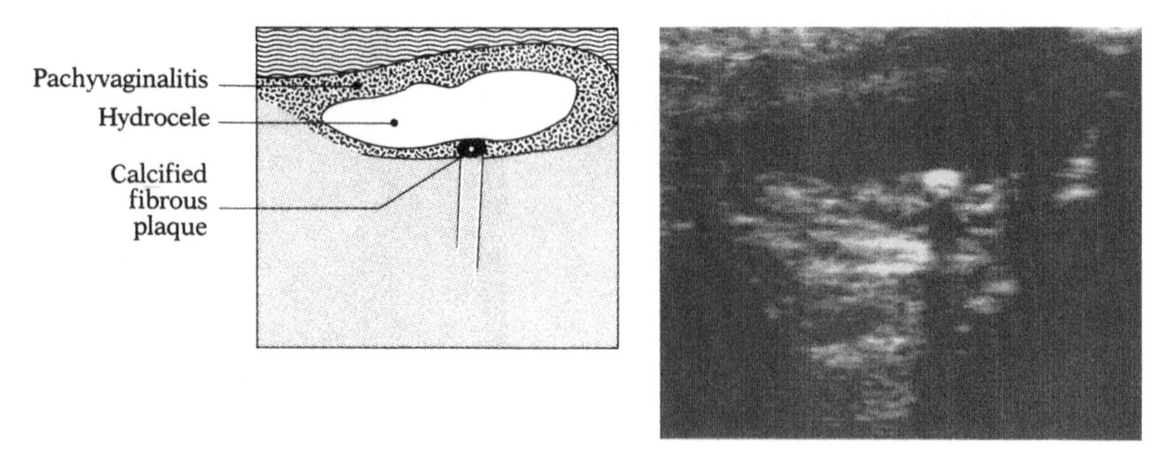

Fig. 24. ***Calcified hydrocele.*** Transverse section of the inferior pole. The collection in the tunica vaginalis is associated with a highly attenuating echogenic zone: fibro-calcific areas are often present in old hydroceles

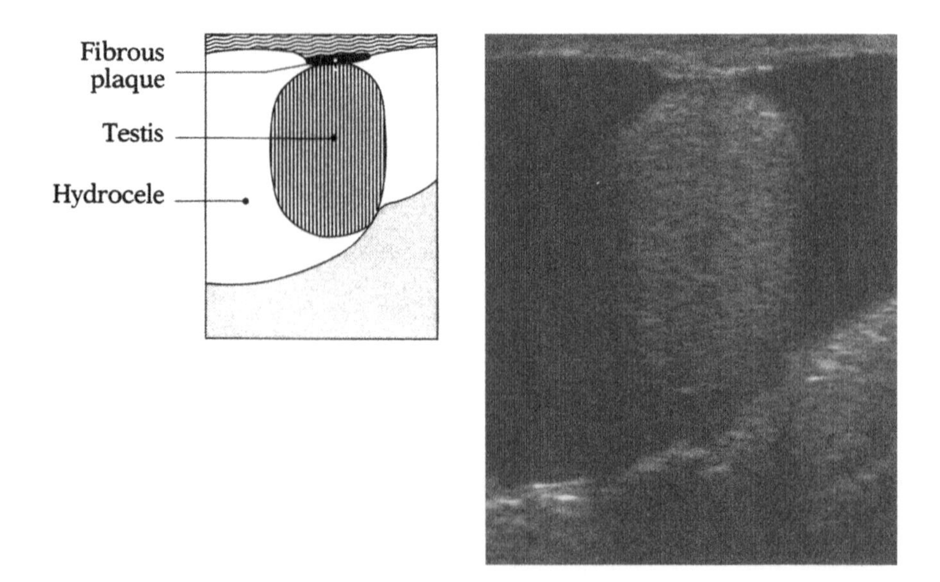

Fig. 25. ***Hydrocele and parietal abnormalities.*** Transverse section: a very large hydrocele which is pushing the testis against the anterior investing layers. There is localised thickening of the parietal layer of the tunica vaginalis appearing echogenic due to fibrosis

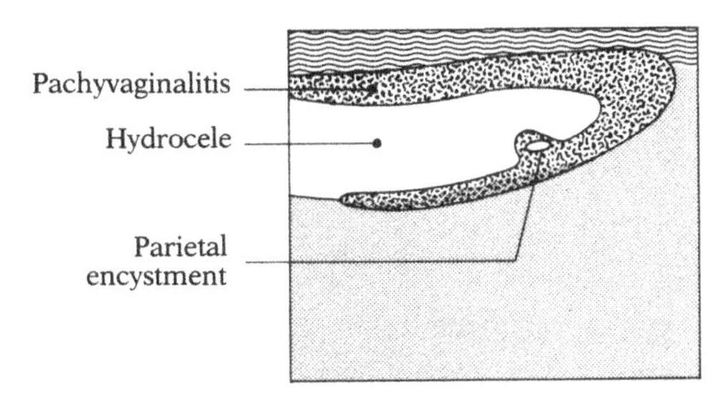

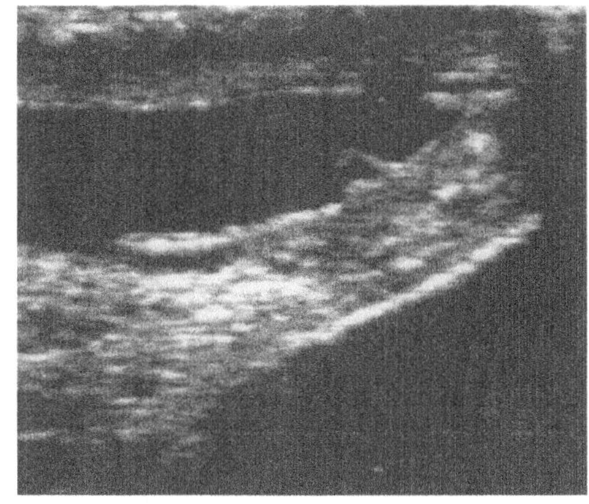

Fig. 26. ***Hydrocele and parietal abnormalities.*** Oblique section of the inferior pole. Vesicular lesion of a few millimetres projecting into the hydrocele, arising from the parietal layer of the tunica vaginalis: intra-parietal microcyst arising in an old adherent hydrocele

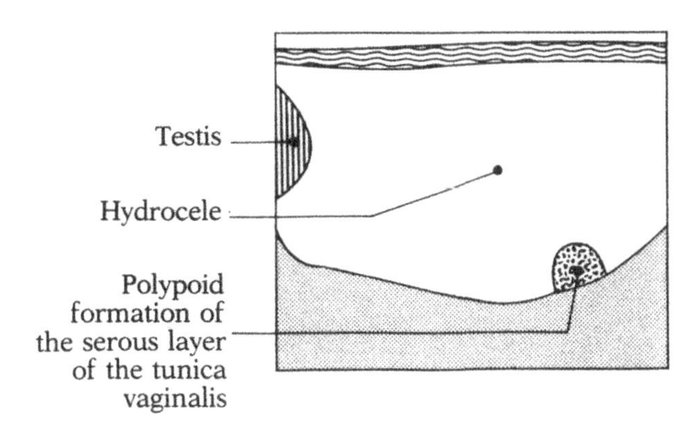

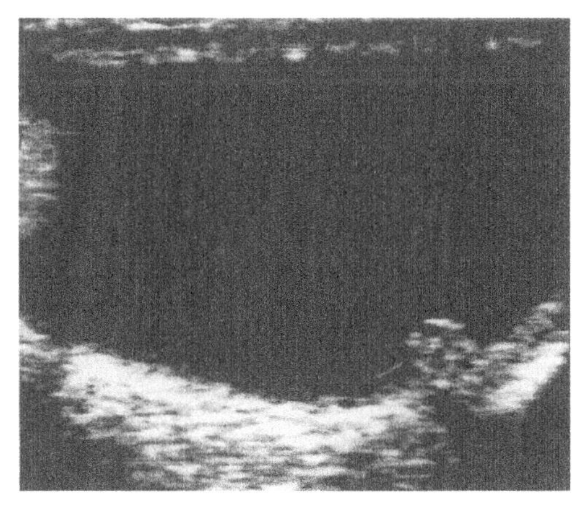

Fig. 27. ***Hydrocele and parietal abnormalities.*** Transverse section. Barely visible testis which is displaced medially against the median raphe by a large hydrocele. On the deep surface of the investing layers is a regular solitary nodule of a few millimetres: hyperplastic nodule of the parietal layer of the tunica vaginalis. This single, small and regular structure has a benign appearance, thus differentiating it from a mesothelioma

Testicular tumours

Germinal Tumours

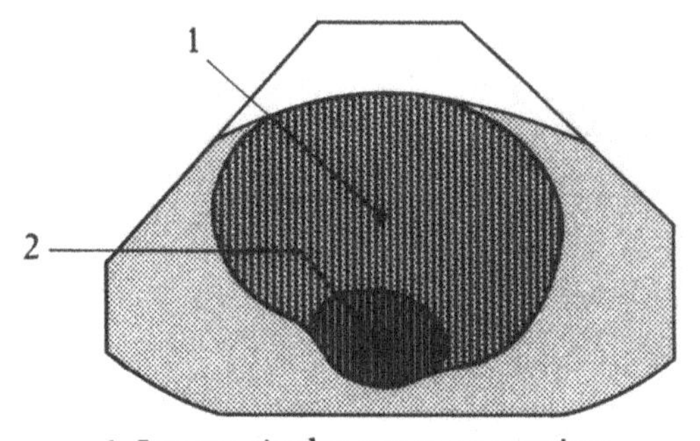

1 Intratesticular space-occupying lesion
2 Perihilar hypoechoic zone

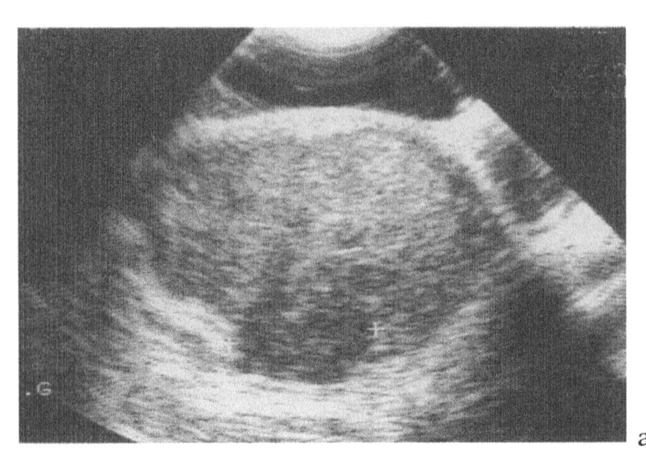

a

1
2
3
4

1 Tunica albuginea
2 Normal parenchyma
3 Tumour
4 Tumour invasion of the rete testis

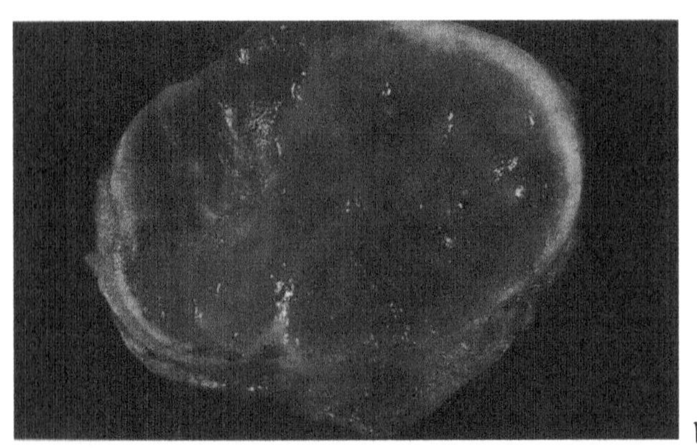

b

Fig. 28a, b. ***Seminoma; infiltrating form.*** Progressive painless enlargement of a testis in a 65 year old man. **a** Sagittal section: enlarged testis whose parenchyma is almost totally replaced by an expansile, fairly homogenous and echogenic process. At the level of the hilum there is a deformity of the contour by a more hypoechoic area. **b** Section of the orchidectomy specimen: the whole of the testis is replaced by tumour apart from a small anterior band of healthy tissue at the superior pole. Invasion of the rete testis corresponding to the projecting structure from the hilum. However, the rest of the tunica albuginea is intact. Histology: seminoma extending into the rete testis

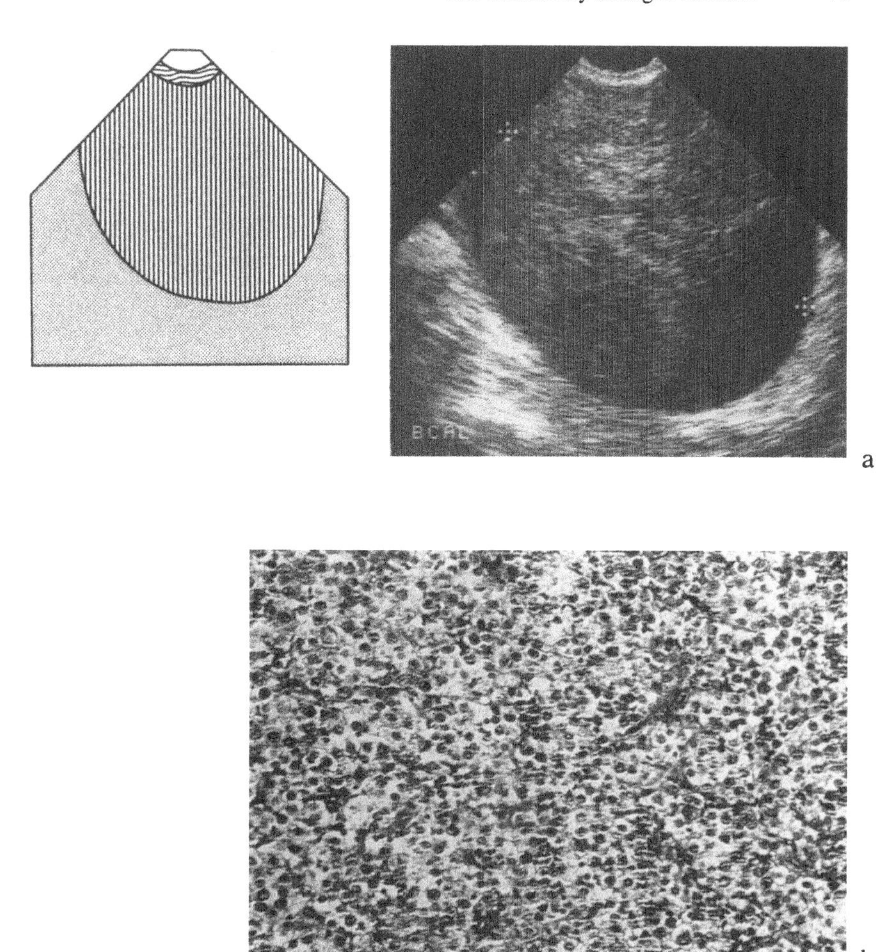

Fig. 29a, b. ***Seminoma; infiltrating form.*** Same clinical picture in a 45 year old man. **a** Sagittal section: marked enlargement of the testis, measuring nearly 8 cm, by solid homogenous tissue. This homogenous appearance, which persists despite the very large size, is very suggestive of a seminoma. **b** Histological section: seminomatous cells, small size and regular in a sheet with a slight associated inflammatory reaction as indicated by narrow fibro- connective tissue bands

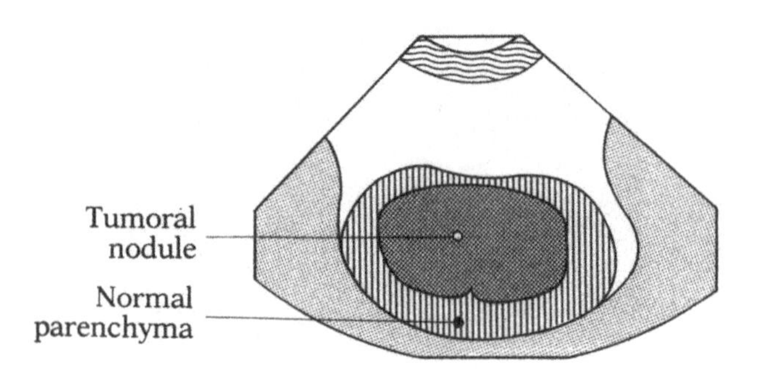

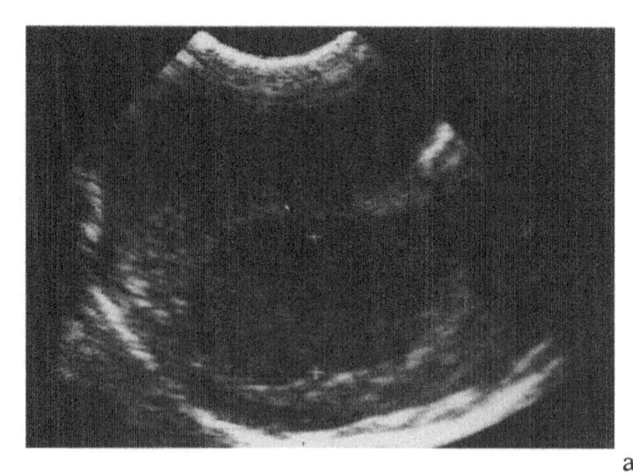

a

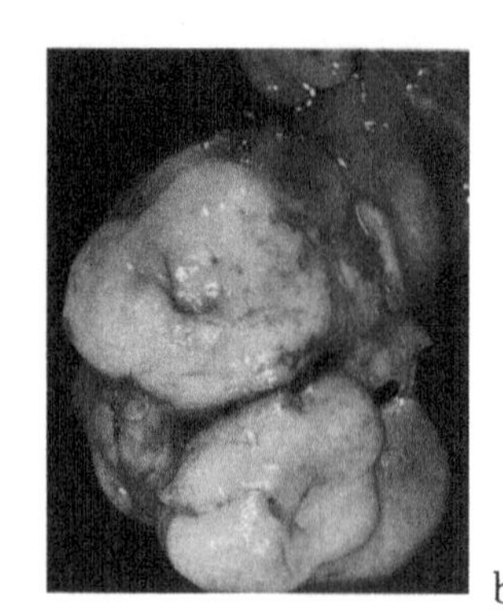

b

Fig. 30a, b. ***Seminoma; nodular form.*** Painless enlargement of the testis in a 30 year old man, HIV positive. a Sagittal section: well-defined, homogenous and hypoechoic oval mass bordered by a tongue of normal testicular tissue. Taking into account the position, age and ultrasonic appearances, the differential diagnosis is seminoma or lymphoma. The latter is less likely due to the absence of tumour nodules in the contralateral testis and the absence of abdominal lymphadenopathy. b Orchidectomy specimen cut in two: the tumour has a lobulated outline and is clearly separate from the band of normal parenchyma. The cord and epididymis are not involved. Histology: seminoma

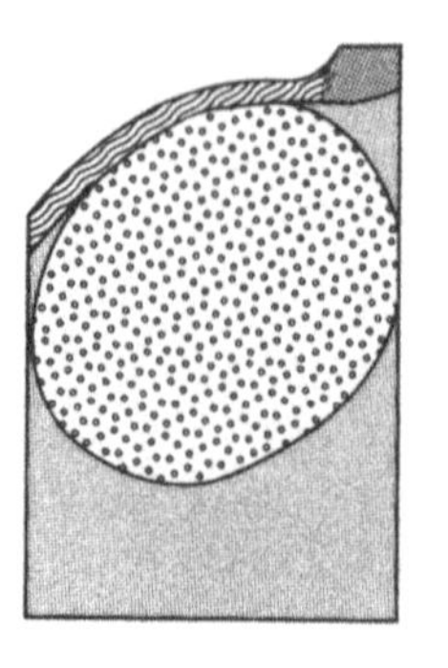

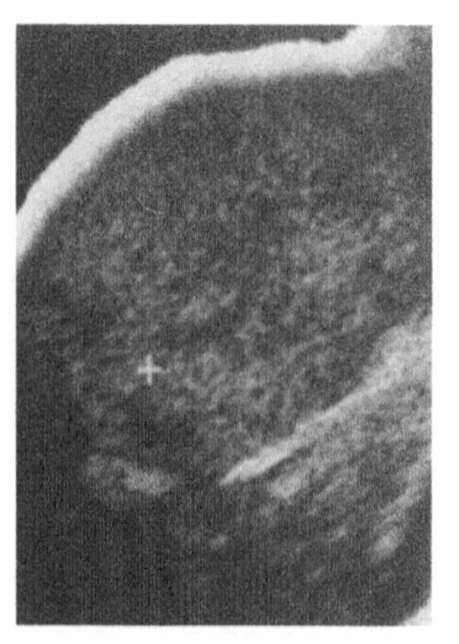

Fig. 31. ***Seminoma with extension into the epididymis.*** The testis is replaced by the tumour which is seen as a fairly discrete heterogeneity within the parenchyma. The junction with the body of the epididymis is indistinct

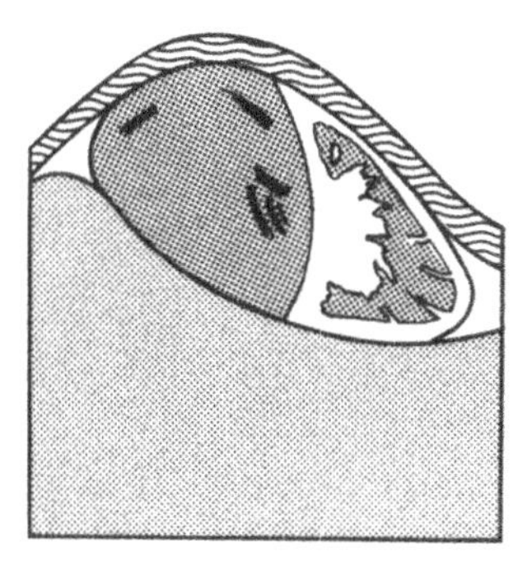

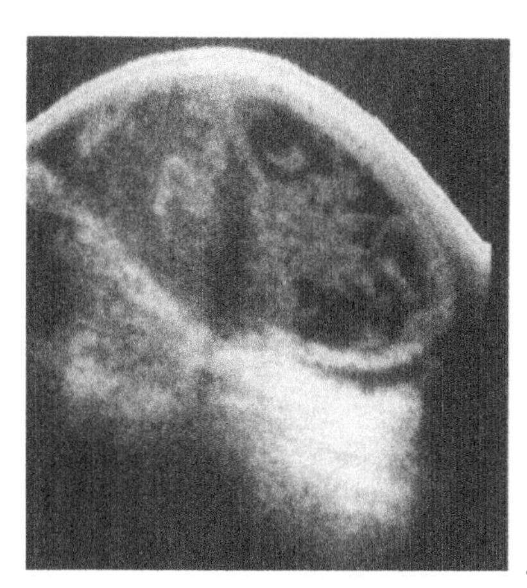

a

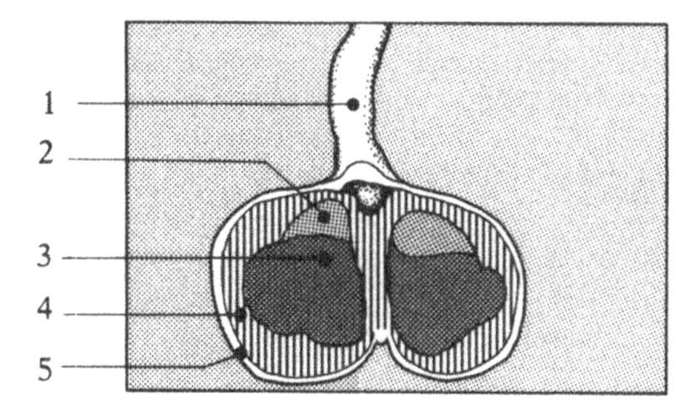

1 Spermatic cord
2 Solid tumour component
3 Necrotic tumour
4 Normal parenchyma
5 Tunica albuginea

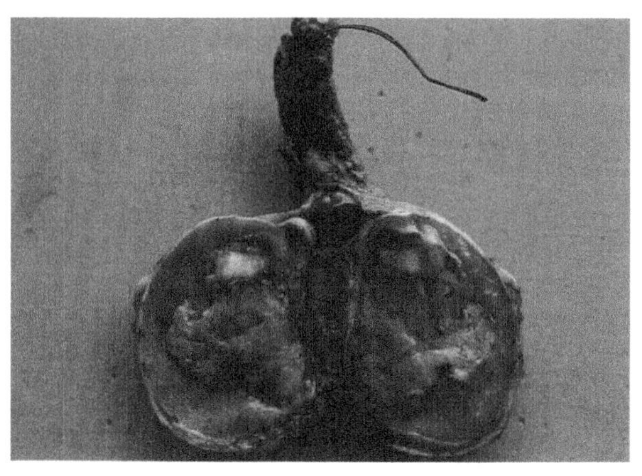

b

Fig. 32a, b. ***Necrotic seminoma.*** **a** Sagittal section: testis with evidence of tumour, enlarged to almost twice the normal size, with a very heterogenous echo pattern and very different appearances in the two halves. In the superior part, the tumour is solid with several echogenic areas, undoubtedly haemorrhagic. In the inferior part, there is solid, central tissue surrounded by a semi-liquid, transonic halo. **b** Orchidectomy specimen cut in two with the spermatic cord above: the main part of the tumour is necrotic and corresponds to the inferior portion ultrasonically. The upper half is solid and fleshy in appearance. A normal strip of tissue separates the tumour from the tunica albuginea

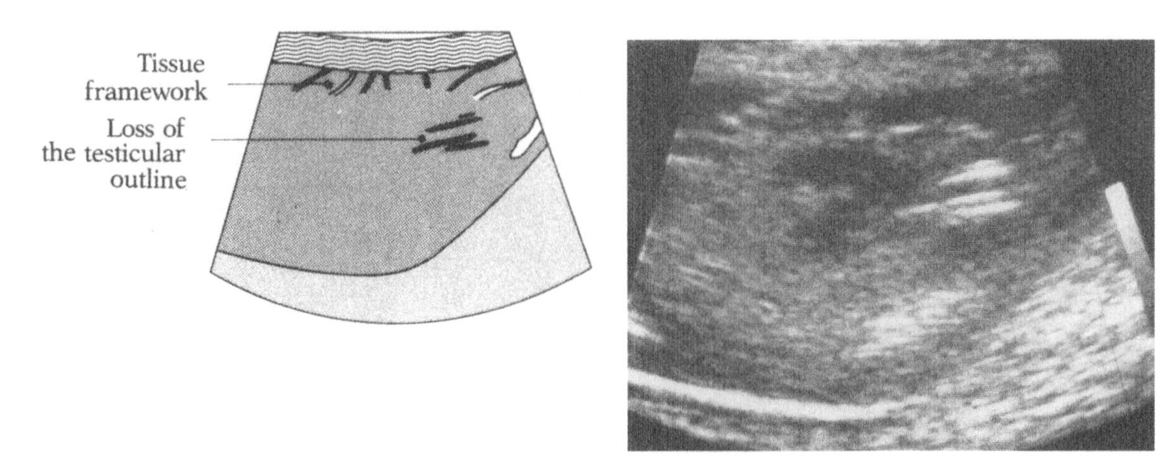

Fig. 33. ***Seminoma with extension in the investing layers of the testis.*** Transverse section: heterogenous testis, obviously tumour with a pseudo-encapsulated appearance antero-inferiorly. The tissue appears adherent to the deep surface of the investing layers and there is loss of regularity of the inferior pole of the testis.These signs indicate tumour invasion of the tunica vaginalis and of the investing layers. In fact, at histopathological examination, a simple seminoma was demonstrated with no evidence of invasion or of extension beyond the tunica albuginea. However, there was a peri-testicular inflammatory reaction responsible for the fibrinous adhesions which explains the ultrasound appearances

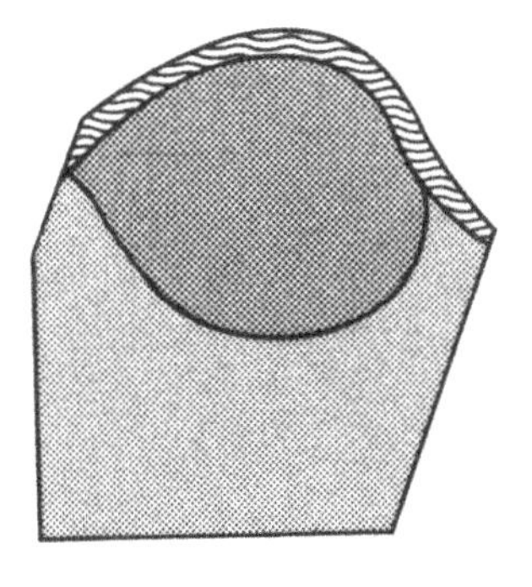

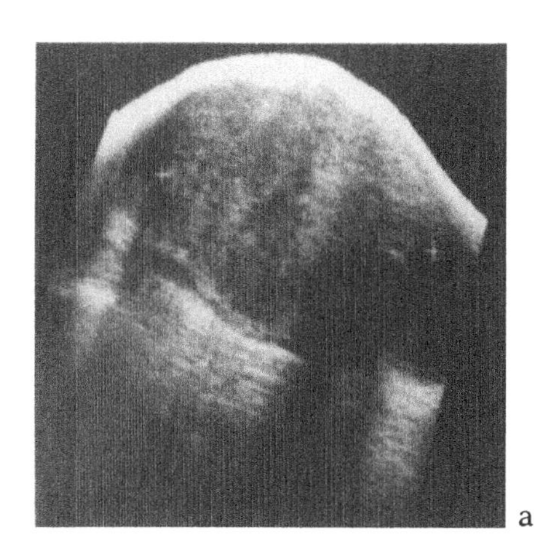

a

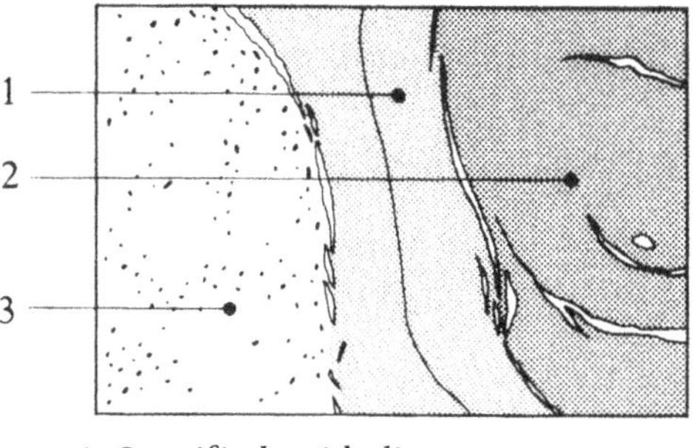

1 Stratified epithelium
2 Keratinised cyst
3 Cartilagenous area

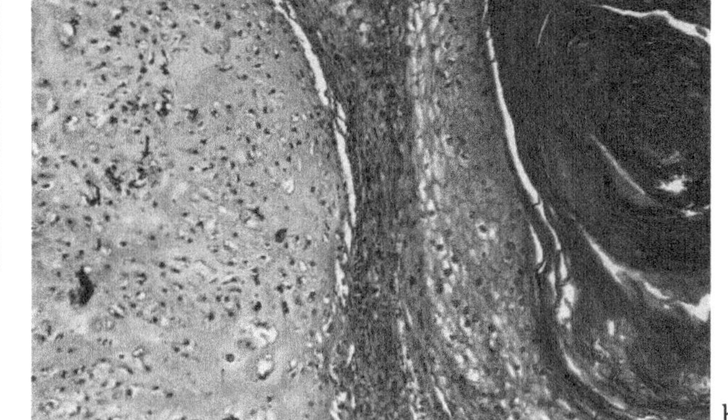

b

Fig. 34a, b. ***Non-seminomatous germinal tumour-embryonic carcinoma with complex malignant dysembryogenesis.*** **a** Sagittal section: a very large heterogenous testis, definitely tumour. Orchidectomy. **b** Histological section through a zone of dysembryoplastic tumour which contains cartilaginous elements and a cyst lined with stratified epithelium. There are no ultrasonic features (calcification) which could predict this dysembryoplastic composition

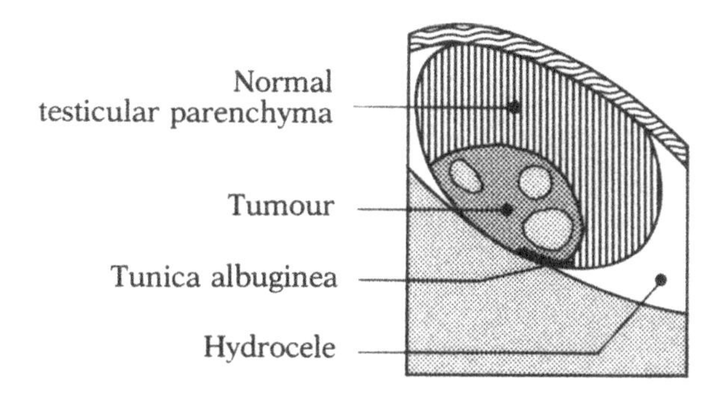

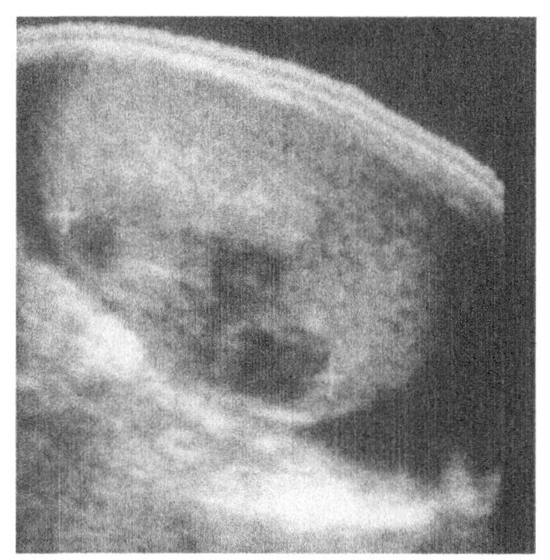

Fig. 35. ***Non-seminomatous germinal tumour; choriocarcinoma and immature teratoma.*** Moderately enlarged, slightly sensitive testis in a 25 year old man. Sagittal section: the morphology of the testis is virtually normal. The region of the tumour is at the hilum. It appears heterogenous and punctuated by three very hypoechoic nodules. Intact albuginea surrounded by a hydrocele

Non-germinal tumours

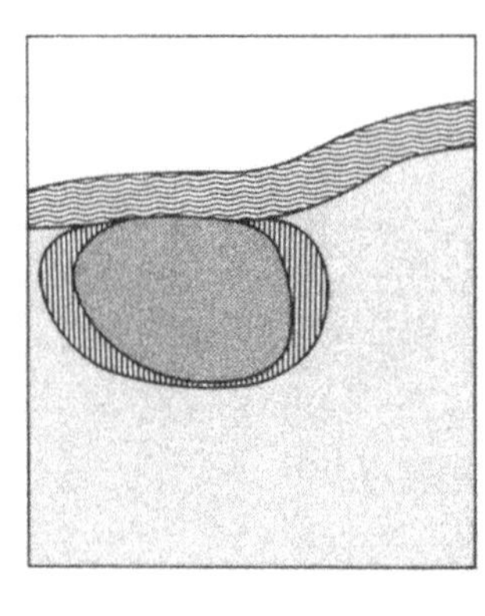

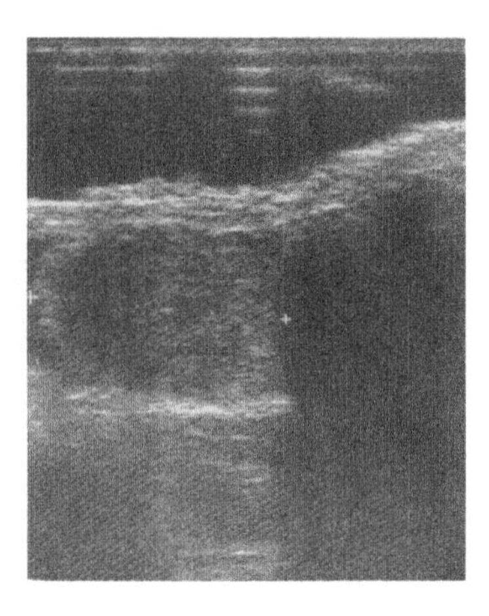

Fig. 36. ***Tumour of the stroma of the gonad; Leydig cell tumour.*** A 33 year old man with bilateral gynaecomastia for 8 years. Slightly elevated serum oestradiol level. Indurated testis on palpation. Sagittal section: large hypoechoic mass (greater than 3 cm) arising within the testis. The association of longstanding gynaecomastia with the slow evolution of the process suggests a Leydig cell tumour. This was confirmed histologically and also demonstrated tumour cells within the capsule of the mass: this is one of the features which suggest a malignant potential of the lesion

Secondary tumours

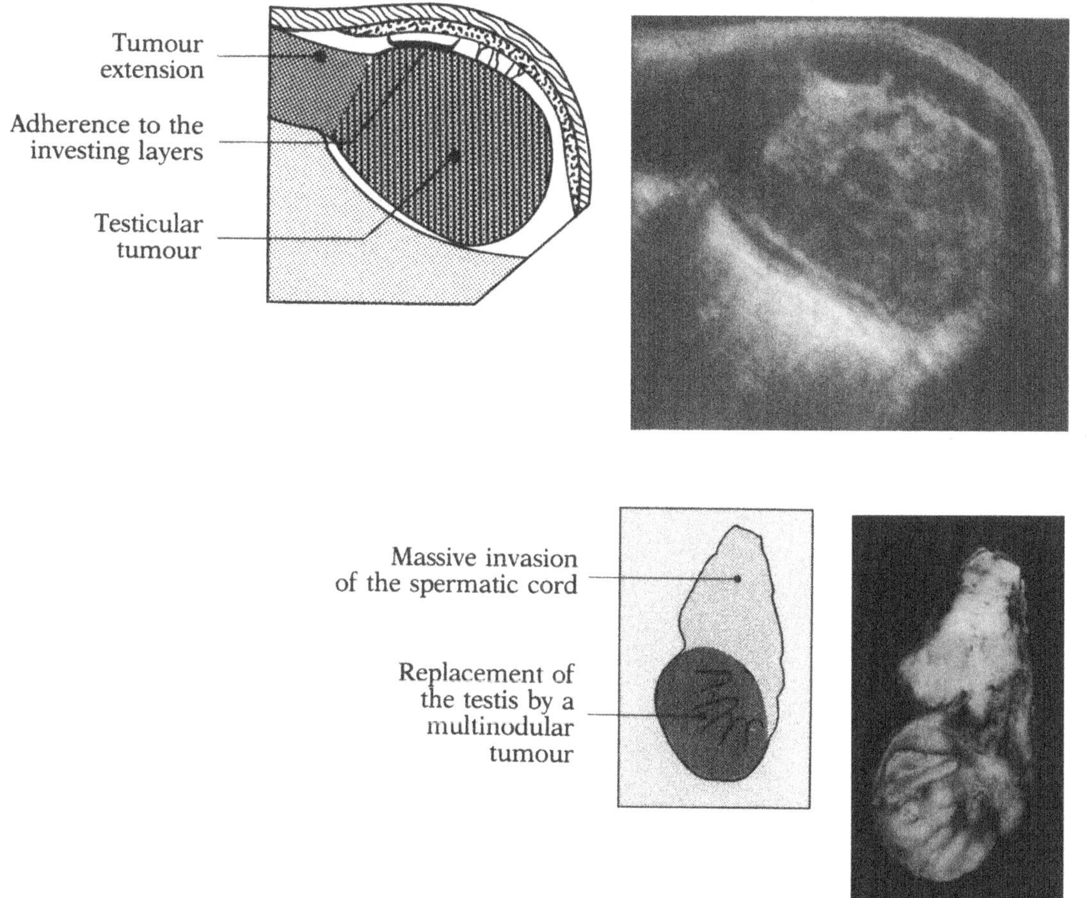

Fig. 37a, b. ***Malignant lymphoma.*** Large indurated testis in elderly man. **a** Sagittal section: the testis is totally replaced by a heterogenous solid tumour which is invading the head of the epididymis and the cord. A more hypoechoic mass is seen extending towards the external orifice of the inguinal canal. **b** Part of a section of the orchidectomy specimen: tumour is occupying all the testis (which is definitely enlarged) and there is extensive invasion of the spermatic cord. Extension of the ultrasound examination to include the abdomen revealed gross intra-abdominal lymphadenopathy

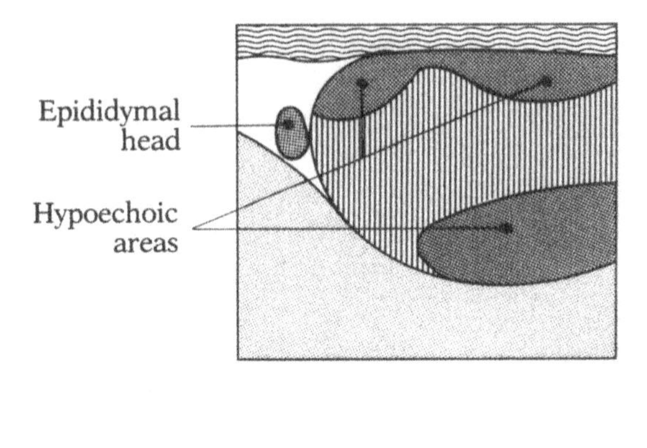

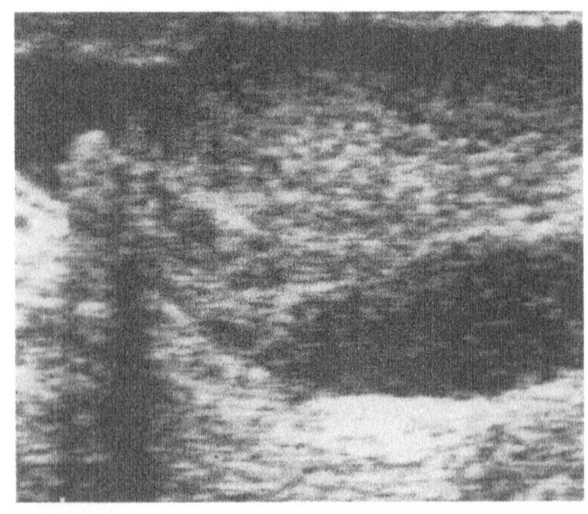

a

Hypoechoic tumour nodules

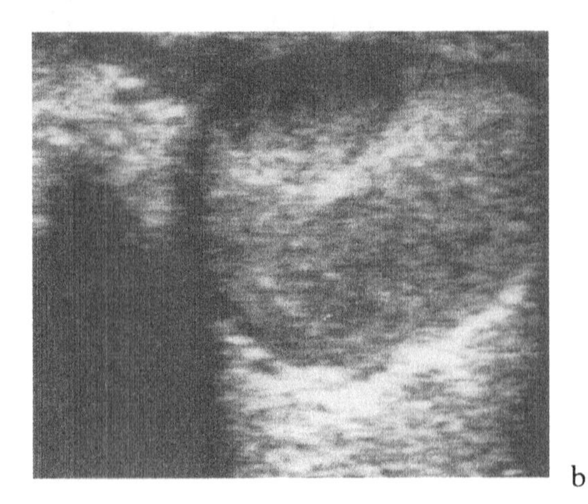

b

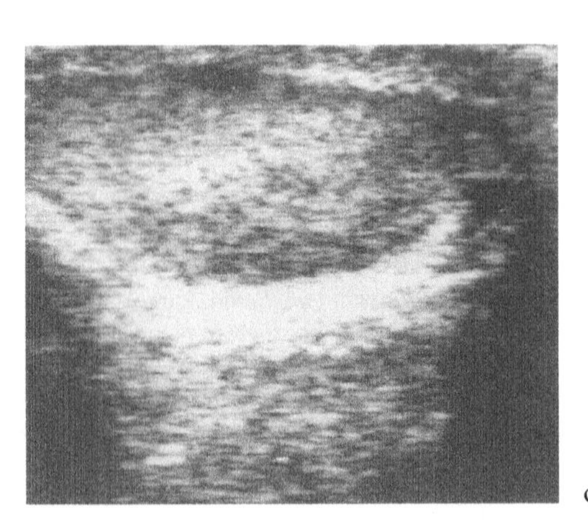

c

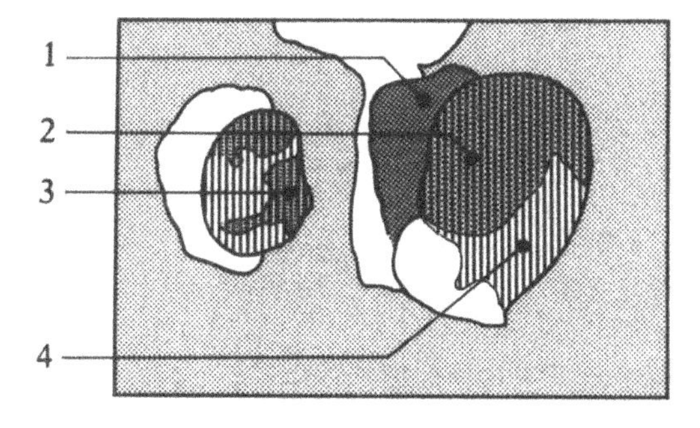

1 Epididymal invasion
2 Enlarged left testis due to tumour
3 Areas of tumour in the hypotrophic right testis
4 Area of normal parenchyma

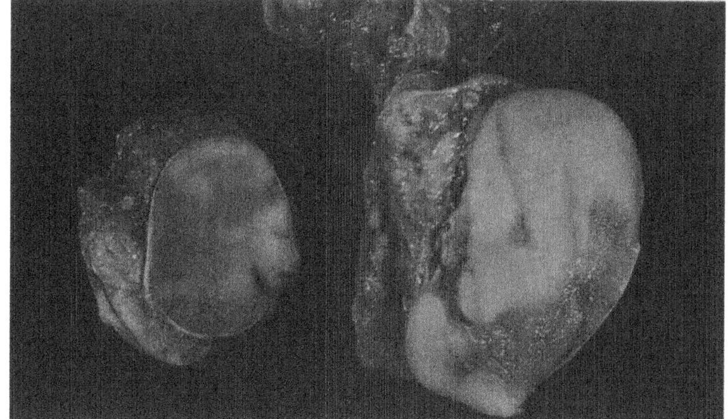

Fig. 38a-d. ***Bilateral malignant lymphoma.*** Enlarged left testis in a 47 year old man treated for supra diaphragmatic Hodgkin's disease 14 years previously. **a** Sagittal section of the left testis: large testis containing obvious tumour with hypoechoic areas. At the most posterior convexity peripherally, there is the suspicion of invasion into the rete testis and body of the epididymis (the head appears normal). **b** Transverse section: the multi-nodular structure of the tumour is apparent. **c** Sagittal section of the contra lateral testis: the testis appears slightly hypotrophic but more importantly heterogenous with hypoechoic areas less well visualised compared to the left. In summary: bilateral multi-nodular tumour in a patient who has previously undergone aggressive chemotherapy. Histological examination revealed non-Hodgkin lymphoma of a high grade malignancy. **d** The castration specimens: large left testis almost entirely replaced by tumour and infiltrating the epididymis; right testis rather small with several areas of tumour peripherally without involvement of the appendages

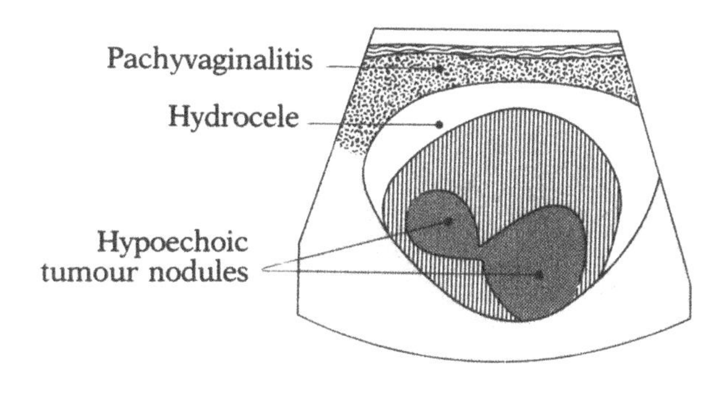

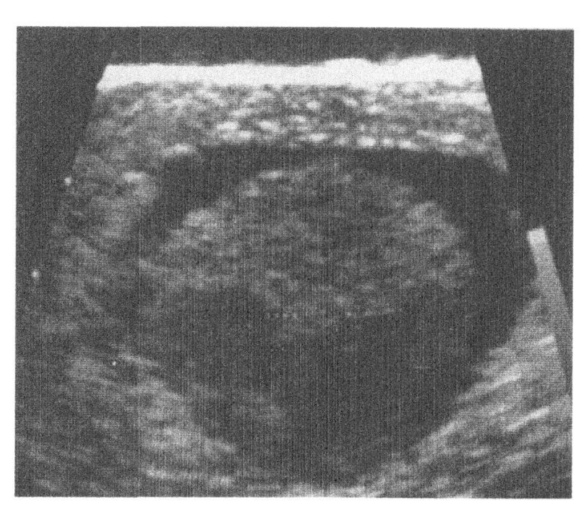

Fig. 39. ***Metastasis from an urothelial carcinoma.*** Enlarged testis noted after several months following a homolateral inguinal hernia repair in a 53 year old man. Clinically suspected post-operative hydrocele. Previous history of total cystectomy and bladder reconstruction due to tumour. Sagittal section: deep to the small hydrocele and the pachyvaginalitis, the testis is abnormal and replaced in its posterior half by hypoechoic zones with confluent nodules; at orchidectomy, metastases from a bladder carcinoma

Tumours and pseudotumours of the testicular appendages

Tumours of the testicular appendages

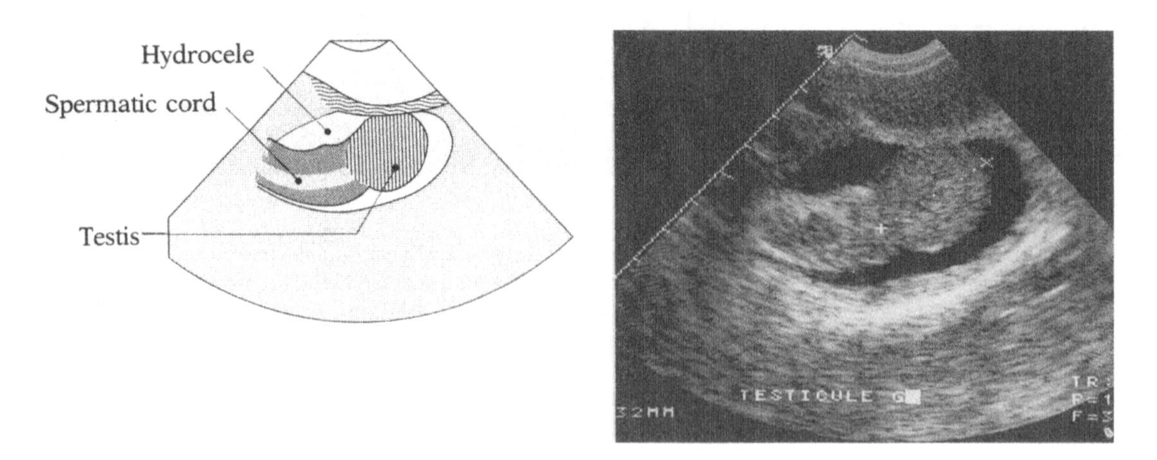

Fig. 40. Leiomyosarcoma of the cord. Progressive painless enlargement of the left testis in a man of about 50. Presumed clinical diagnosis of a hydrocele with chronic epididymitis. Sagittal section: medium sized hydrocele surrounding a pathological spermatic cord: a very large, elongated structure with a heterogenous echopattern and notably a slightly echogenic centre suggesting its nature. No contained vascular elements. These characteristics exclude the possibility of a torsion or a varicocele. Therefore, it is a tumour of the cord. It is not echogenic enough to be purely fatty. The testis, with a "ringing-bell" appearance, is intrinsically normal. At operation: a primitive leiomyosarcoma with involvement of the iliac and inguinal lymph nodes

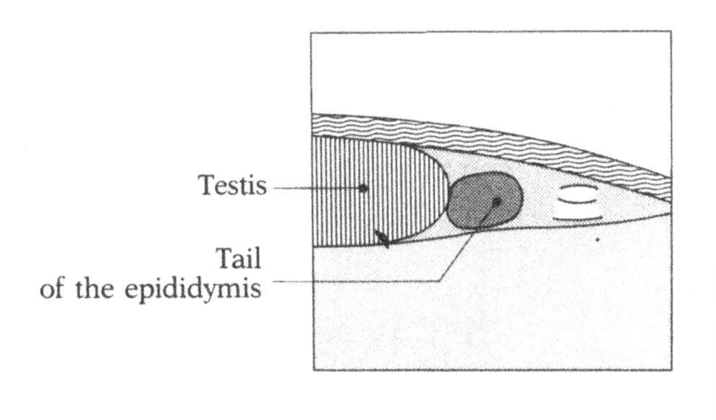

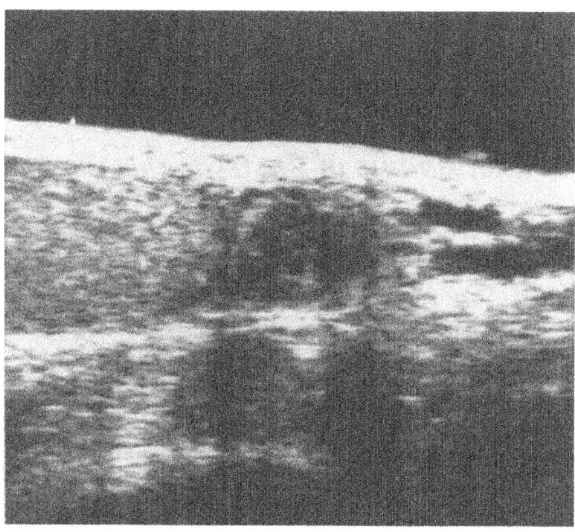

a

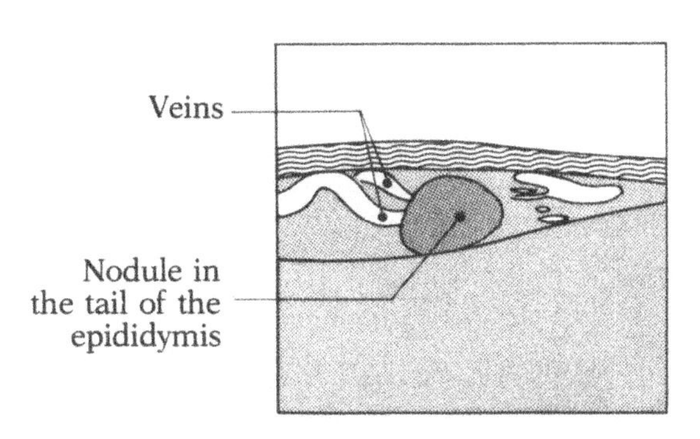

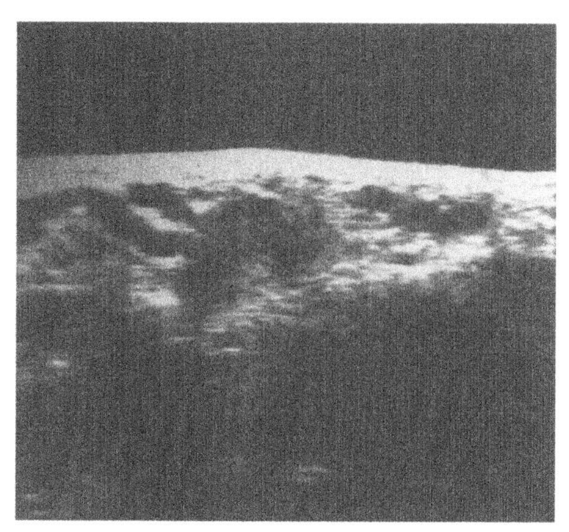

b

Fig. 41a, b. ***Adenomatoid tumour of the epididymis.*** A 20 year old young man presenting with a painless nodule in the left testis. **a** Sagittal section of the inferior pole: there is an extra testicular nodule which is clearly separate from the intact inferior pole of the testis. It is a small, regular,well-defined structure of greater than 1 cm diameter situated in the tail of the epididymis. **b** Transverse section through the inferior pole: the nodule is homogenous, hypoechoic, non-attenuating and therefore solid, with vessels converging towards it. Its size, homogeneity and hypo echogenicity do not suggest a chronic epididymitis. It is more likely to be an adenomatoid tumour (a benign lesion), particularly with its position. Simple clinical follow-up is all that is required

Pseudotumours of the testicular appendages

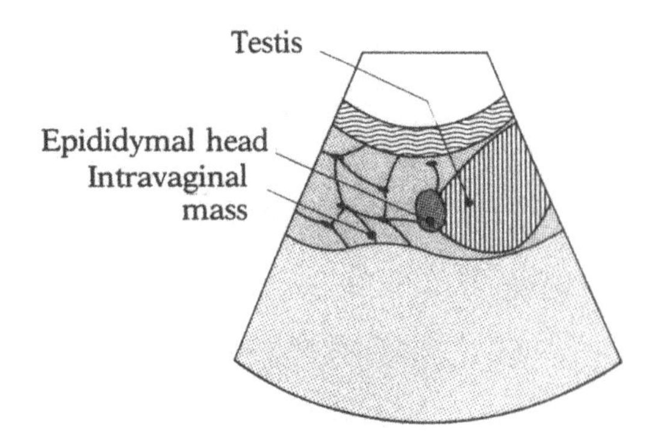

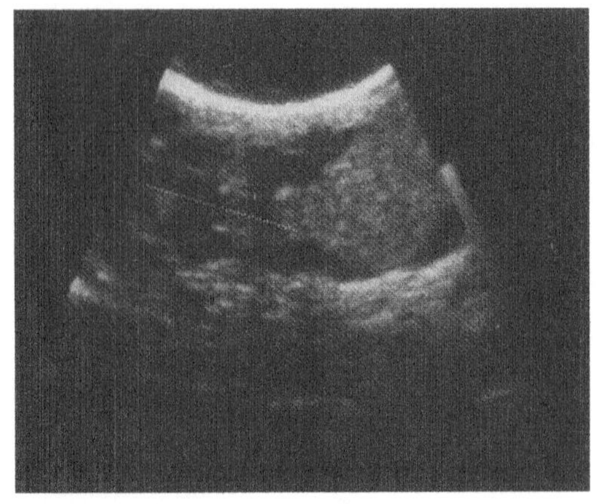

a

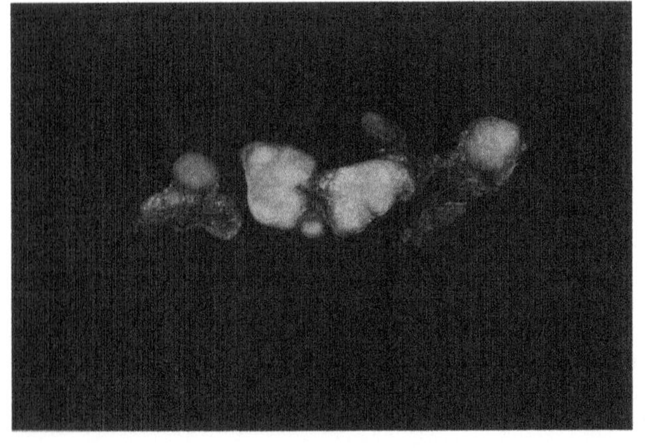

b

Fig. 42a, b. ***Fibrous pseudotumour of the testicular appendages; multinodular form.*** Progressive enlargement of the right testis with a feeling of heaviness in a 32 year old man. Clinically, the spermatic cord is indurated. **a** Sagittal section: large mass arising in the spermatic cord but also involving the tunica vaginalis since it is encasing the superior part of the testis which is deformed but retains its normal echo pattern. The lesion has a discrete hyoechoic and multinodular structure with echoes within the pseuocapsules of the nodules. **b** Macroscopic specimen of the mass which was simply excised with preservation of the testis. The fibrous tumour was made up of several well-defined nodules which appear white or yellow on the cut surface. It is encasing the spermatic cord and tunica vaginalis

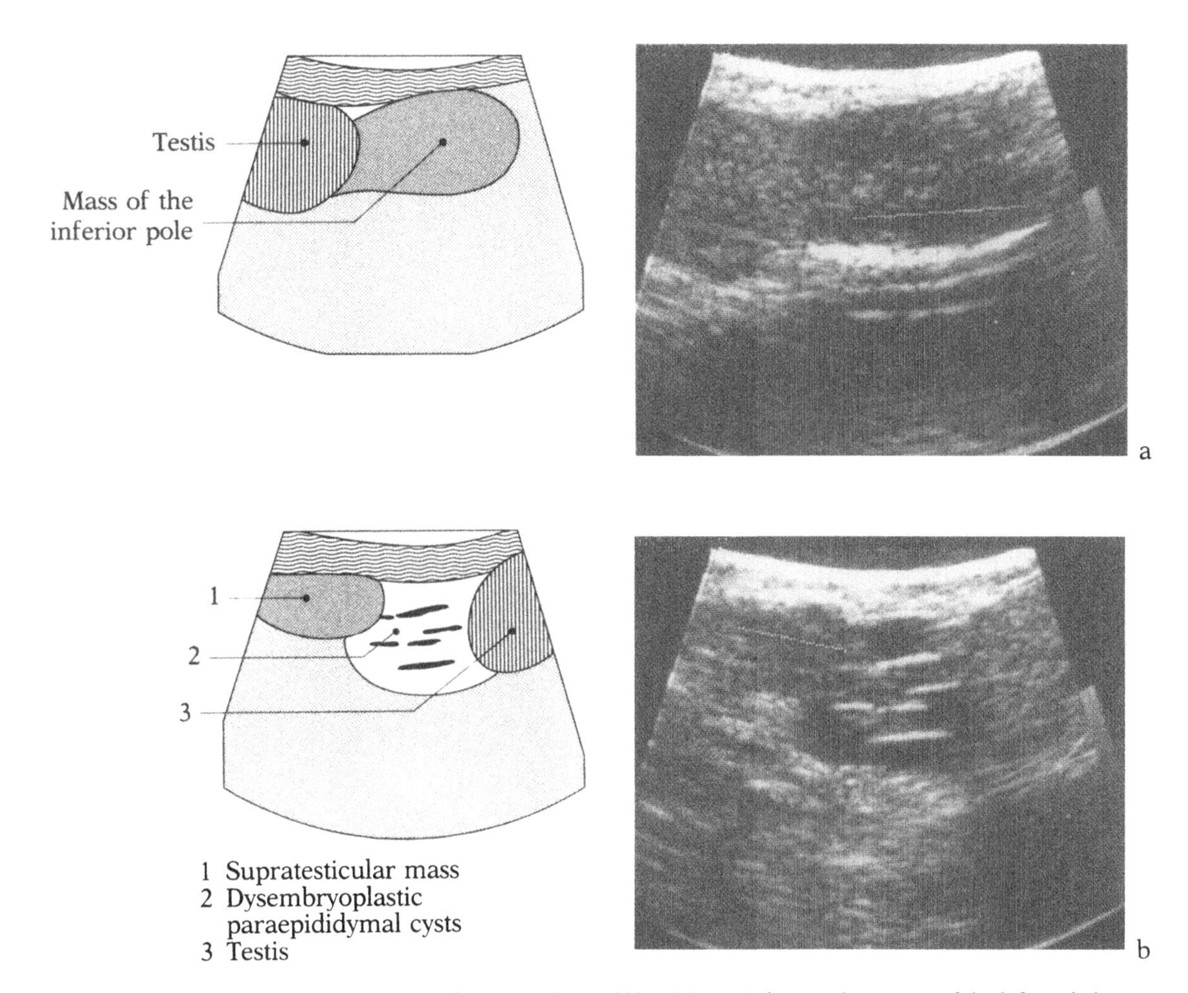

Fig. 43a, b. ***Fibrous pseudotumour of the testicular appendages; bifocal form.*** Painess enlargement of the left testis in a 45 year old man. Ipsilateral epididymo-orchitis 2 years previously, medically treated. **a** Sagittal section of the inferior pole: oval , well-defined solid hypoechoic mass beneath the testis. **b** Oblique section of the superior pole: another identical but smaller nodule in the spermatic cord is separated from the testis by a small varicocele as indicated by fine transonic tubular structures. Despite the diagnosis of an extra-testicular tumour suggesting benign disease, an orchidectomy was nevertheless performed with insertion of a prosthesis. Histologically: fibrous bifocal pseudotumour of the spermatic cord and tunica vaginalis

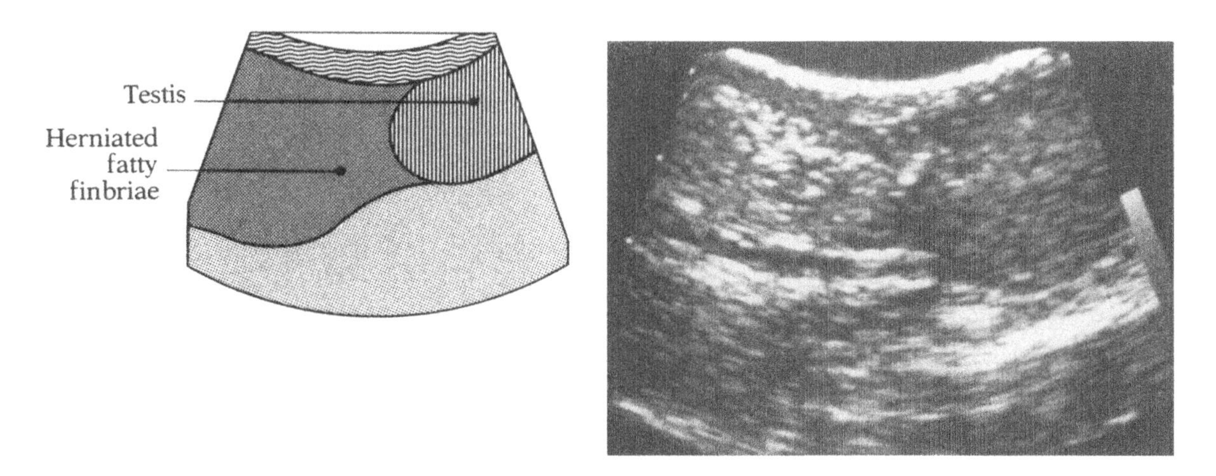

Fig. 44. ***Purely fatty inguino- scrotal hernia.*** Sagittal section of the inguino-scrotal region: above the normal testis is a poorly defined, fairly homogenous and echogenic structure which is extending superiorly: mesenteric fat which has herniated through the inguinal canal into the scrotum

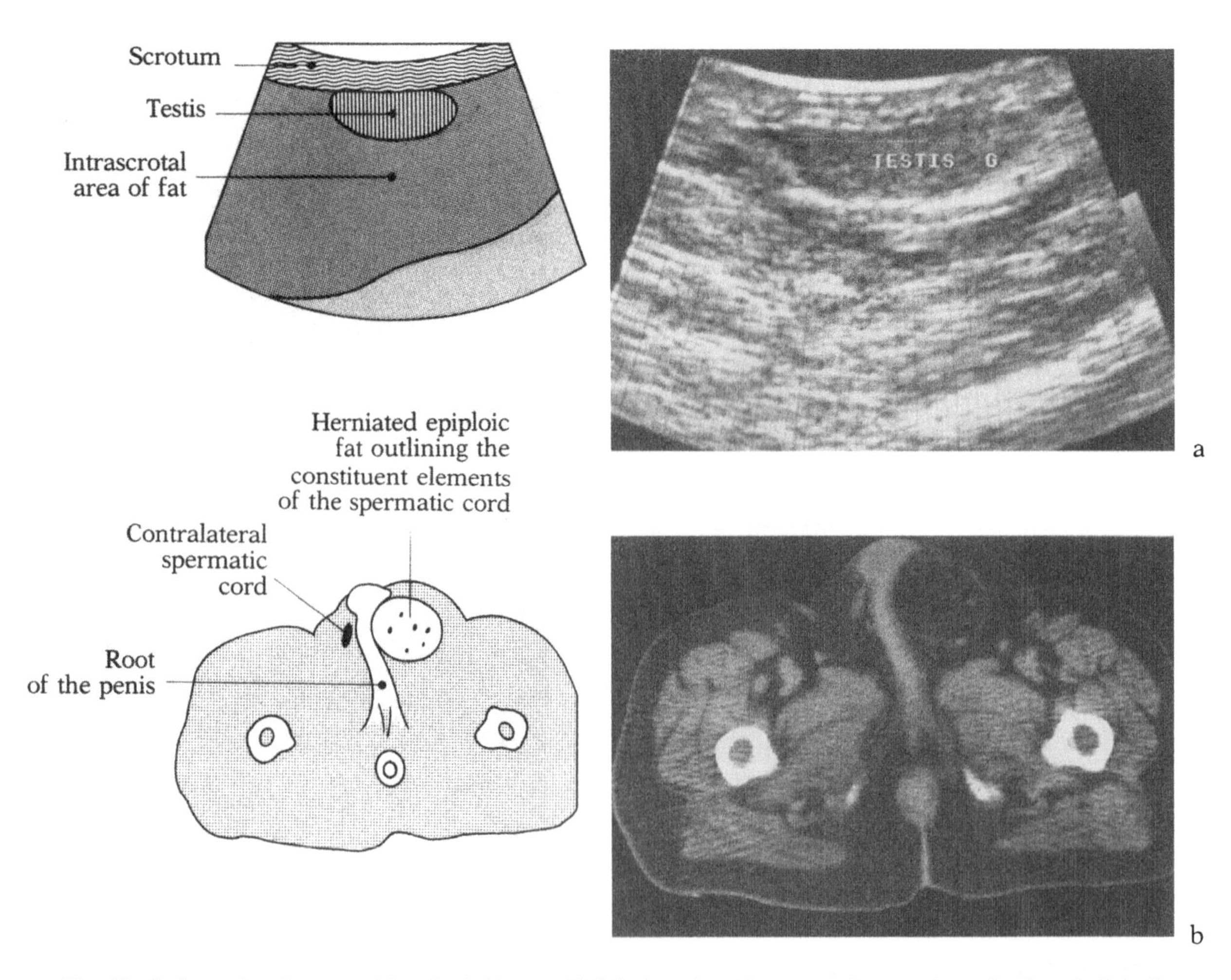

Fig. 45a, b. ***Large inguino-scrotal hernia.*** A 63 year old diabetic patient. Scrotum and spermatic cord enlarged clinically. **a** Sagittal section: very atrophic testis (thickness less than 1 cm) pushed anteriorly by a large, very echogenic structure situated posteriorly and extending in a sheet from the orifice of the inguinal canal. **b** A single slice on CT confirmed the fatty nature of this mass which is separating the different elements in the spermatic cord

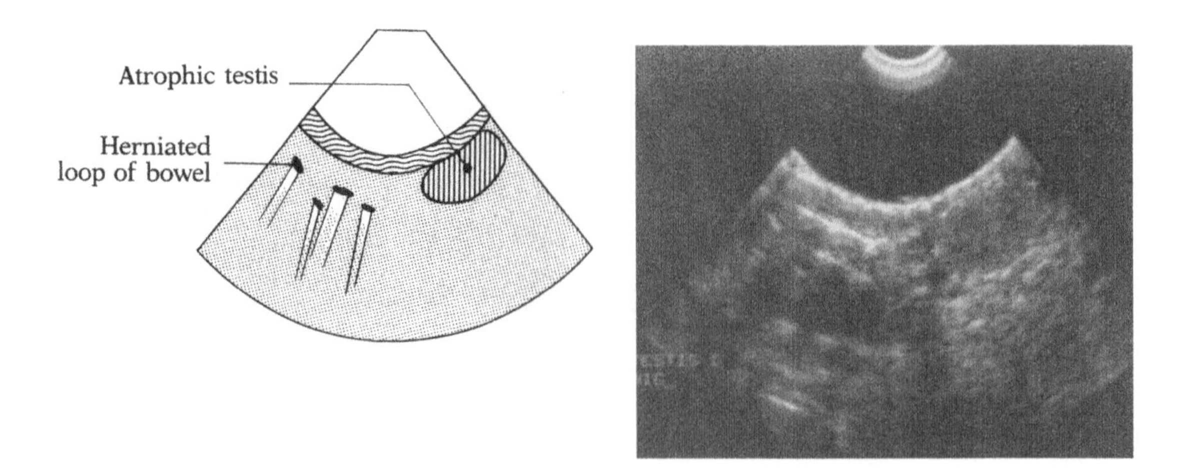

Fig. 46. ***Mixed inguino-scrotal hernia.*** Sagittal section: slightly hypotrophic testis. Heterogenous mass above and posteriorly, poorly defined and continuous with the inguinal canal. Its heterogeneity with highly attenuating echogenic areas is due to two components within the hernia: mesenteric fat and ileum. In doubtful cases a plain x-ray with a soft tissue exposure centred on this region is useful to look for the presence of bowel gas within the hernia

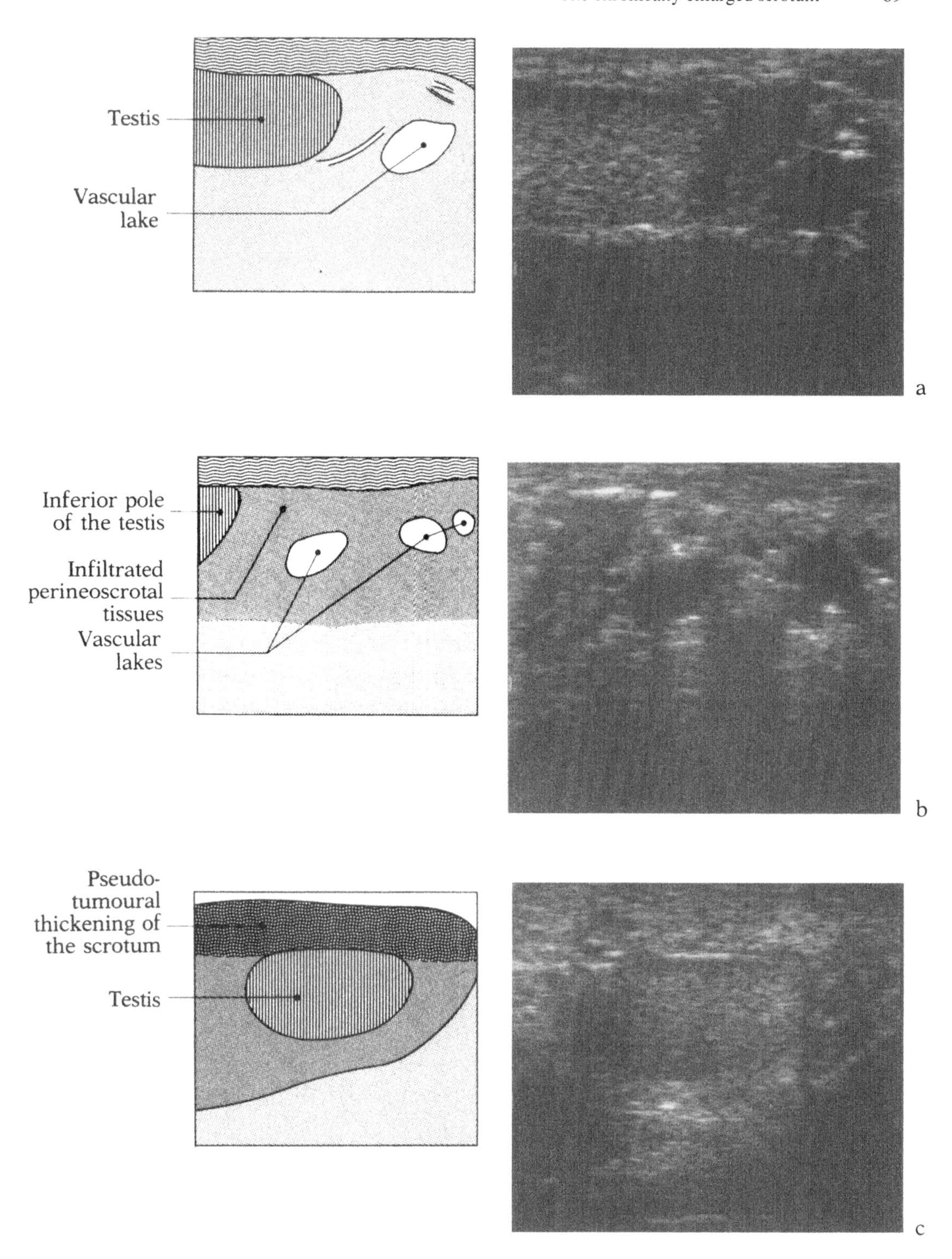

Fig. 47a-c. ***Congenital lymphangiomatosis of the scrotum.*** **a** Sagittal section of the inferior pole: a vascular lake of greater than 1 cm diameter, indicated by a transonic area in the inferior part of the scrotum. Normal testis. **b** Transverse section of the inferior part of the scrotum: several ectatic vessels seen as pockets of fluid within thickened layers of the scrotum. **c** Sagittal section: significant infiltration of all the layers of the scrotum due to venous and lymphatic stasis

Impalpable testicular tumours within a clinically normal scrotal sac

Although scrotal examination is normal, the Clinician suspects underlying intrascrotal pathology, particularly tumour. Ultrasound examination is invaluable in 3 circumstances:

- investigation of the aetiology of lymphadenopathy, particularly retroperitoneal, in a young adult male;
- investigation of the aetiology of gynaecomastia;
- investigation of unexplained, persistent scrotal pain, particularly in a young man.

Investigation of the aetiology of lymphadenopathy

It is important to exclude a subclinical germinal tumour of the testis. Twenty per cent of germinal tumours present with metastases, 10% of which have lymphadenopathy, mainly retroperitoneal and occurring in young men.

In the staging of germinal tumours, two appearances are observed:

- A *rounded expansile intratesticular structure*, often hypoechoic and small, which has already spread via the lymphatic system. This is a rare finding.
- *Or more often an echogenic area, always small* (less than or around 1 cm),with a variable attenuation, deep within the parenchyma of a normal or small testis. It is an almost characteristic appearance and suggests a fibrous, sometimes calcified scar from a germinal tumour which has totally or partially involuted due to necrosis or very early haemorrhage. Active tumour cells can still persist within this scar. More importantly, there can also be tumour foci within the tubules which are definitely not visible ultrasonically.

Therefore, in both cases an orchidectomy is necessary.

Investigation of the aetiology of gynaecomastia

Gynaecomastia can be uni- or bi-lateral. It can be recent or longstanding, present for several years, or can disappear then reappear. It may be an isolated finding or associated with other signs of oestrogen activity (e.g. impotence) which,when present,will necessitate an ultrasound examination in association with further biochemical tests.

The aim of the ultrasound examination is to exclude:

- *Primarily a Leydig cell tumour*. The ultrasound appearances, although non-specific, in this clinical context suggest a tumour: expansile, intra-testicular, invasive and hypoechoic process, often small. This is a non-germinal tumour since it originates from the stroma of the gonad, the Leydig cells. It accounts for about 3% of testicular tumours, more than 20% are associated with gynaecomastia: 10% are bilateral and 10% malignant. It is a slow growing tumour with an uncertain prognosis, particularly in the adult. The presence of metastatic disease is the only way of confirming the malignant nature of the lesion (mainly to the lungs, liver and lymph nodes). This malignant potential may also be suggested histopathologically by the presence of tumour cells in the pseudo-capsule around the lesion.
- *A complex germinal tumour (much rarer)* : In practice, in the presence of gynaecomastia, the lesion is of such a size that it is palpable. Ultrasonically, it is

seen as a small solid mass of variable homogeneity within the parenchyma of the testis.

In both cases the diagnosis of a tumour and precise histology can only be determined by histopathological examination following orchidectomy.

Unexplained and persistent scrotal pain in a young adult

This is a less well recognized and often neglected clinical situation. In no case is there any real clinical indication for an ultrasound examination, such as severe pain or a feeling of heaviness in the scrotum. However, if the pain persists and remains unexplained, it is reasonable (including from a medico legal point of view) to perform a scrotal ultrasound.

The aim of this examination is to detect an impalpable testicular tumour which by definition is small (usually less than 5-10 mm). It is often subcapsular in position and this possibly explains the early presentation with pain caused by stretching of the tunica albuginea of the testis.

The prognosis of the small tumours is excellent if there is early operative intervention. Treatment consists of orchidectomy, follow-up is by clinical examination and non-invasive imaging techniques.

Impalpable testicular tumours within a clinically normal scrotum sac

Investigation of the aetiology of lymphadenopathy, especially retroperitoneal

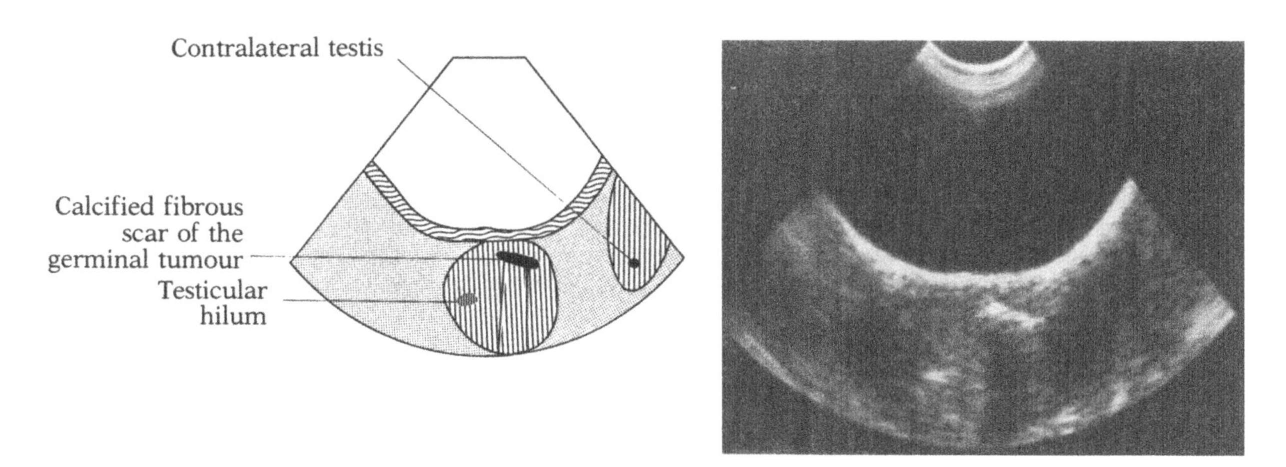

Fig.1. ***Impalpable tumours of the testis. Scar from a germinal tumour.*** Detected in a 31 year old man with acute abdominal pain due to necrotic retroperitoneal lymphadenopathy. Transverse scan: highly attenuating,linear hyperechogenicity measuring 13 mm within the testicular parenchyma antero inferiorly. It is easily distinguishable from the hilum which is also seen as an echogenic linear area, but is thinner, non attenuating and postero-superior in position. The ultrasonic appearance is typical of a fibrous scar, in this instance calcified, from a germinal tumour. This was confirmed histopathologically which also revealed micro-foci of tubular seminoma in the rest of the testicular parenchyma

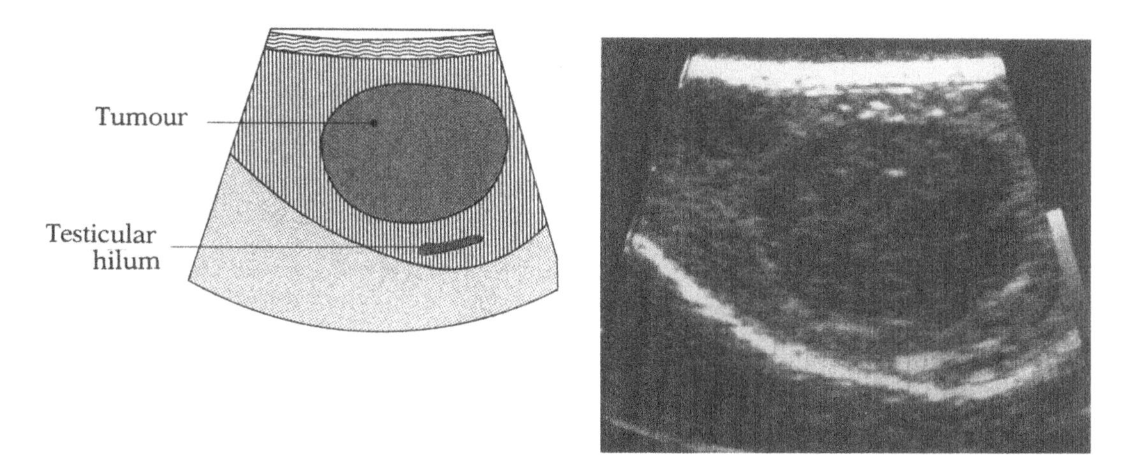

Fig. 2. ***Impalpable testicular tumours. Seminoma.*** Identical clinical picture. Previous history of surgical correction of ectopic testes in childhood. Sagittal section: rounded hypoechoic and homogenous mass, greater than 1 cm in size. Its development centrally within the testis may explain why the lesion is impalpable

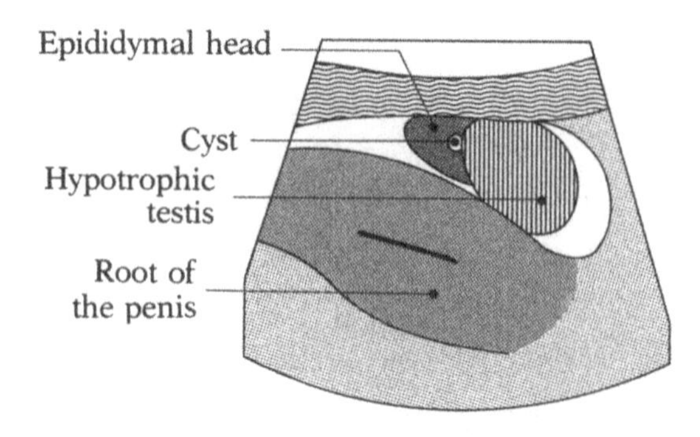

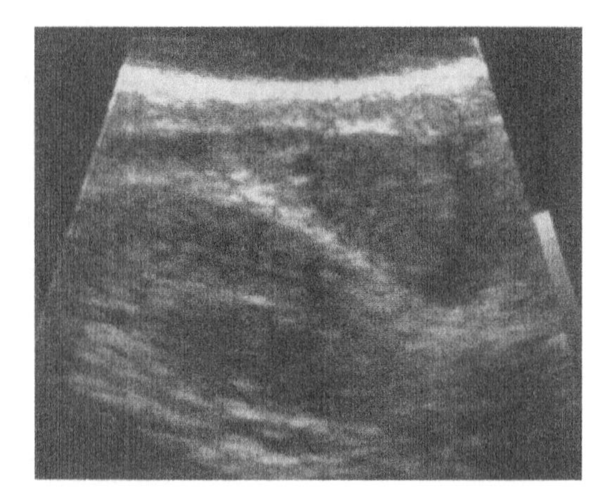

Fig. 3. ***Impalpable testicular tumours, misleading image.*** Same clinical picture. Lymph node biopsy revealed a seminoma. For this reason scrotal ultrasound was performed. Sagittal section of the testis: atrophic testis. Cystic structure of less than 1 cm at the epididymo-testicular junction: despite the clinical context, the appearances do not suggest a testicular lesion, but rather are those of a simple small dystrophic vestigial cyst. The retroperitoneal mass is an intra-abdominal seminoma

Investigation of the aetiology of gynaecomastia

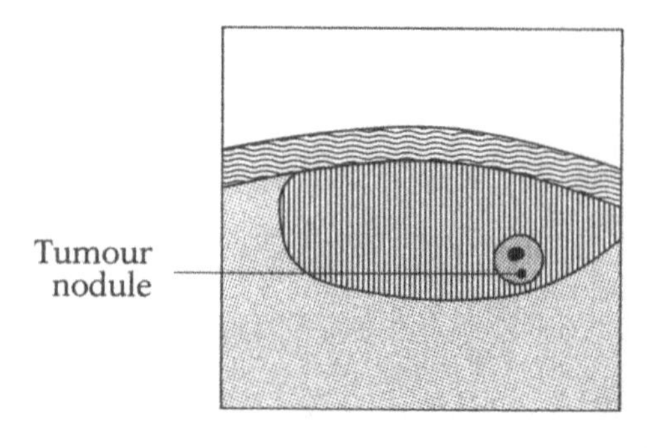

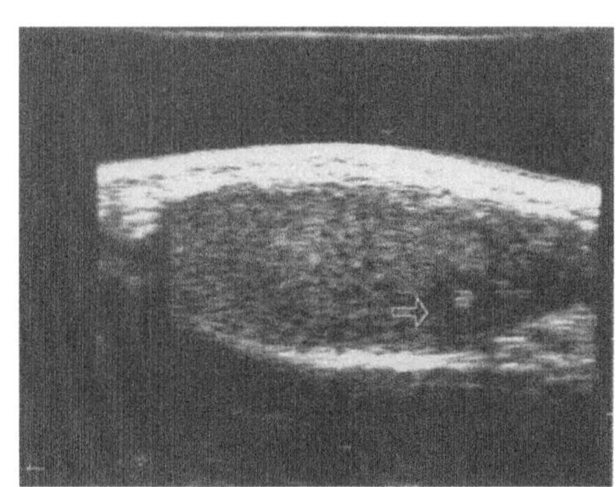

Fig. 4. ***Mixed germinal tumour.*** Bilateral gynaecomastia for 4 months in a 26 year old man. Elevated serum testosterone and oestradiol levels. Sagittal section of the right testis: 8 mm nodule detected in the inferior pole of the testis, hypoechoic with an echogenic centre and no posterior attenuation. Orchidectomy revealed a chorio-carcinoma associated with an intra-tubular seminoma. Further investigation revealed retroperitoneal lymphadenopathy

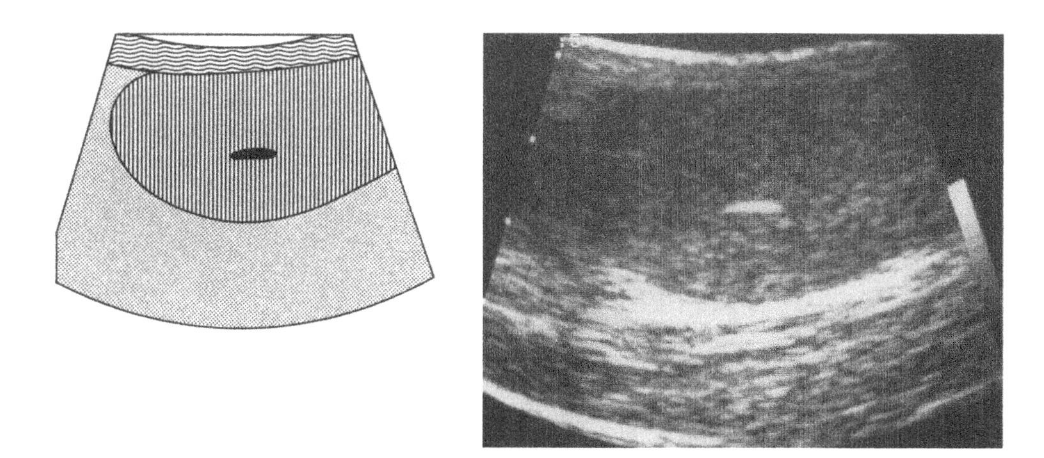

Fig. 5. ***Misleading image.*** Bilateral gynaecomastia in a 55 year old man with no abnormal serum hormone levels. Sagittal section: the testis is not atrophic. Linear, hyperechogenicity of a few millimetres, non-attenuating and not hilar in position. This abnormality is not dissimilar to a fibrous scar from a germinal tumour (c.f. Case 1) but in the absence of hormonal disturbance and lymphadenopathy, simple follow-up is sufficient. No change two years later: probable testicular granuloma

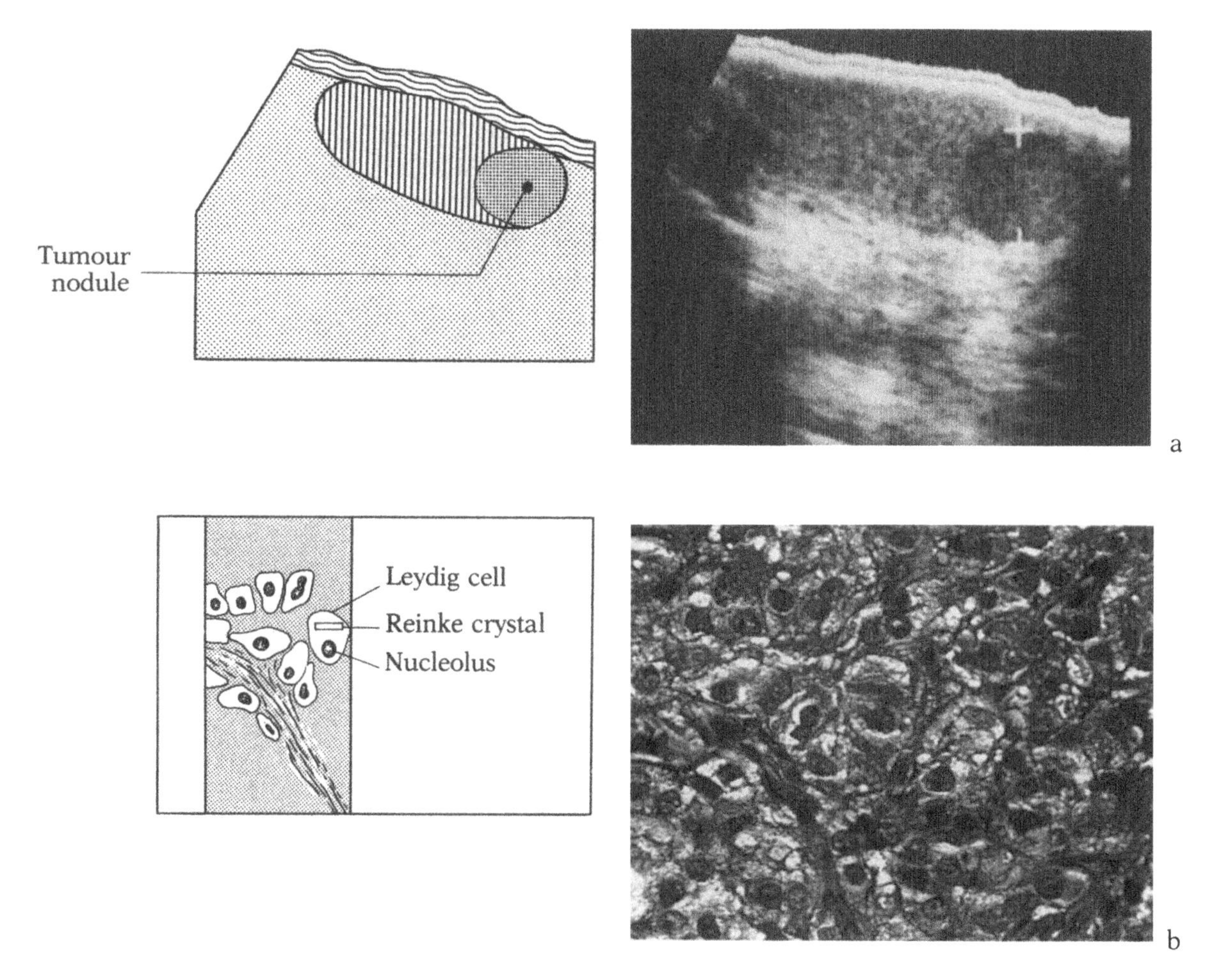

Fig. 6a, b. ***Leydig cell tumour.*** Bilateral gynaecomastia developing successively in each breast over several years, bilateral operative intervention. Recent onset of impotence. **a** Sagittal section: oval,very regular, hypoechoic, expansile lesion slightly less than 1 cm. totally excised. **b** Histological section of the excised specimen: evidence of Reinke crystals which are pathognomonic for Leydig cell tumours. These are cystoplasmic inclusion bodies in the shape of a sugar loaf within a sheet of fairly regular cells with rounded nucleoli

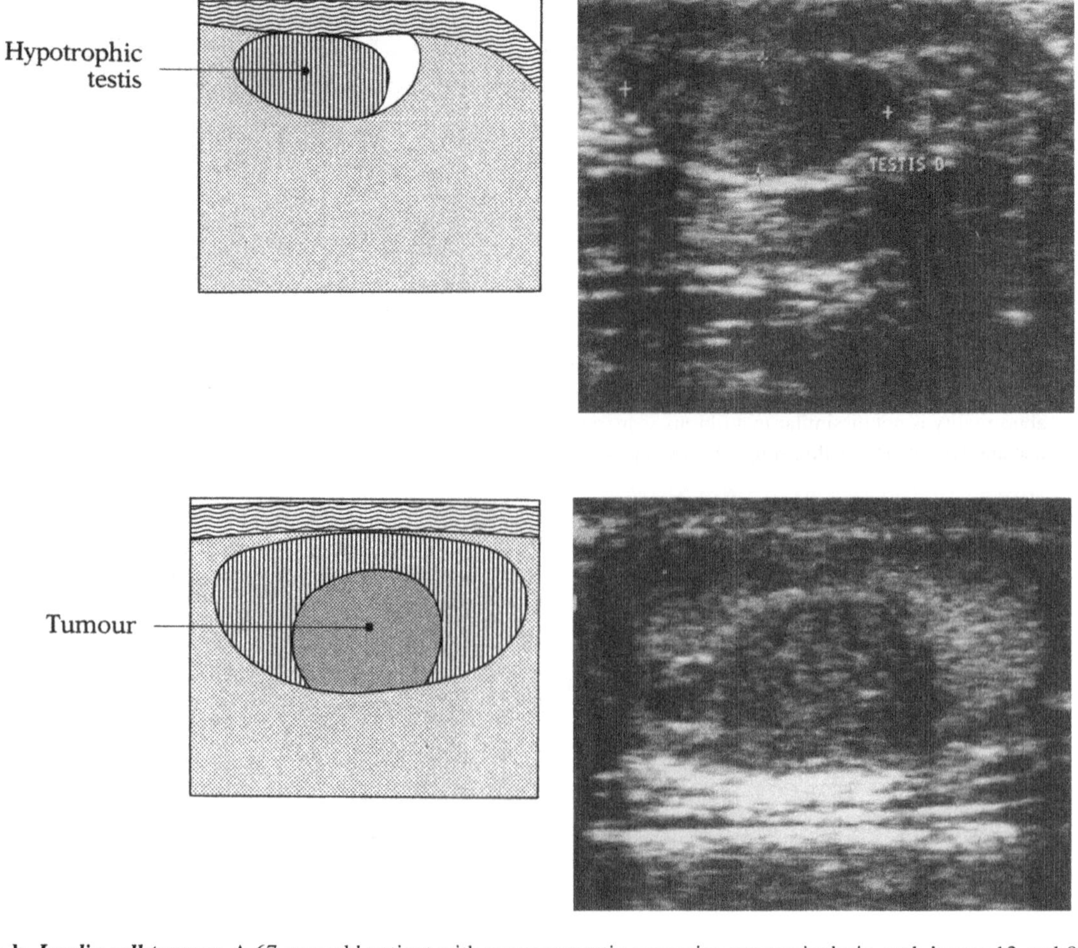

Fig. 7a, b. ***Leydig cell tumour.*** A 67 year old patient with gynaecomastia appearing successively in each breast 13 and 8 years previously, having disappeared on medical treatment. Recent unilateral recurrence. Ultrasound requested to examine an atrophic right testis and a clinically normal left testis. **a** Sagittal section of the right testis: frankly atrophic, hypoechoic right testis (thickness barely more than 1 cm). No focal abnormality. **b** Sagittal section of the left testis: a solid hypoechoic mass of about 2 cms. is seen in the hilar region of the testis. At orchidectomy: Leydig cell tumour

Unexplained scrotal pain in a young man

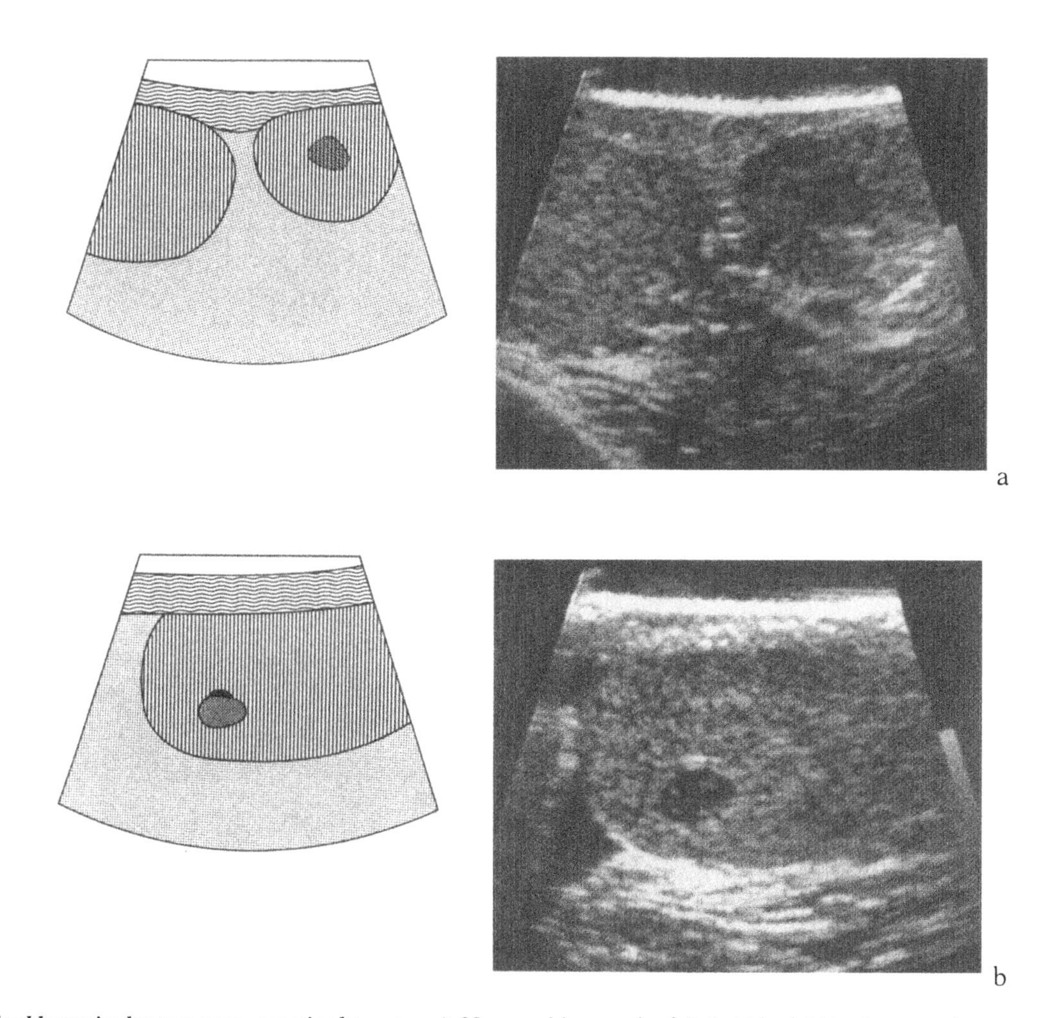

Fig. 8a, b. ***Impalpable testicular tumours; germinal tumour.*** A 38 year old man who felt that his right testis was enlarged. No abnormality clinically apart from a doubtful asymmetry in testicular size. Ultrasound advised to reassure the patient. **a** Transverse scan of both testes: the right testis definitely larger than the left but perfectly homogenous; by contrast there is a nodule in the left testis. **b** Sagittal section of the left testis: the nodule measures 8 mm x 6 mm, is hypoechoic with a discrete echogenic line on its anterior surface: expansile solid lesion, probably tumour. Orchidectomy and insertion of a prosthesis; seminoma with a small area containing embryonic carcinoma. Further investigation negative. Simple follow-up

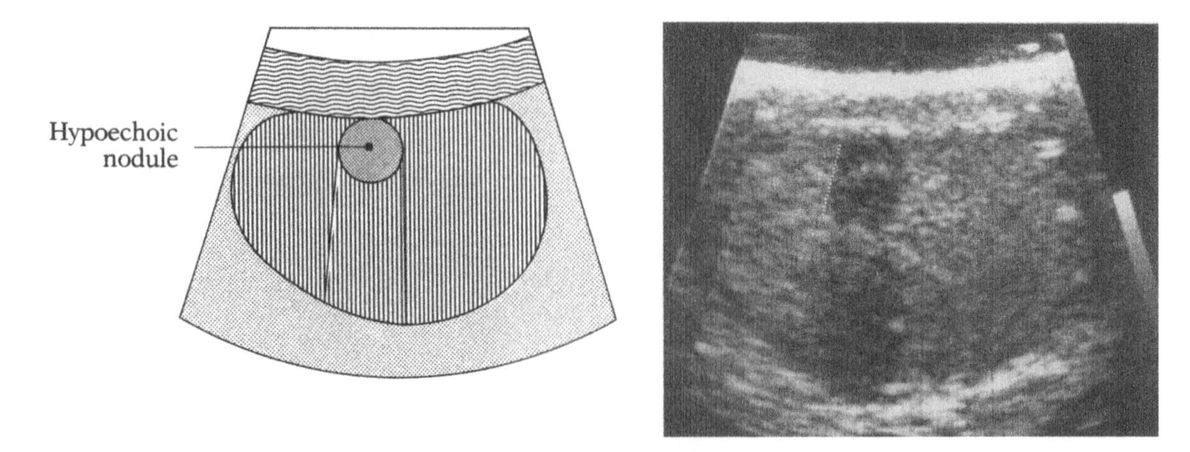

Fig. 9. ***Impalpable testicular tumours; germinal tumour.*** A 35 year old man presenting with persistent pain in the right testis. Sagittal section: normal sized testis. 8 mm subcapsular hypoechoic nodule with posterior accoustic shadowing. Exploratory surgery: seminoma discovered on the unfixed specimen leading to orchidectomy. Pure seminoma

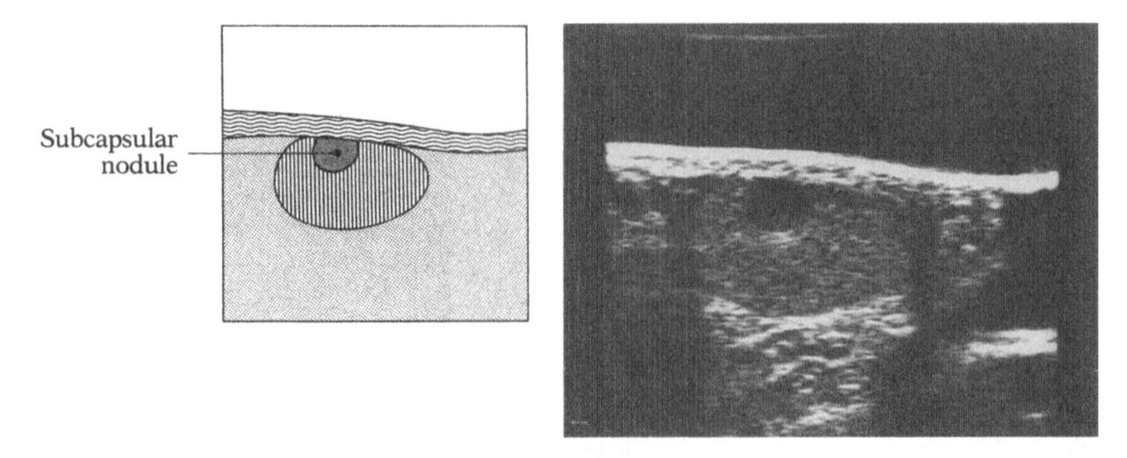

Fig. 10. ***Impalpable testicular tumours; benign fibroma of the tunica albuginea.*** A 26 year old man. Same clinical picture. Sagittal section (Image courtesy of Drs. Tordjmann and Lachand): 6 mm subcapsular hypoechoic nodule. Exploratory scrototomy. Benign fibroma of the tunica albuginea suggested by examination of the unfixed specimen and confirmed on the locally excised specimen thus allowing conservation of the testis

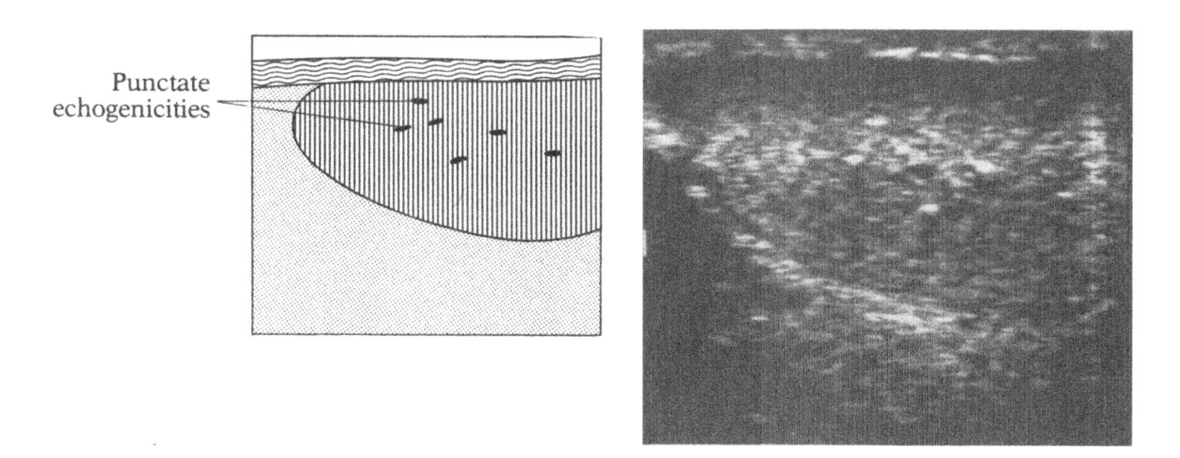

Fig. 11. ***Testicular hyperechogenicities.*** A 34 year old man. Same clinical picture. Sagittal section of a testis: multiple punctate echogenic flecks, some of which are attenuating throughout the testicular parenchyma. Bilateral abnormalities of unknown aetiology, no biopsy performed (?fibrosis) but are benign since there has been no change over a period of time since the initial ultrasound examination

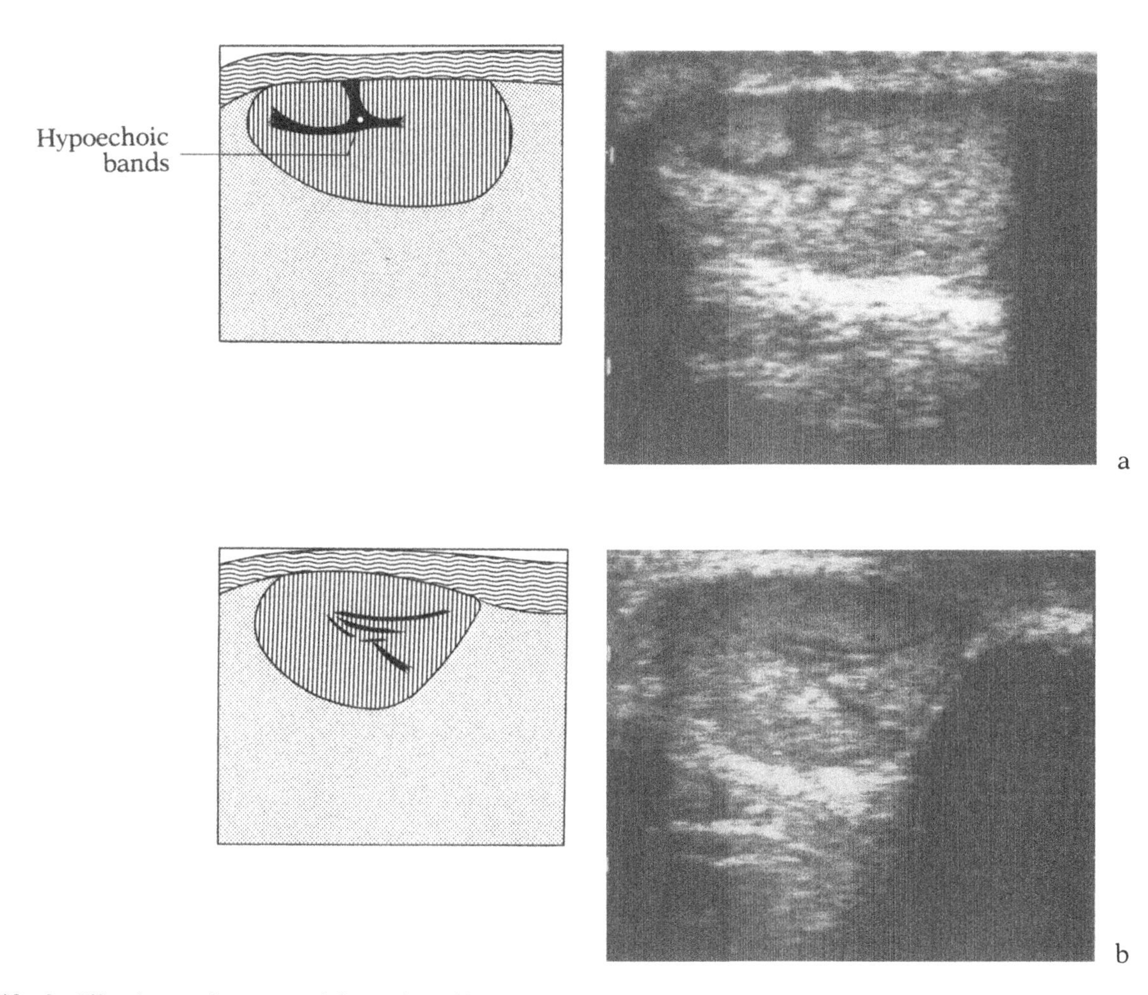

Fig.12a, b. ***Fibrotic pseudotumour of the testis.*** A 30 year old patient complaining of pains in the right testis for several months. No significant clinical abnormality. **a** Sagittal section: slightly hypotrophic testis (thickness less than 20 mm) through which run hypoechogenic bands of a few millimetres in a star-like configuration from the periphery towards the centre. **b** Transverse section. Radial appearances with normal adjacent testicular tissue. Despite their linear morphology, these are not vascular structures (absence of Doppler signal), no change in size on standing up or with Valsalva manoeuvre. At orchidotomy: diffuse fibrous scarring. No evidence of tumour

Male infertility

The concept of genital ultrasound
(Table 1)

The ultrasound examination, in this clinical context, should cover the whole of the genital tract, including internal organs. Therefore, a *genital ultrasound* should include an examination of the scrotum, followed by a study of the junctional region of the prostate, seminal vesicles and the vas deferens. This latter part is performed initially by a suprapubic scan. If this gives insufficient detail, a complimentary endorectal scan is indicated.

In addition, in cases of agenesis of the seminal vesicles and vas deferentia, ultrasound of the kidneys is mandatory.

Indications for genital ultrasound

Ultrasound is not routinely performed in the investigation of male infertility. It is indicated in well defined circumstances, and should never be performed as an initial test before the results of the other tests are available, including sperm analysis and, if necessary, the FSH level.

The main indications are:

- *Exclusion of a testicular tumour:* Leydig cell tumour or germinal tumour in cases of an ectopic testis (whether operatively corrected or not).

- *Suspicion of a unilateral epididymal abnormality in cases of oligospermia.*

- *Exclusion of epididymal abnormalities, often bilateral in cases of azoospermia thought to be due to an excretory problem* (normal or low FSH level).

- *To confirm the presence of a varicocele* which was only suspected during a difficult or doubtful clinical examination.

These different indications concern a group of conditions causing infertility which are potentially curable surgically.

In fact, in addition to these indications, ultrasound can be useful in the assessment of testes which are abnormally soft on examination.

It is possible that there will be new indications in the future with refinements in the performance of ultrasound and improvements in surgical and histological techniques.

Table 1. ***The concept of genital ultrasound***

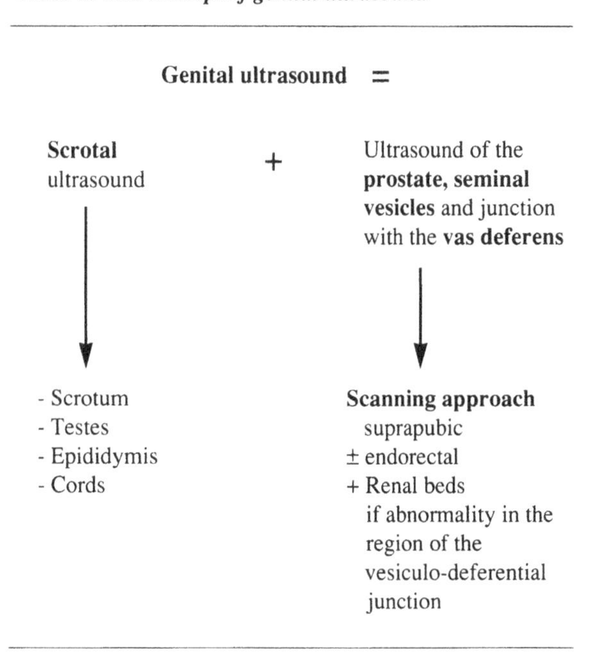

Table 2. ***Investigation of hypofertility and sterility. The principal ultrasound findings***

	Ultrasound signs	Complimentary investigations possibly indicated
Varicocele	- Calibre of veins > 3mm - Enlarged principal vein of the cord - Bi- or unilateral - + testicular hypotrophy if thickness < 15 mm	- Phlebography of the spermatic veins ± embolisation
Enlarged epididymis, distal obstruction	- Enlarged head - diameter > 12 mm - Several central micro cyst - Bi- or unilateral Distal obstruction ?	- FSH level prior to ultrasound - Vesicular markers (fructose) and epididymal markers (carnitine) - Detection of anti-spermatozoal antibodies - Finally, cystoscopy with catheterisation of the ejaculatory duct (stenosis)
Abnormalities of the prostate and seminal vesicles	- Heterogenous + enlarged prostate - Asymmetrical heterogenous seminal vesicles ; ± abcess	- Sperm cultures

The important steps in the performance of genital ultrasound

It is a very detailed examination, time consuming and should be conducted in a methodical manner.

Examination of the scrotum

Each element is examined.

- *Scrotum :*
  - measurement of its thickness. It would appear that the thickness of the scrotum in hypofertile individuals is often larger than in the general population (?effect on the thermoregulation of the testes).

- *Testis:*
  - position; a testis high in position, inguino-scrotal or mobile, should be noted. This position may contribute to an elevation in temperature,
  - measurement of 3 dimensions (length, depth and thickness) and approximate volume, obtained directly in the majority of ultrasound studies, assuming that the testis is essentially an ellipse,
  - volume,
  - echopattern.

- *Epididymis:*
  - visualisation of each part: in practice only the head, sometimes the tail and virtually never the body,
  - comparative size of the head and tail,
  - analysis of the echopattern.

- *Spermatic venous plexus:*
  - measurement of the calibre of several veins, during normal respiration, following the Valsalva manoeuvre and particularly after standing for long enough to appreciate any significant valvular insufficiency. Duplex Doppler ultrasound may also be of value.

Examination of the pelvis

- *Prostate:*
  - dimension,
  - weight,
  - echopattern.

- *Seminal vesicles:*
  - visibility,
  - dimensions (base, extremities),
  - symmetry,
  - comparative echopattern.

- *Ampullae of the vas deferentia:*
  - Sometimes visible
  - The principal abnormalities detected by genital ultrasound are summarized in Table 2.

Male infertility

The concept of genital ultrasound

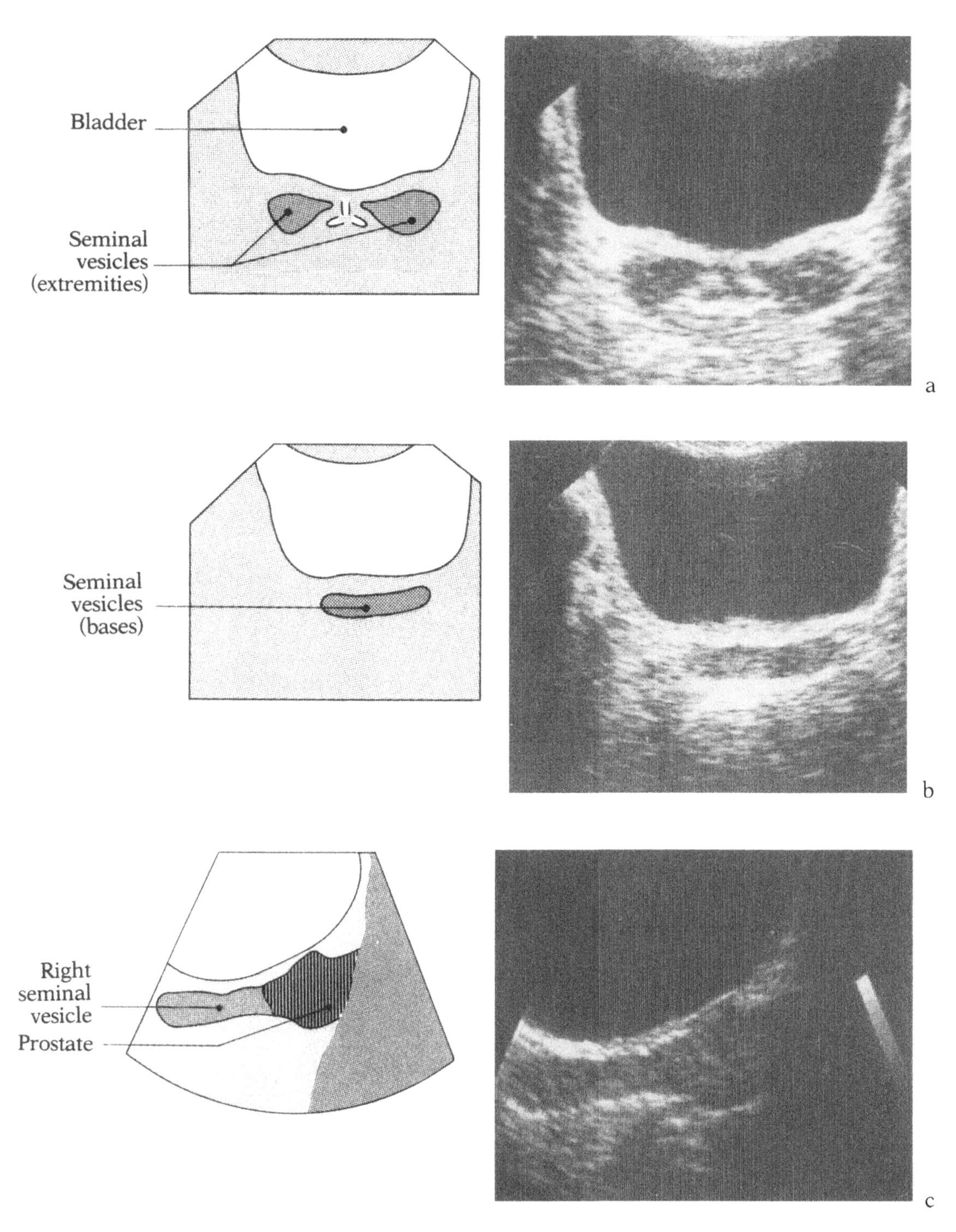

Fig. 1a-c. ***Seminal vesicles.*** Suprapubic scan. **a** Tranverse section through the postero-lateral extremities of the seminal vesicles. Bulging, symmetrical and hypoechoic appearance of both organs. **b** Transverse section through the base (or neck): appear as hypoechoic bars. **c** Sagittal section of the right seminal vesicle: regular contour, enlarging progressively from the neck to the extremity

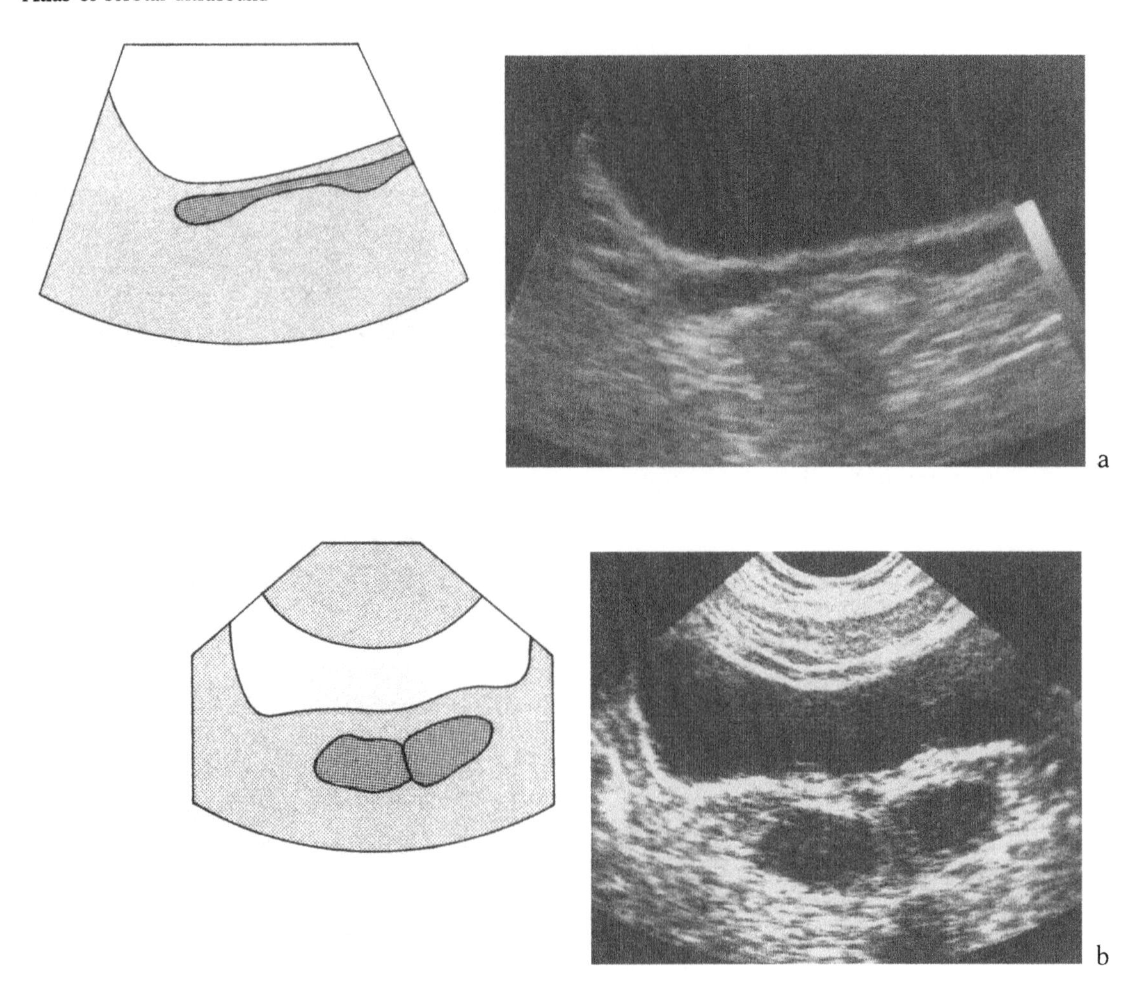

Fig. 2a, b. ***Seminal vesicles. Morphological variation.*** Suprapubic scan. **a** Transverse section: narrow seminal vesicles. **b** Transverse section: large, full seminal vesicles, some time since an ejaculation

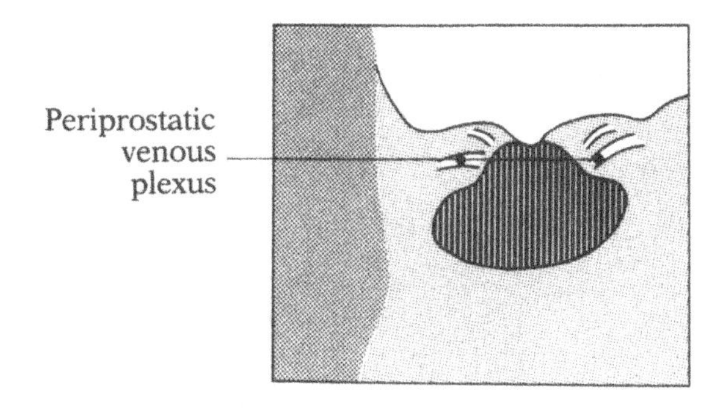

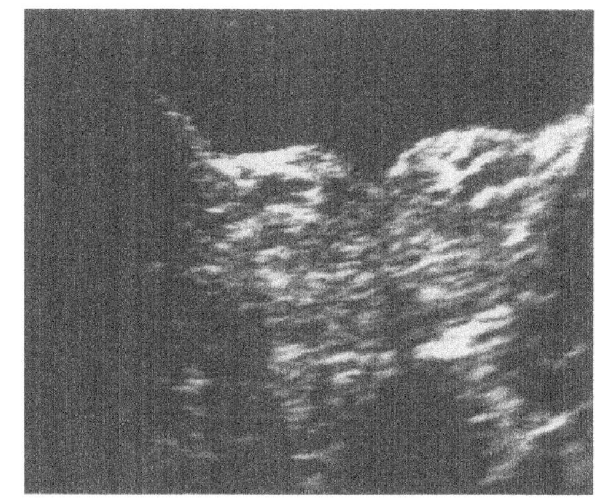

a

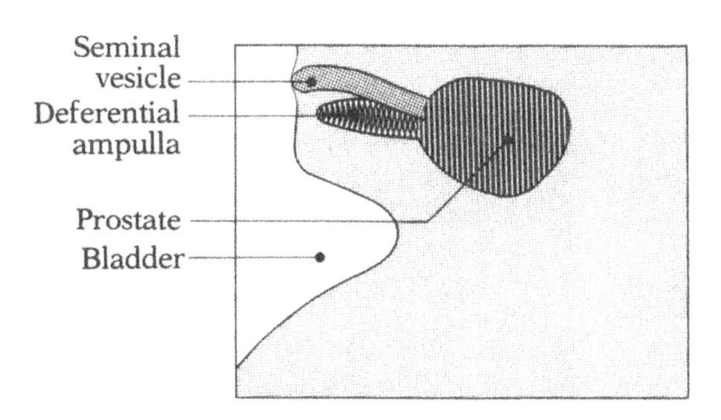

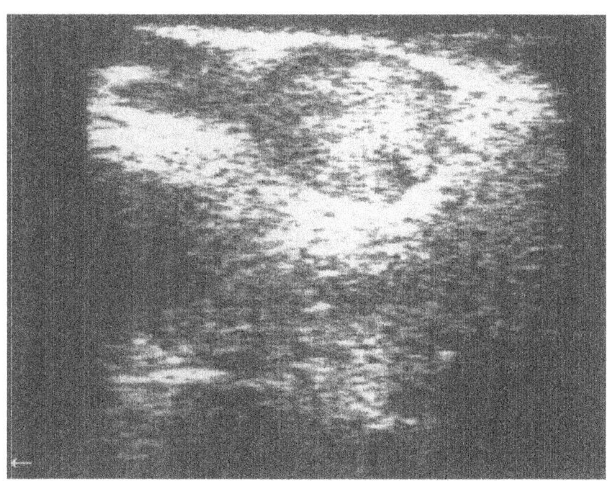

b

Fig. 3a, b. ***Prostate and ampullae of the vas deferentia.*** **a** Transverse suprapubic section. The bladder neck is clearly defined as a V-shape. Anterior to the prostate, the ampullae of the vas deferentia are visualised. Further anteriorly and thinner are the veins of the seminal venous plexus. **b** Sagittal section: endorectal scan (linear array). Good detail of the morphology and topography of the seminal vesicle and deferential ampulla;an endorectal scan is indicated if there is the suspicion of an abnormal implantation of the vas deferens or an ectopic insertion of the ureter

Varicoceles

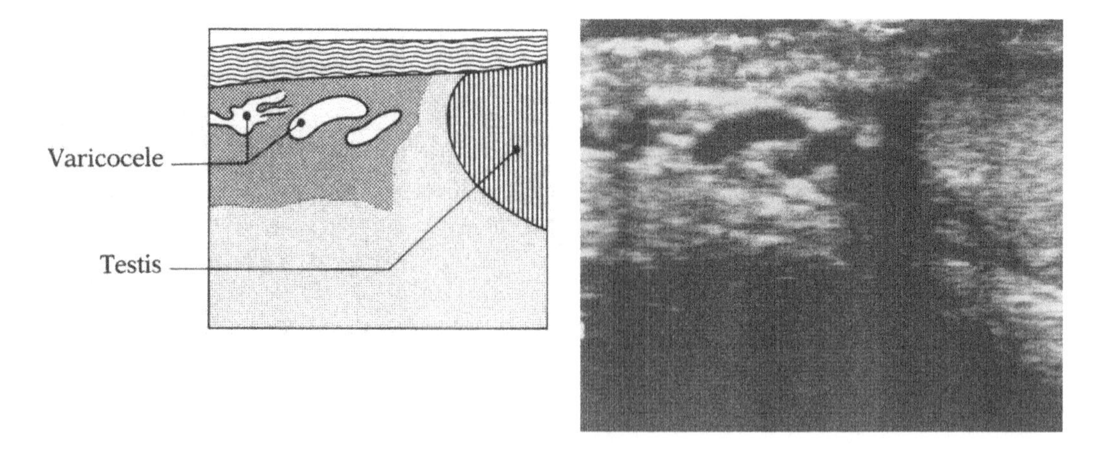

Fig. 4. ***Varicoceles. Spermatic cord.*** Primary sterility. Oligoasthenospermia (markedly reduced sperm count with poor motility). Bilateral varicoceles. Sagittal section: large dilated and tortuous veins in the spermatic cord

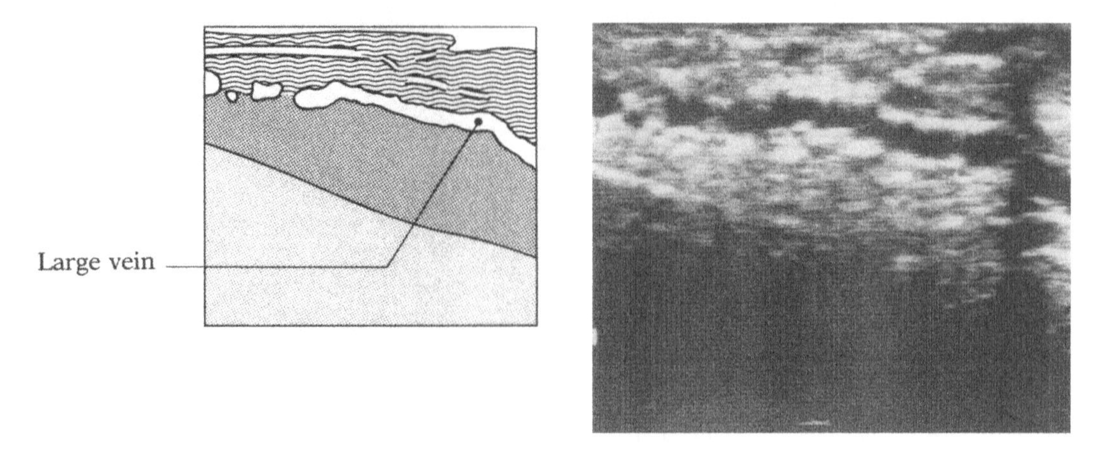

Fig. 5. ***Varicoceles. Spermatic cord.*** Sagittal section through the cord: large principal draining vein which is not very tortuous when followed along almost its entire length

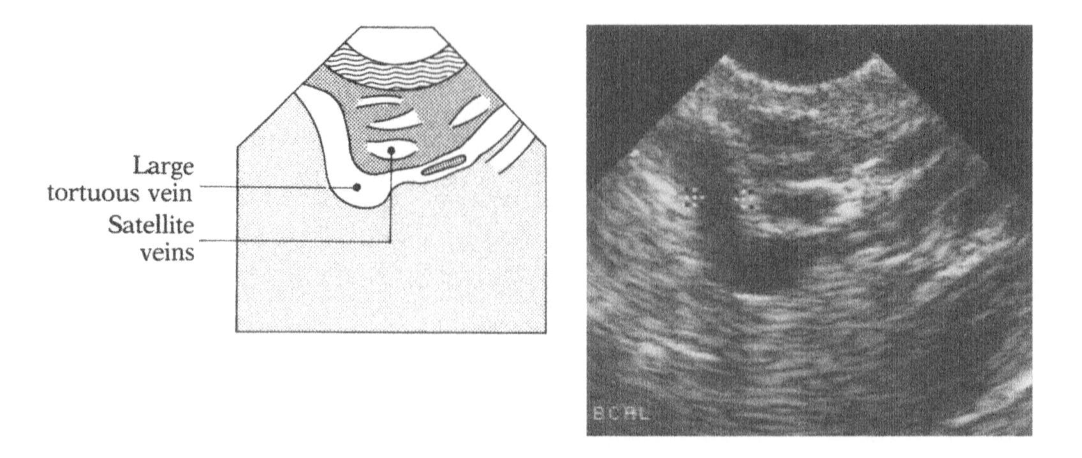

Fig. 6. ***Varicoceles. Spermatic cord.*** Large idiopathic left varicocele in a young 19 year old man. Oblique section through the cord. Principal draining vein greater than 5 mm in calibre forming a loop. There are also other dilated veins of slightly smaller calibre

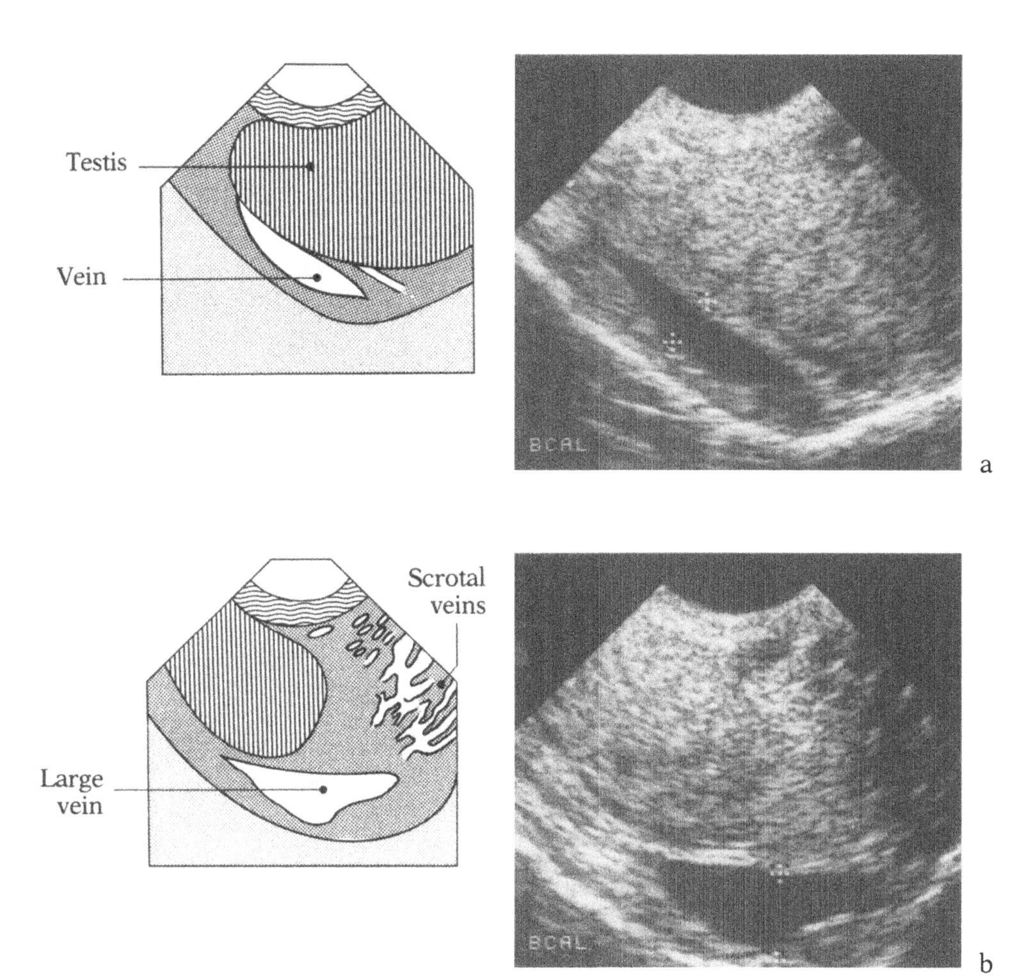

Fig. 7a, b. ***Varicoceles. Dynamic manoeuvres.*** **a** Sagittal section. Patient supine, normal respiration. Posterior to the testis there is a large transonic tubular structure whose calibre is greater than 5mm. **b** Sagittal section. After standing the patient for several minutes, there is definite enlargement of the structure to around 1 cm demonstrating that it is venous in nature. Below the inferior pole of the testis a dilated network of scrotal veins is discernible. Massive global varicocele

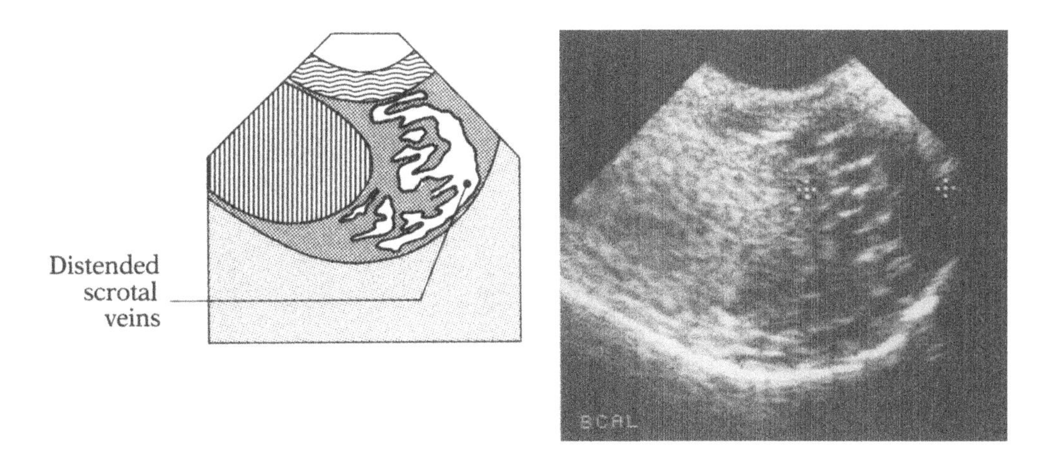

Fig. 8. ***Varicoceles. Dynamic maneouvres.*** Oblique section of the inferior pole. Markedly varicosed dilatation of the deep scrotal veins, difficult to appreciate clinically. They become more evident after standing the patient up for some time. Network of fine, linear transonic structures, separated from each other by echogenic interfaces

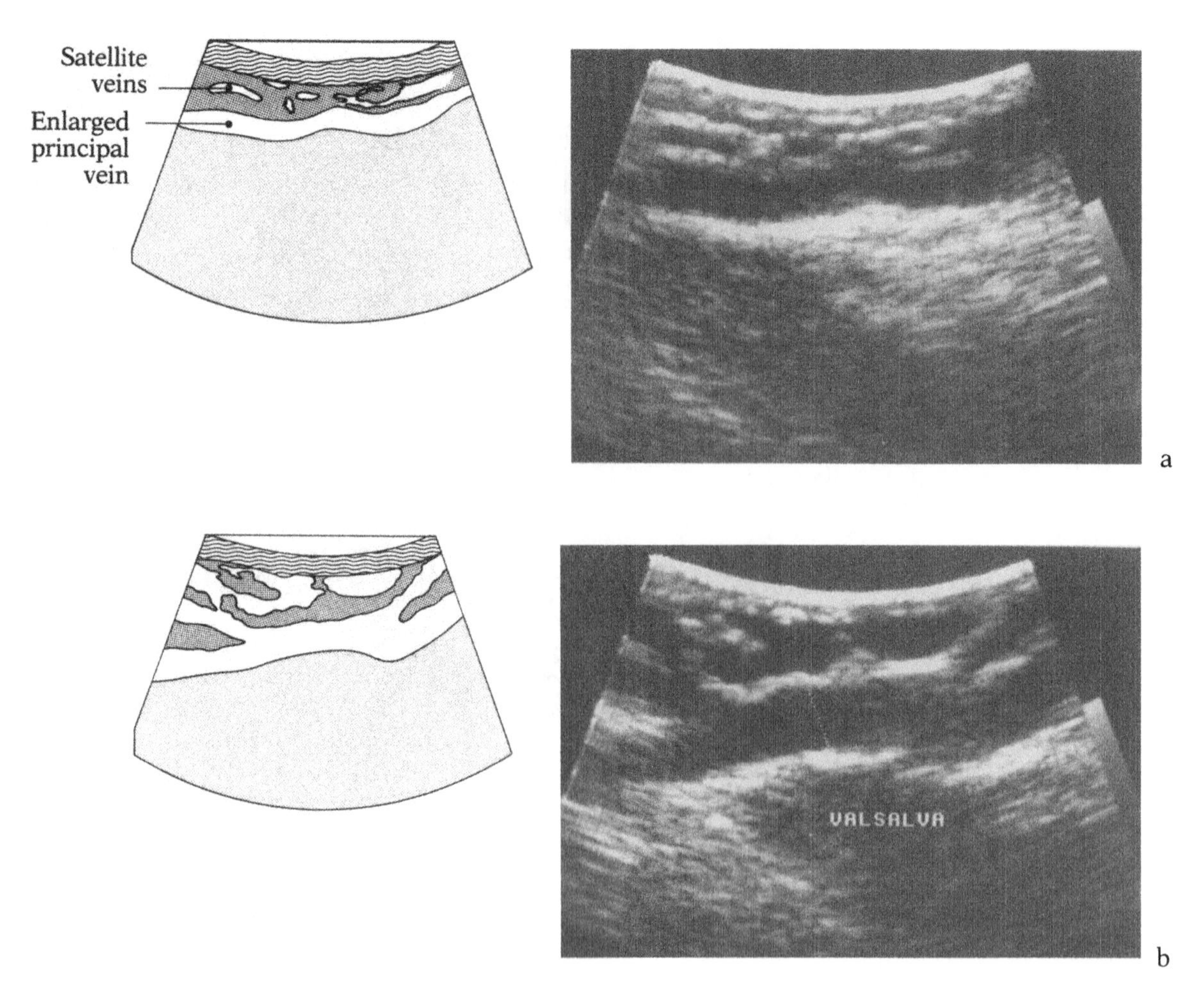

Fig. 9a, b. ***Varicoceles. Dynamic manoeuvres.*** **a** Sagittal sections of the spermatic cord. Large principal vein accompanied by less dilated veins anteriorly. **b** Same section after Valsalva manoeuvre. The distension of all the tubular structures is clear and confirms their venous nature. Sometimes this can be difficult to confirm in cases of a more discrete varicocele

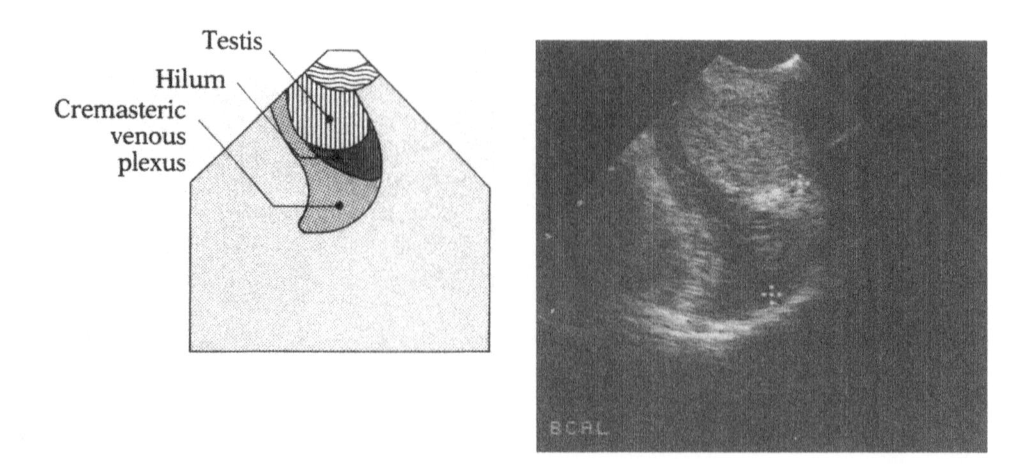

Fig. 10. ***Varicoceles. Cremasteric plexus.*** Oblique section. Beneath the testis, a 2.5 cm hypoechoic area enlarging during Valsalva manoeuvre: network of dilated veins of the posterior spermatic or cremasteric plexus which was difficult to feel clinically, all that could be noted was simply a thickening. In fact, it was a varicocele involving, rather unusually, the cremasteric plexus

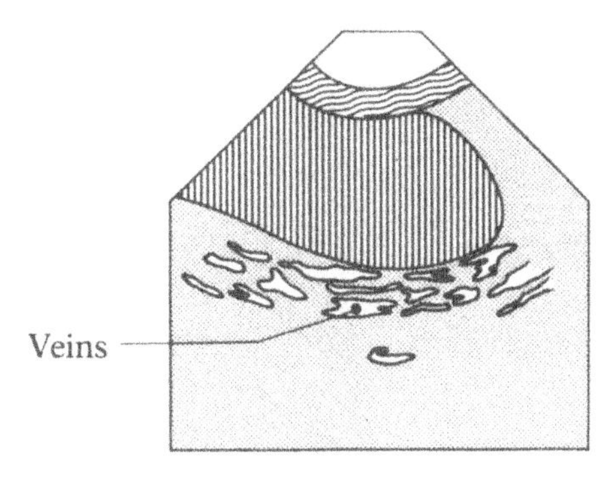

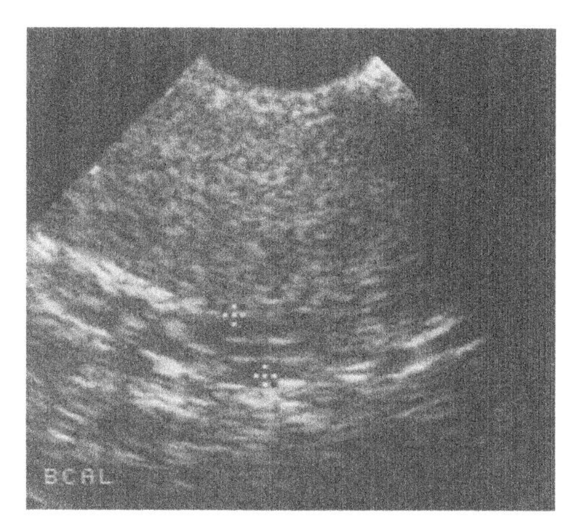

Fig. 11. ***Varicoceles. Subclinical form.*** Hypofertility with oligoasthenospermia. No abnormality clinically. Sagittal section of the left testis. Posterior to the testis are fine tubular transonic structures in groups of 2-3 mms: in the absence of intercurrent inflammation, the veins are too numerous and too prominent. The incompetence of the veins would perhaps be more apparent with dynamic manoeuvres

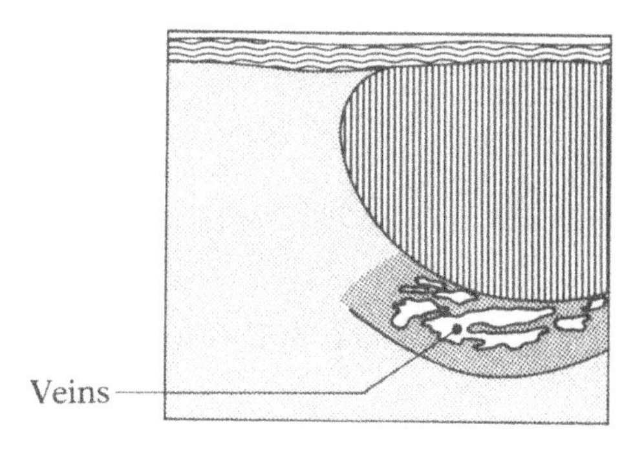

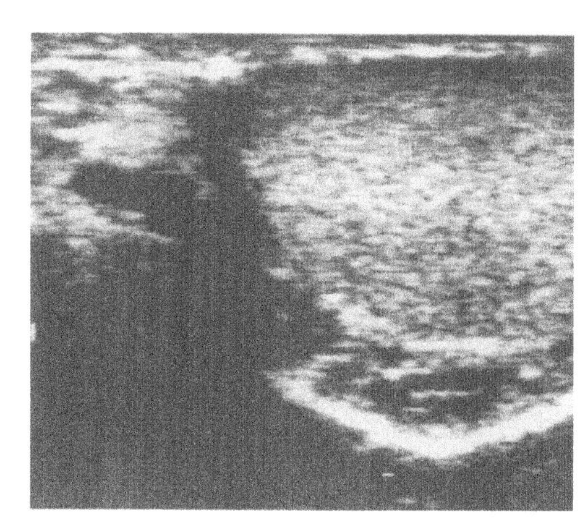

Fig. 12. ***Varicoceles. Subclinical form.*** Transverse section. Posterior to the testis is an abnormal area rather like a honeycomb which explains the dilatation of the veins of the anterior spermatic plexus. In the mild or moderate form the hilar varicocele is more easily visualised on the transverse rather than sagittal section

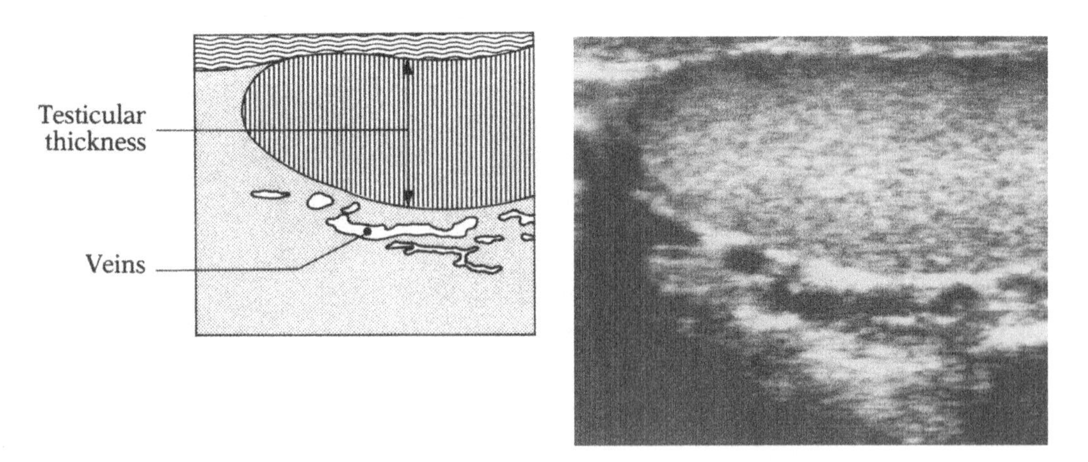

Fig. 13. ***Varicoceles. Measurements of the testis.*** Sagittal section. Definite varicocele indicated by dilated veins in the spermatic pedicle and posterior to the testis. Testicular measurements should include length, width (transverse scan) and especially thickness (or height). This last parameter would appear to be the first to be reduced in cases of hypotrophy

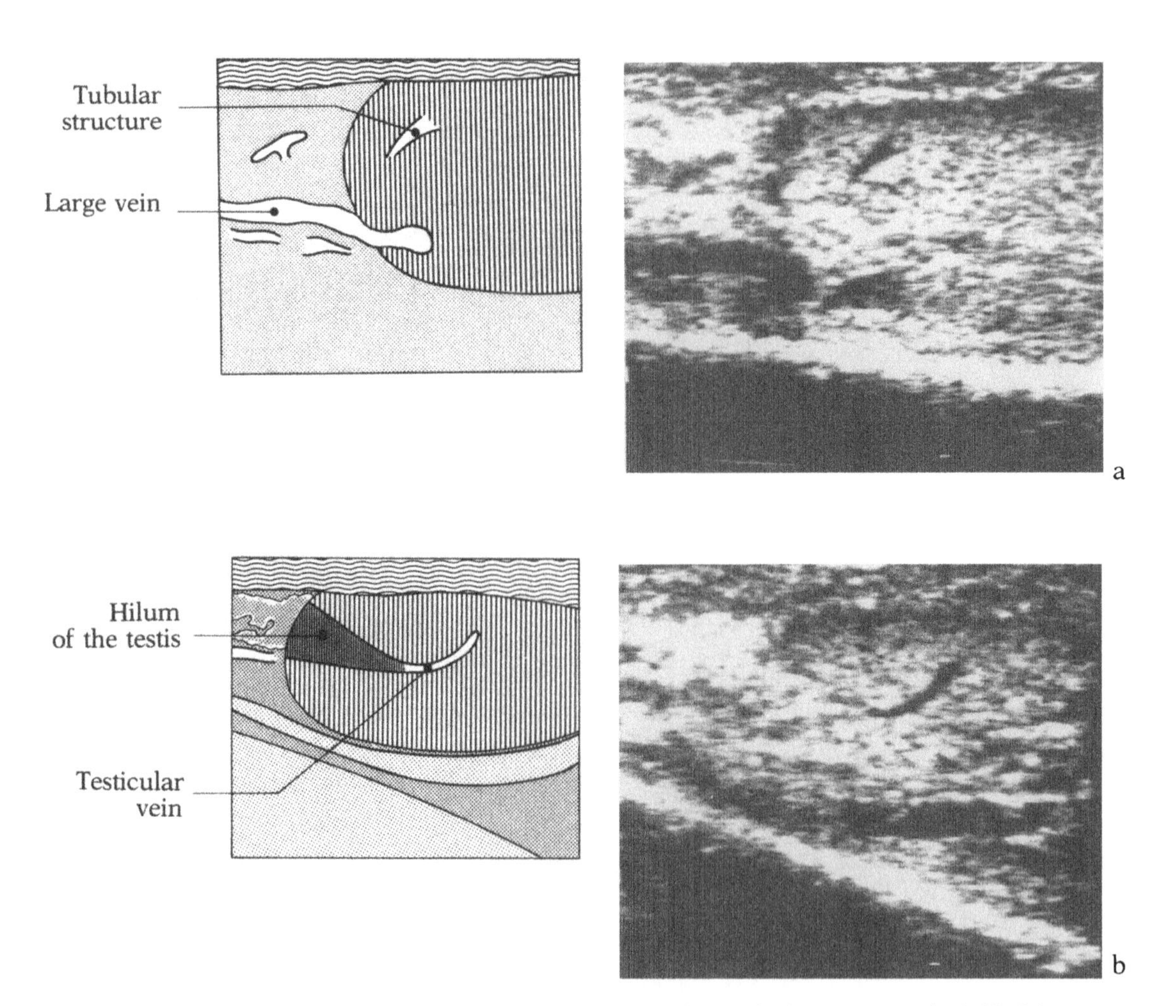

Fig. 14a, b. ***Varicoceles. Misleading images.*** **a** Sagittal section: Hypoechogenic zone in the antero-superior half of the testis which must not be misinterpreted as a tumour. The linearity of its boundaries should lead one to suspect a vascular structure. **b** Section of the inferior pole: markedly distended varicosities of the deep scrotal veins, inferior to the testis, confirming the venous nature of the structure and the non pathological nature of the intratesticular structure

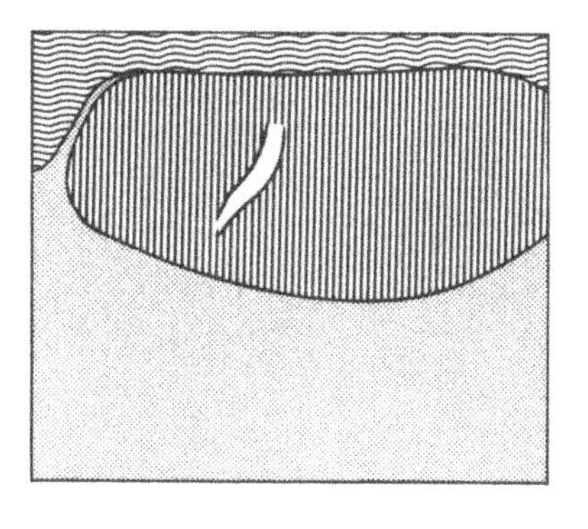

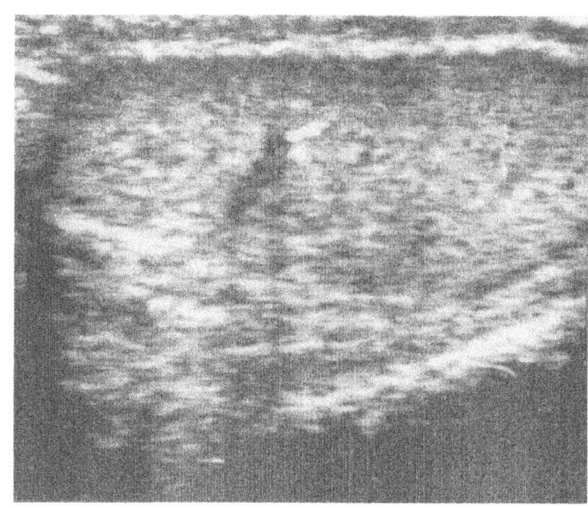

Fig. 15. ***Varicoceles. Misleading images.*** Sagittal section. Another morphological variant of a dilated superficial testicular vein in the presence of a global varicocele: narrow hypoechoic triangular structure at the postero-superior base (towards the hilum) crossing testis

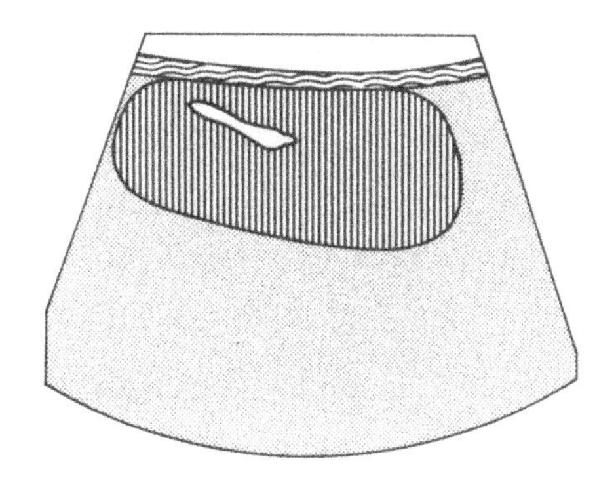

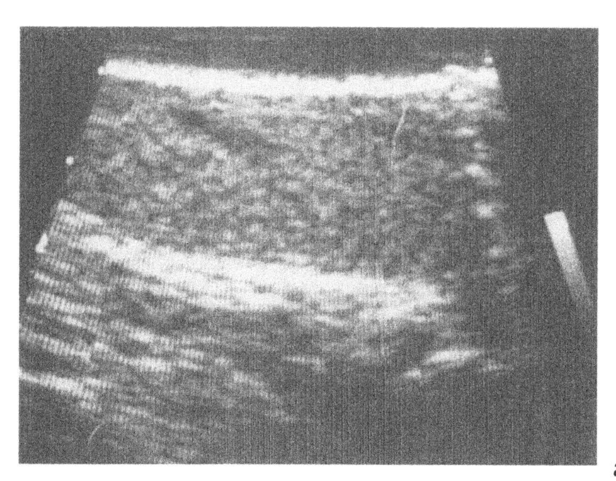

a

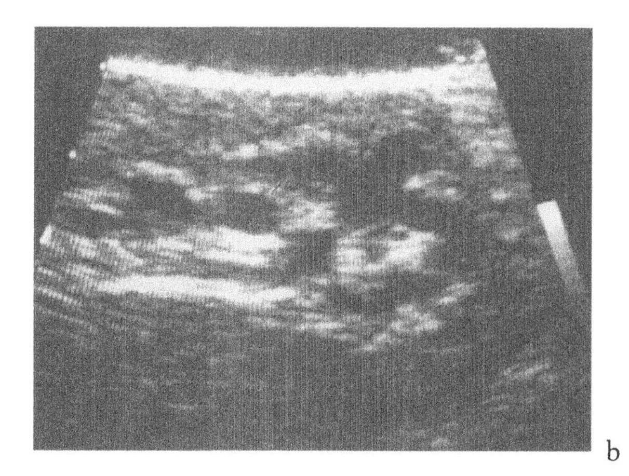

b

Fig. 16a, b. ***Varicoceles. Misleading images.*** **a** Sagittal section. Hypoechoic structure, appearing tubular, crossing the anterior half of the testis. **b** Oblique section of the inferior pole. Frankly dilated varicosity of the deep scrotal veins. The superficial vein is involved therefore in a varicocele

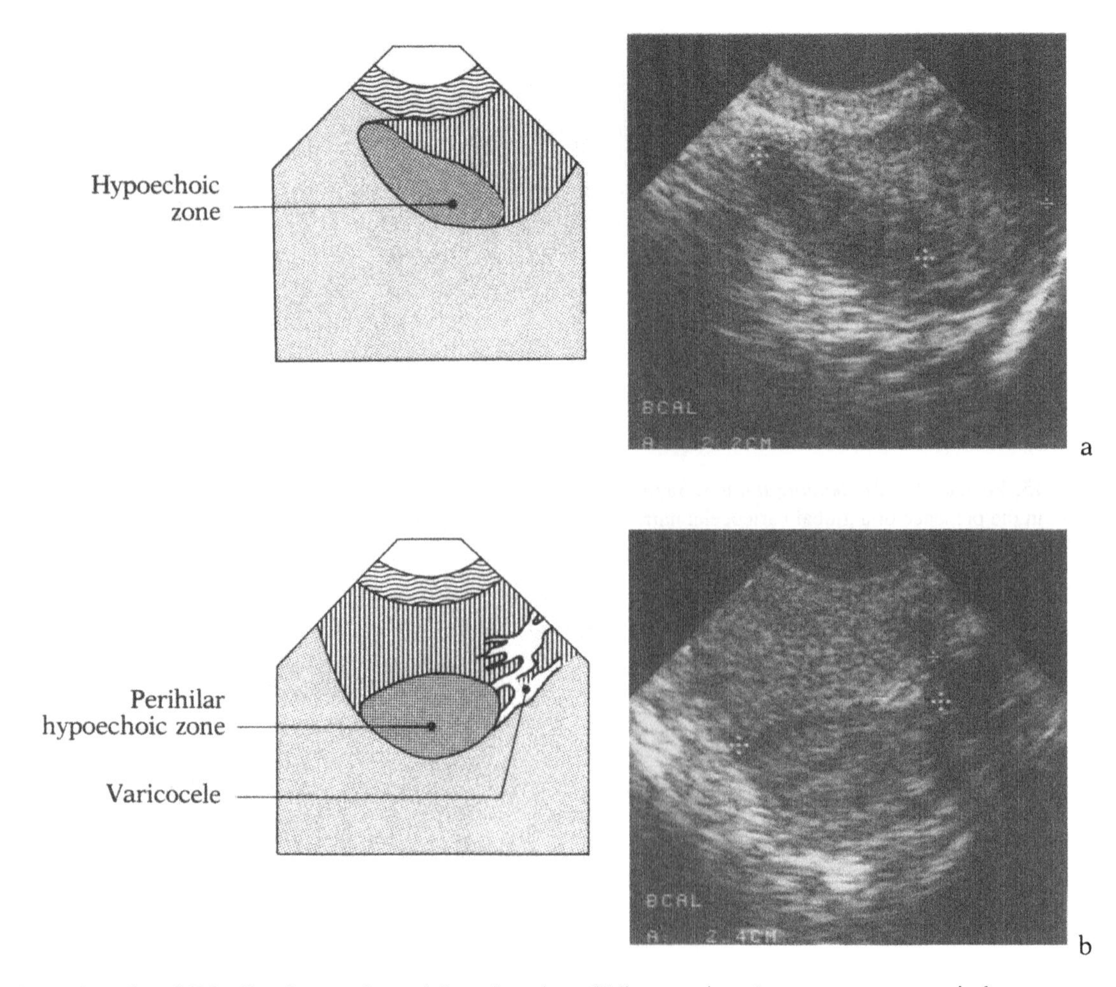

Fig. 17a, b. ***Varicoceles. Misleading images.*** Large left varicocele. **a** Oblique section. An area postero-superiorly appearing less echogenic than the rest of the testis. **b** Transverse section: persistence of the hypoechoic perihilar area in this different plane of section. This alteration in the hilar echo pattern should not be mistaken for a tumour of the rete testis and is seen in cases of a large varicocele: probably represents a degree of interstitial oedema due to venous stasis

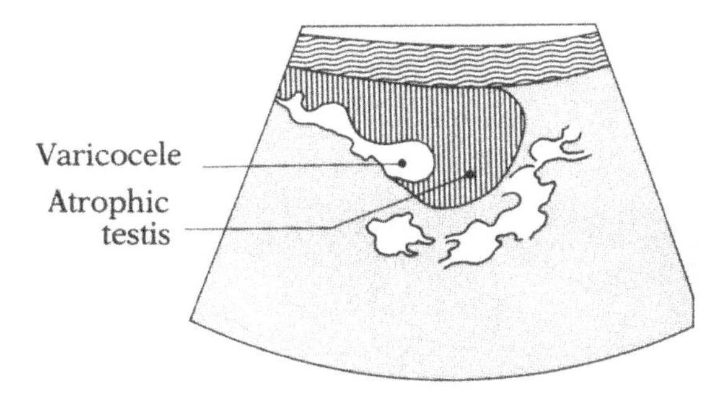

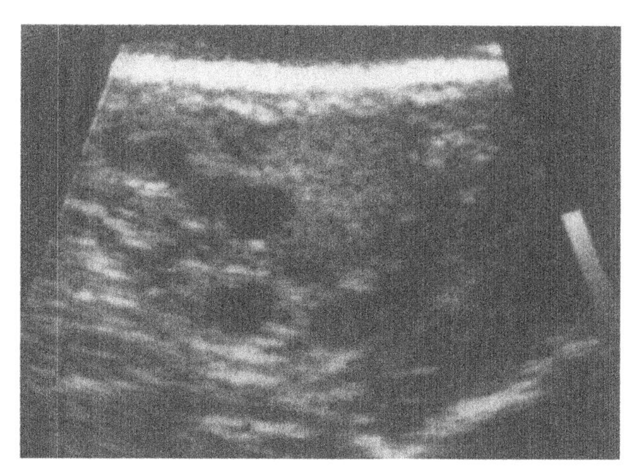

Fig. 18. ***Varicocele. Testicular atrophy.*** Transverse section. Large varicocele shown by serpiginous dilatation of the veins, particularly well seen at the hilum. The echo pattern of the testis is preserved but there is a definite reduction in its breadth and thickness

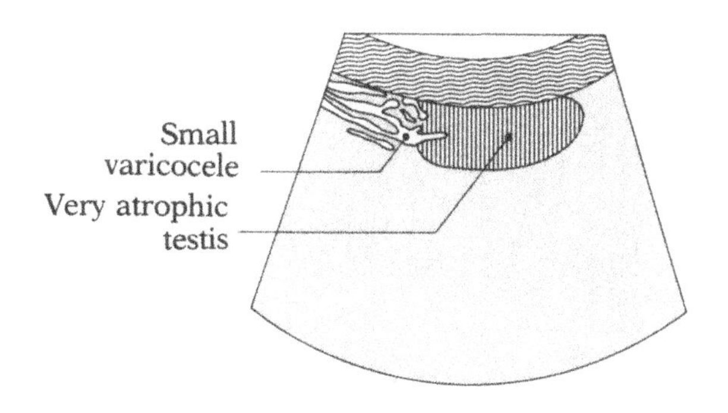

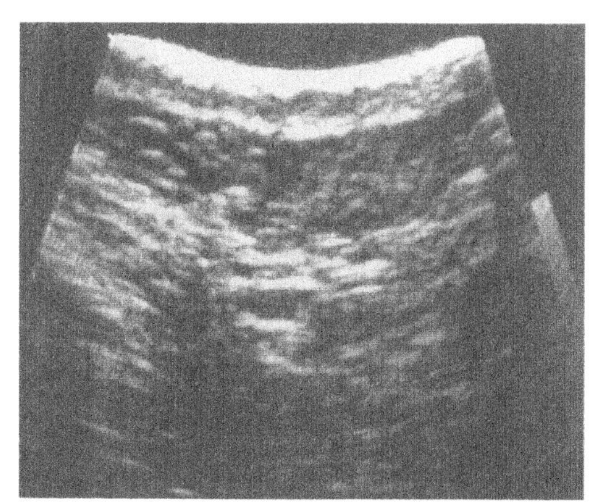

Fig. 19. ***Varicocele. Testicular atrophy.*** Sagittal section. Moderate varicocele associated with marked testicular atrophy (thickness barely 1 cm). These two cases illustrate the fact that the degree of atrophy is not proportional to the size of the varicocele

The epididymis

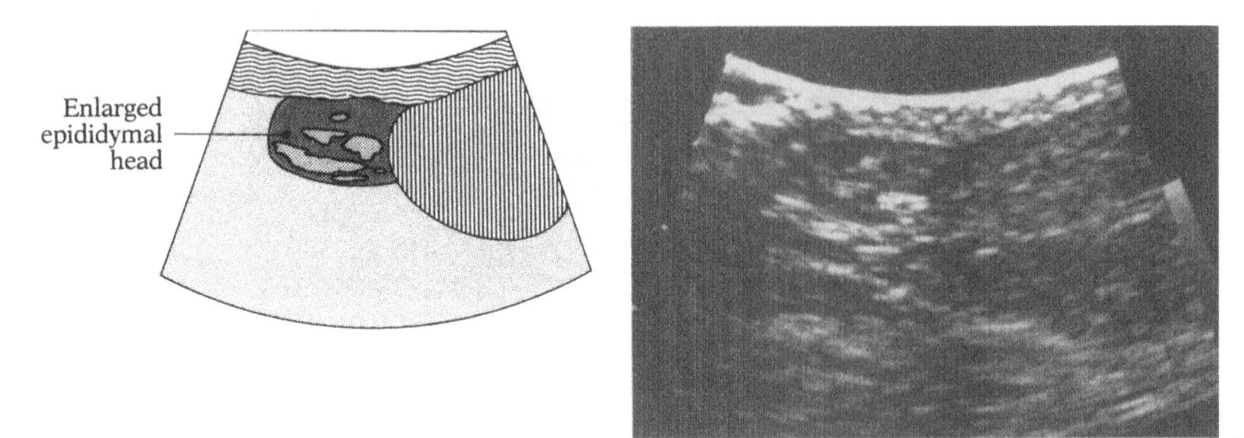

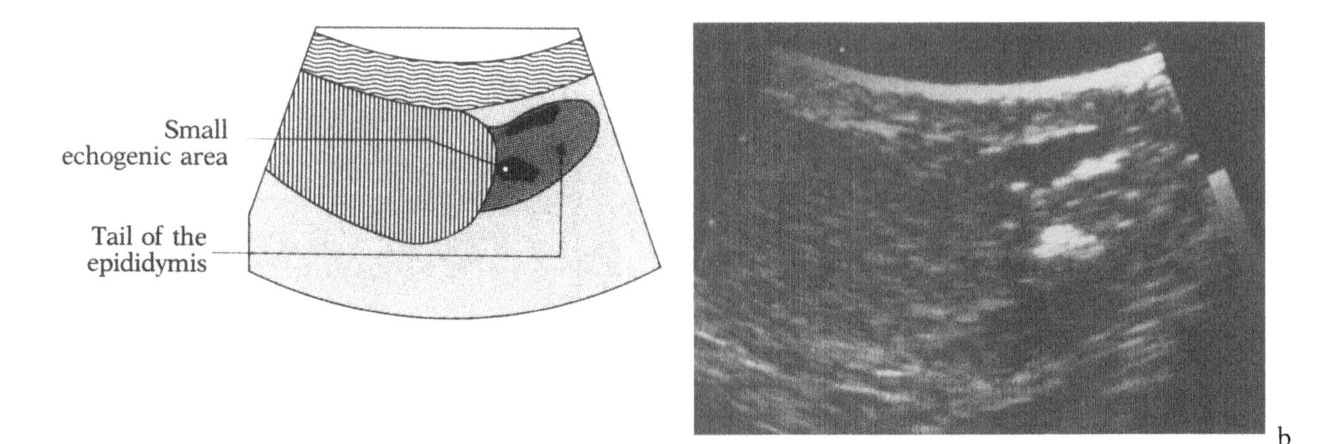

Fig. 20a, b. ***Epididymal abnormalities.*** Secondary sterility. **a** High sagittal section. Above the testis, a large heterogenous epididymal head containing several echogenic areas. **b** Inferior sagittal scan: inferior to the testis, the epididymal tail is abnormally well visualised due to enlargement and definite increased echogenicity within it. Same abnormalities on the contra-lateral side indicating bilateral blockage distally: obstruction of the ejaculatory ducts

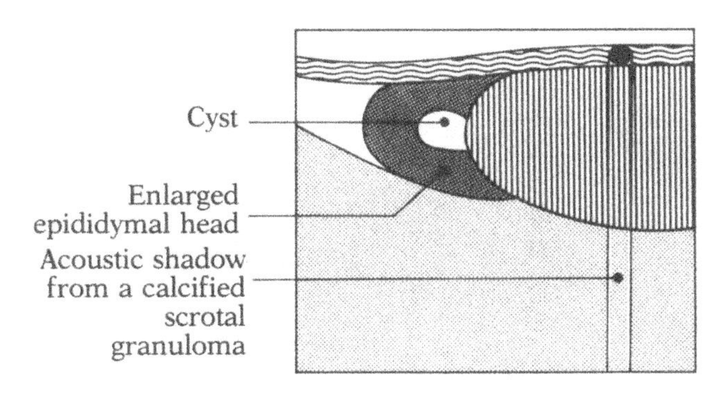

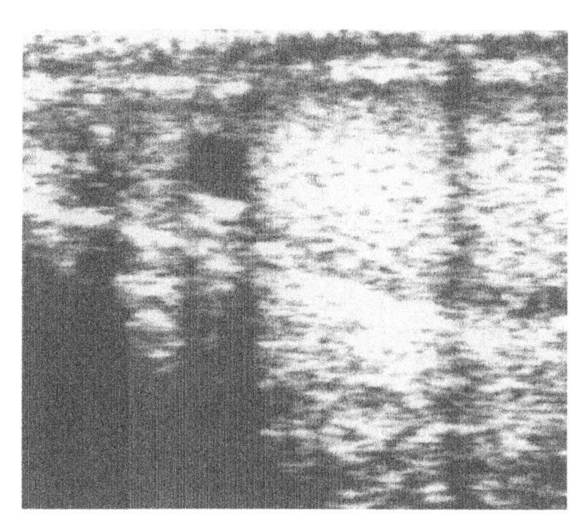

Fig. 21. ***Epididymal abnormalities.*** Primary sterility. Sagittal section. Enlarged epididymal head (greater than 12 mm in two diameters) containing a cyst of a few millimetres. The suggested diagnosis of a distal obstruction must be taken in conjunction with the hormonal status (in particular,the serum FSH level)

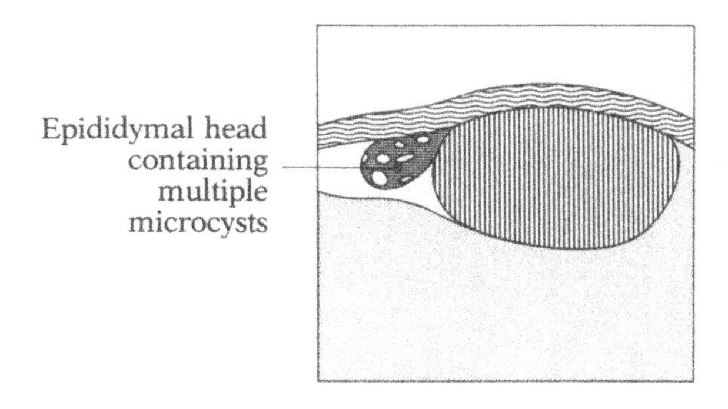

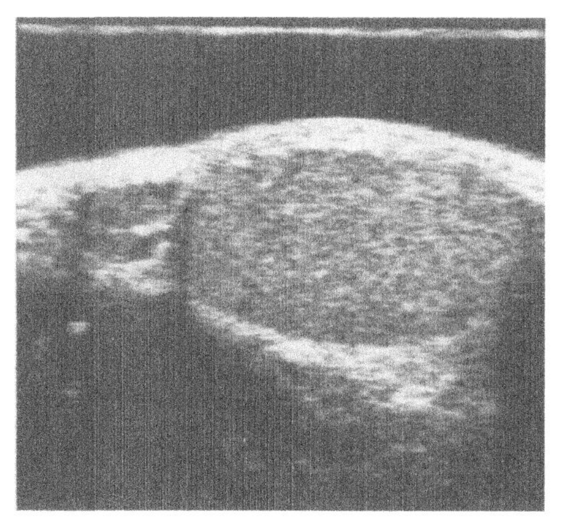

Fig. 22. ***Epididymal abnormalities.*** Primary sterility. Excretory azoospermia. Sagittal section. Normal testis. Slightly enlarged epididymal head. Note particularly the abnormal echopattern with punctate rounded hypoechogenic areas: distal obstruction which proved to be obliterated non-patent ejaculatory ducts

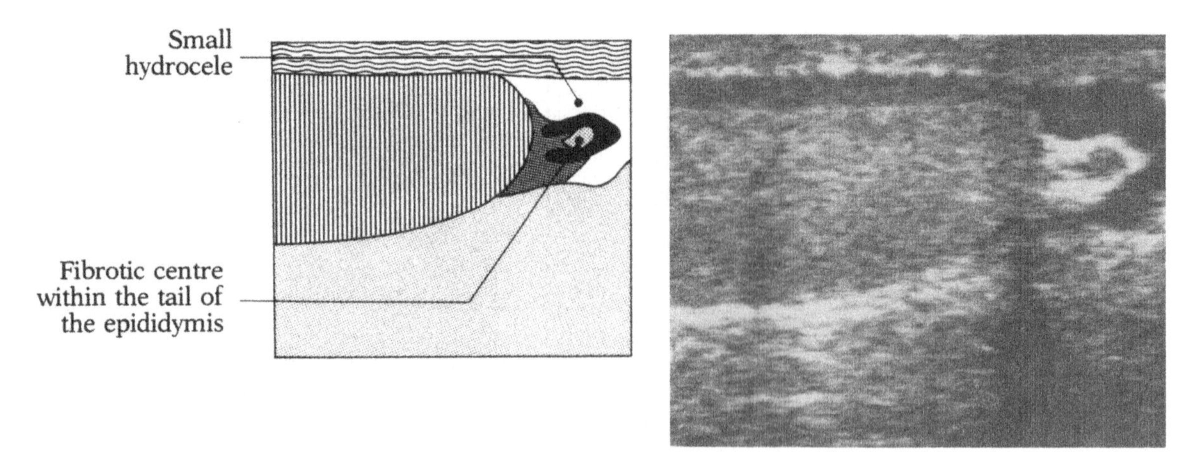

Fig. 23. ***Epididymal abnormalities.*** Same context. Palpable hard nodule at the inferior pole of the testis. Sagittal section. The palpable nodule corresponds to the tail of the epididymis which is enlarged (measures nearly 1 cm) and is surrounded by an echogenic line: sclero-fibrotic nodule, secondary to a previous caudal epididymitis and causing obstruction to the normal passage of spermatozoa

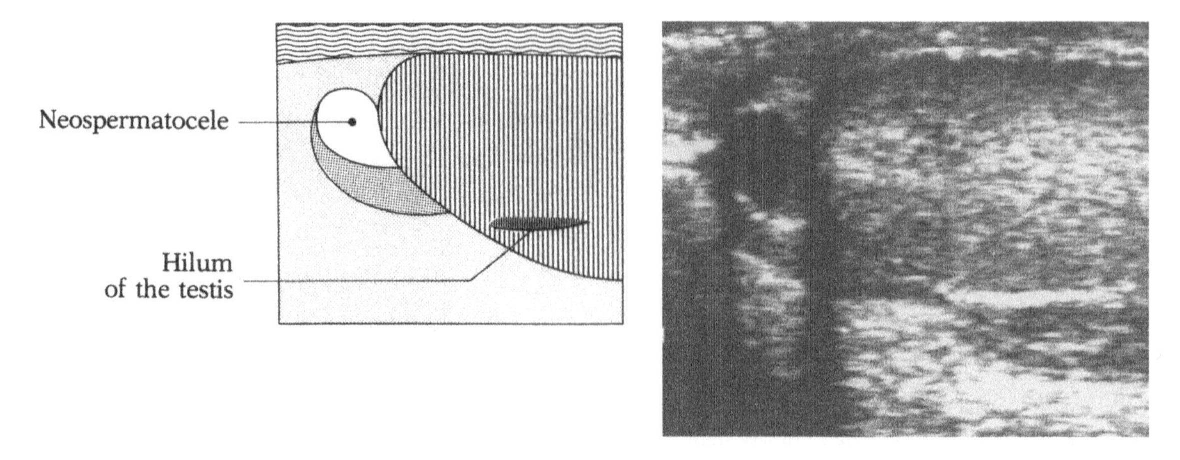

Fig. 24. ***Epididymal abnormalities.*** Post-operative appearance. Sterility due to bilateral agenesis of the vas deferentia. Fashioning of a neo-spermatocele (epididymal fistula and vaginal patch). Control baseline examination on the 8th day. Regular outline of the neo-spermatocele, transonic with no adjacent effusion

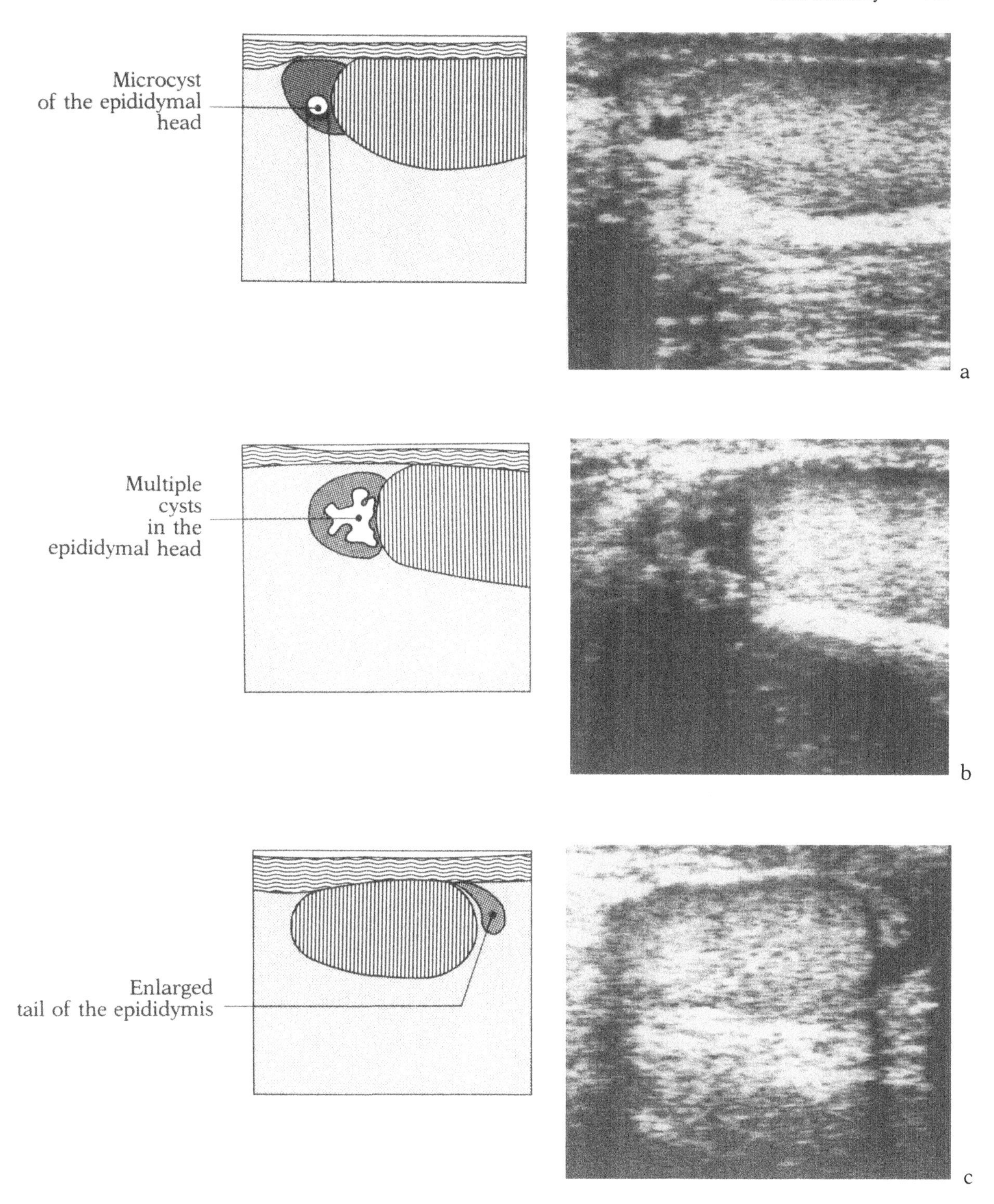

Fig. 25a-c. ***Epididymal abnormalities.*** Secondary sterility. Oligoasthenospermia. **a** Sagittal section of the right testis. Normal size epididymal head (about 1 cm) containing a solitary 2-3 mm diameter cyst in its postero-inferior portion. The size of the cyst and the absence of other cysts in the presence of a normal size epididymis suggest the diagnosis of a small insignificant dystrophic cyst. **b** Sagittal section of the left scrotal sac. The head of the epididymis is enlarged with a cystic pattern due to tiny anechoic areas. **c** Sagittal section of the inferior pole. The tail of the epididymis is abnormal, because too well distinguished but still homogeneous. In conclusion : on the right side, insignificant dystrophic cyst of the epididymis and on the left, cystic epididymal enlargement suggesting distal obstruction

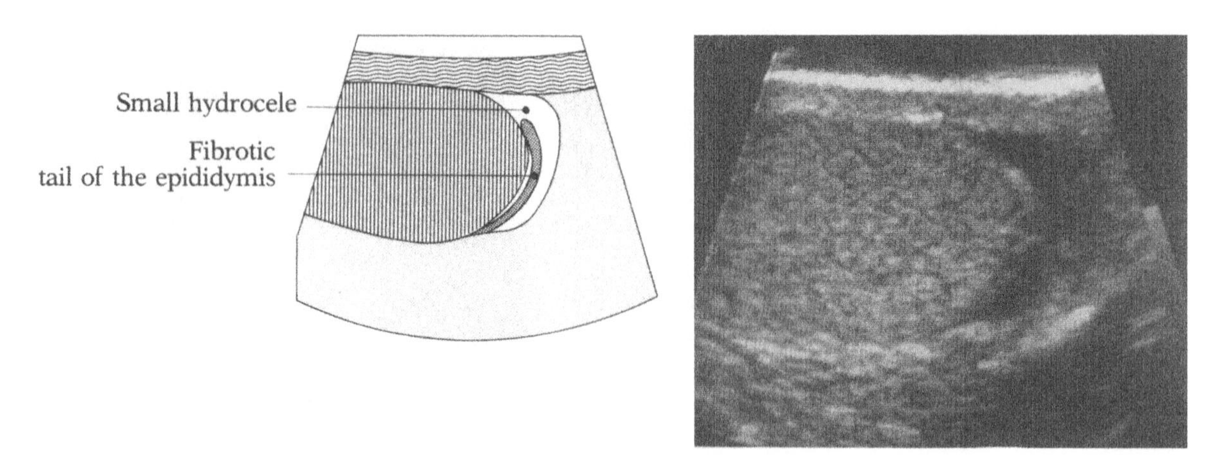

Fig. 26. ***Epididymal abnormalities.*** Secondary sterility. Sagittal section of the inferior pole. Inferior to the normal testis, the epididymal tail is abnormally well visualised in the form of an echogenic tongue separated from the testis by a fine transonic line: sclero-fibrotic changes in the tail causing obstruction to the passage of the spermatozoa

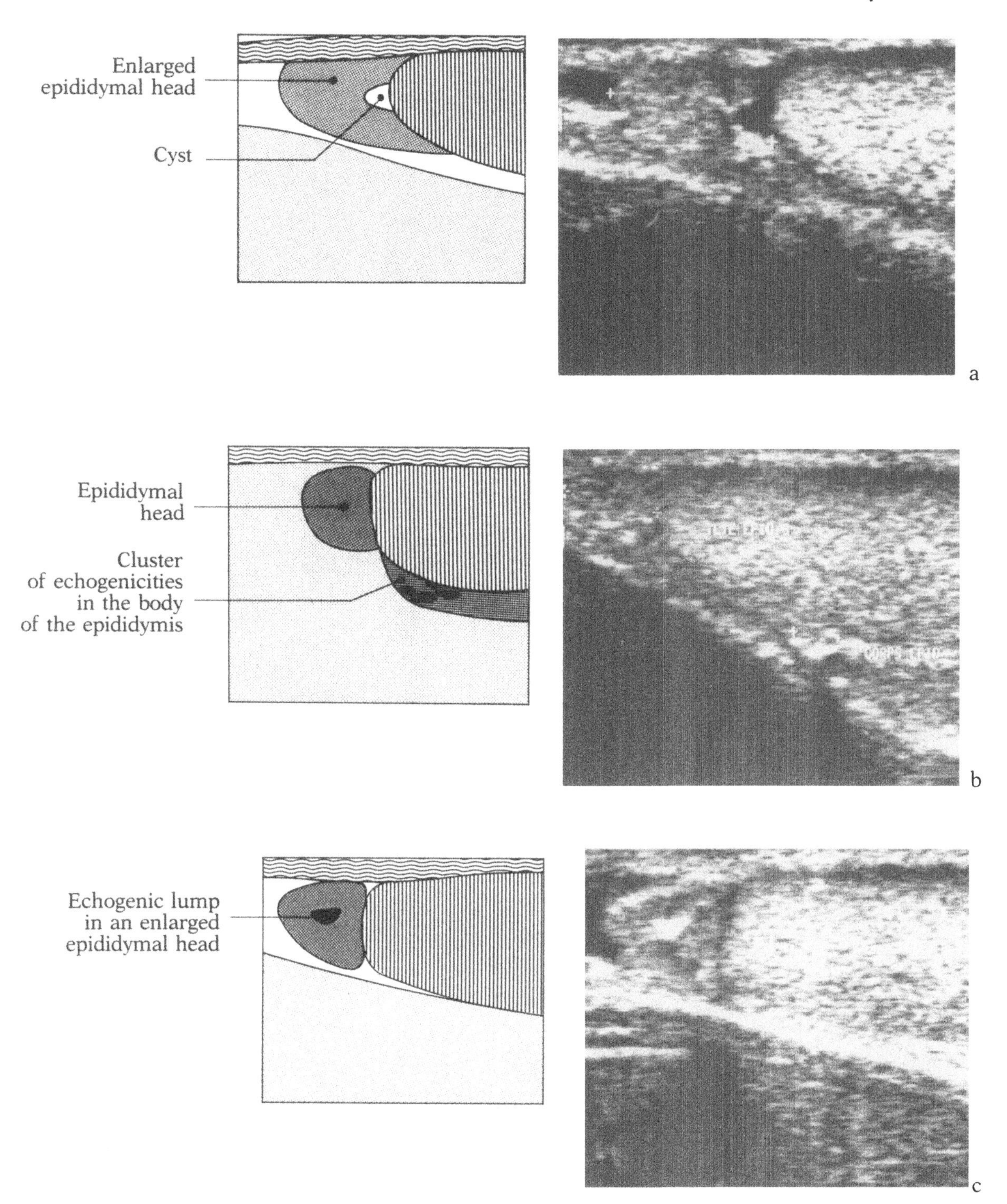

Fig. 27a-c. ***Epididymal abnormalities.*** A 31 year old patient, originating from Mali. Primary sterility: azoospermia with reduced FSH levels, suspected underlying obstructive pathology. **a** Sagittal section of the left testis. Enlarged epididymal head (greater than 2 cm) with a solitary cyst. **b** More oblique section. Several abnormal echogenic linear structures are seen in the body of the epididymis. **c** Section of the right testis. Enlarged epididymal head with an echogenic centre. In conclusion: bilateral abnormalities with enlargement of both epididymal heads suggesting bilateral obstruction at the level of the ejaculatory canals

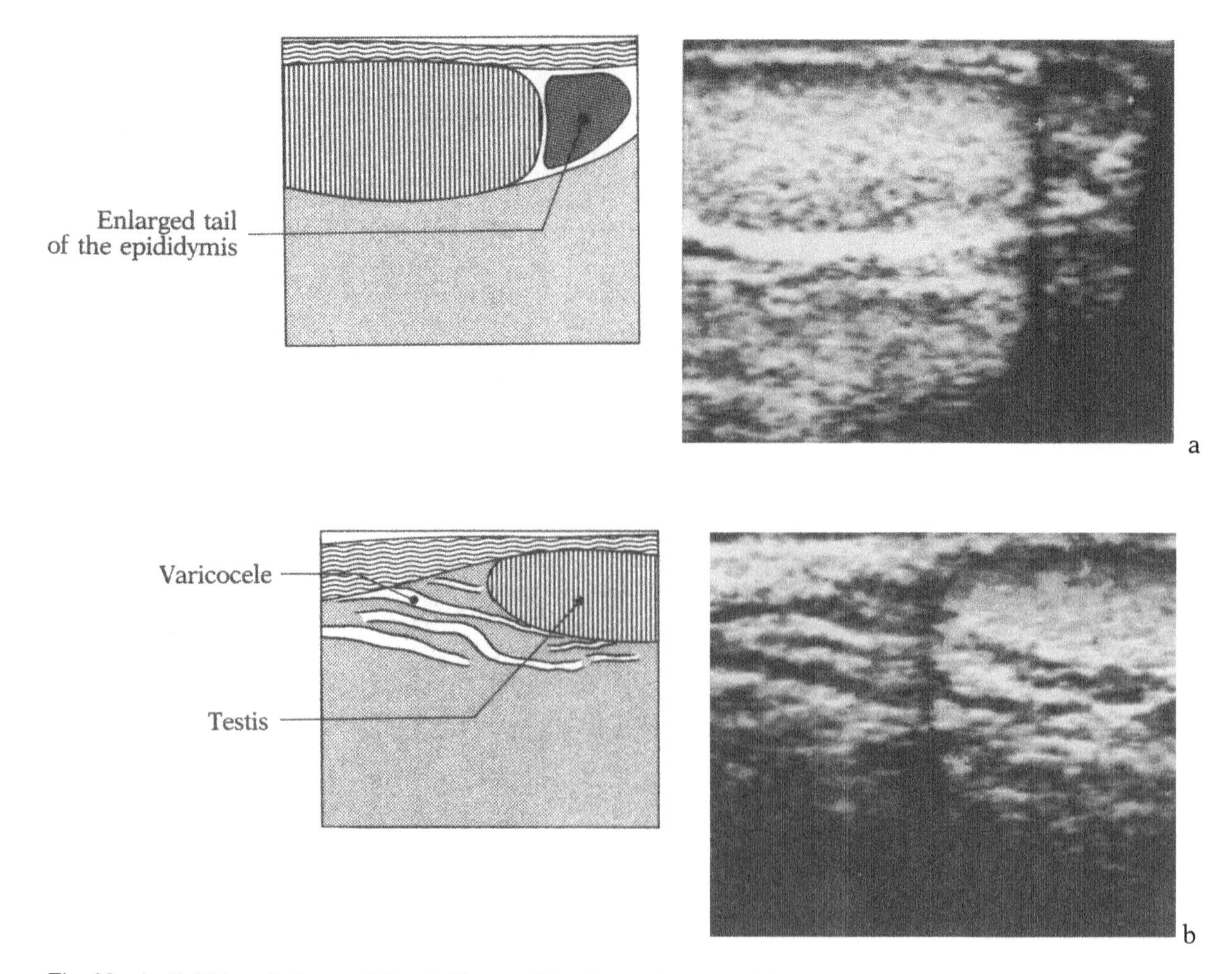

Fig. 28a, b. ***Epididymal abnormalities.*** A 36 year old patient: primary sterility with anti-spermatozoal antibodies in the semen. **a** Sagittal section of the right scrotal sac. Enlarged epididymal tail (almost 10 mm). **b** Oblique section of the superior pole. Associated global varicocele: network of dilated veins posterior to the testis and in the spermatic pedicle. Same appearances on the contra lateral side. This example is a reminder of the frequency of complex abnormalities associated with sterility: in this case bilateral varicoceles with a nodule in the right epididymal tail

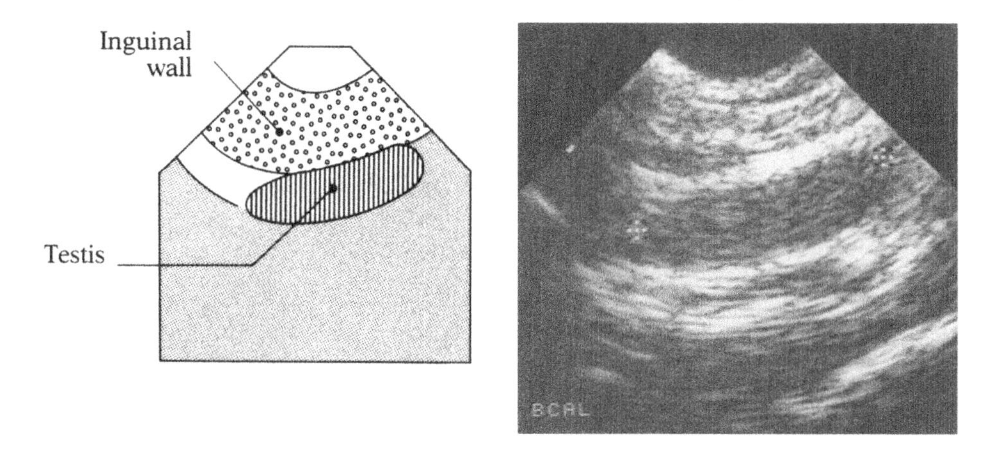

Fig. 29. ***Testicular abnormalities: Position; size.*** Primary sterility. Right side of the scrotum appears empty. Palpable inguinal testis. Ultrasound to assess its echopattern. Sagittal section of the inguinal region. Testis easily recognisable by its shape and normal echopattern, in the inguinal canal. Fusiform shape due to marked reduction in its thickness (barely 5 mm): homogenous but atrophic inguinal testis

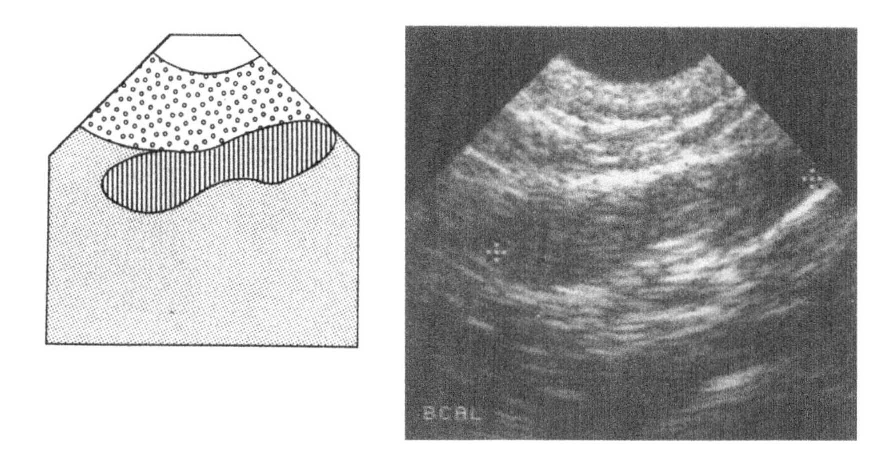

Fig. 30. ***Testicular abnormalities: Position; size.*** Same picture. Same section. Testis easily recognisable but with a central constriction giving an "hour-glass" appearance, due to its position within the inguinal canal. Severe atrophy indicated by marked reduction in thickness

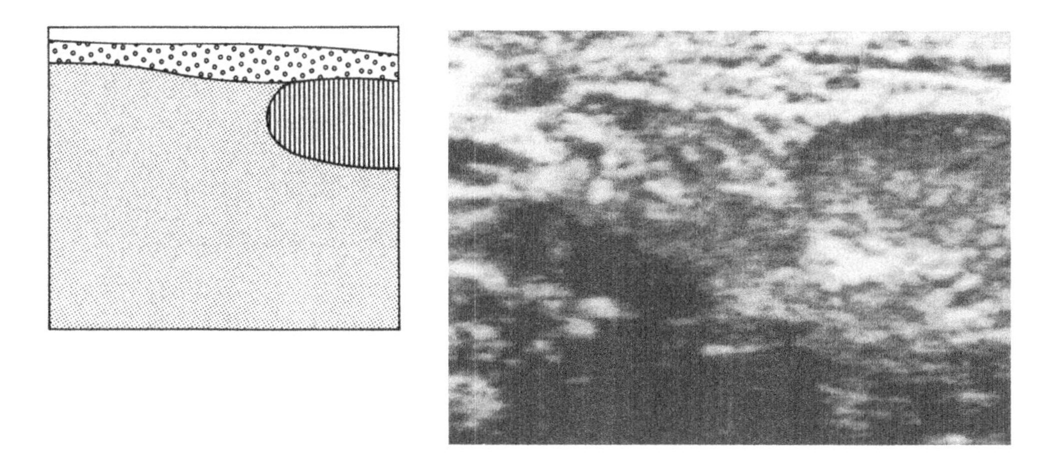

Fig. 31. ***Testicular abnormalities: Position; size.*** Sterility in a 34 year old obese patient with an empty right side of the scrotum and an impalpable testis. Sagittal section of the inguinal region. An homogenous testis is seen which is of reasonable size since its thickness is greater than 1 cm

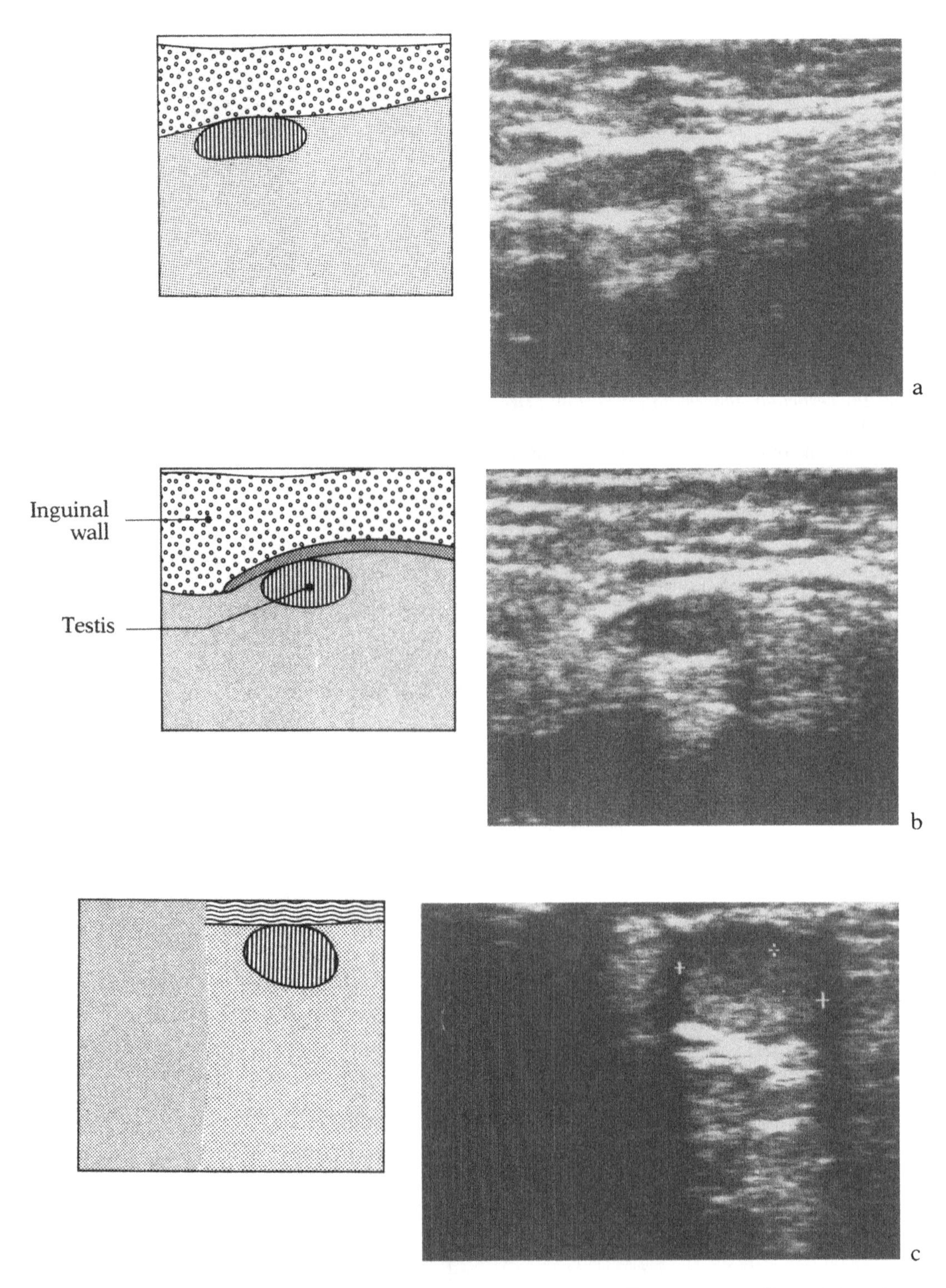

Fig. 32a-c. ***Testicular abnormalities: Position; size.*** A young, obese 11 year old boy. Empty scrotum. Testes felt at the inguinal ring. **a, b** Sagittal sections of the two inguinal regions, in order to obtain a baseline measurement of the testes before starting hormonal treatment. **a** Right: easily recognisable testis, fusiform, lying deep to the cutaneous tissue and inguinal musculature. The testis appears hypoechoic which is normal given the age of the child; there is, however, a definite reduction in its thickness (less than 5 mm). **b** Left: less elongated and slightly thicker testis. **c** Control three months later after a series of nine gonadotrophin injections (each of 1500 units). Sagittal section of the right side of the scrotum. The testis has descended into the scrotum which itself is of normal thickness. There has been an apparent enlargement of the testis (thickness of 10 mm). Same results on the left

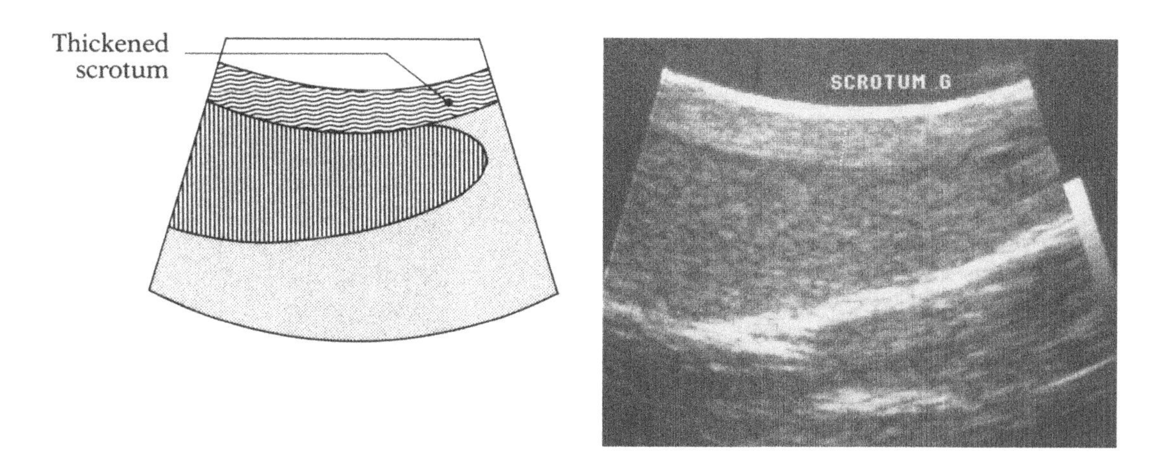

Fig. 33. ***Testicular abnormalities. Investing layer.*** Primary sterility. Sagittal section. Same appearances on both sides: thickening of greater than 5 mm of the investing layers of the testis, no other abnormality. This appearance seems to be more frequently seen in the sterile population

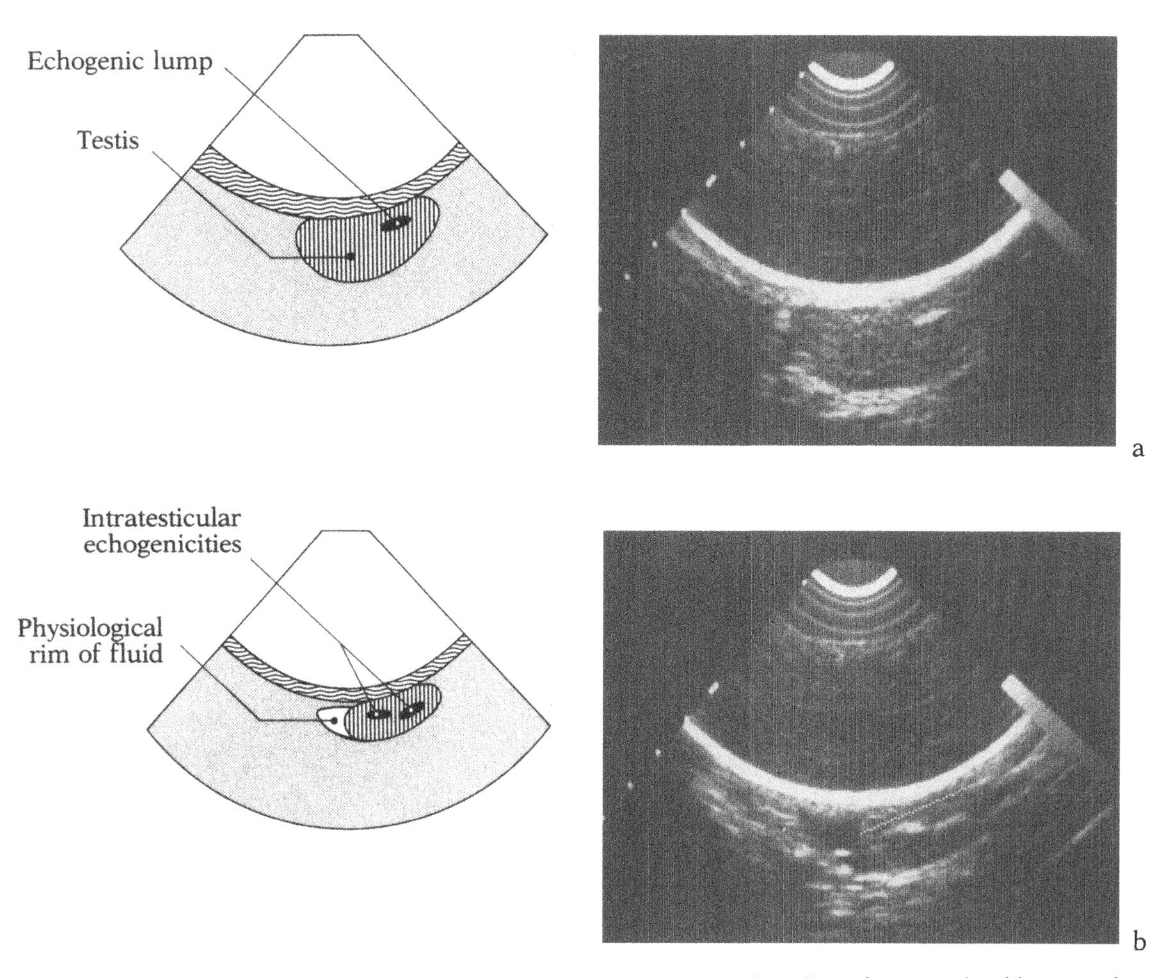

Fig. 34a, b. ***Testicular abnormalities. Echopattern.*** Sterile patient. Association of an oligoasthenospermia with a normal FSH level and chronic bronchitis suggesting Young's syndrome. **a** Sagittal section of the left testis. Atrophic testis containing echogenic fusiform non-attenuating areas of a few millimetres orientated along the long axis of the gland. They are not well seen in the same plane of section. **b** Sagittal section of the right testis. Small testis with identical appearances. Conclusion: Bilateral intratesticular abnormalities, possibly due to abnormal seminiferous tubules

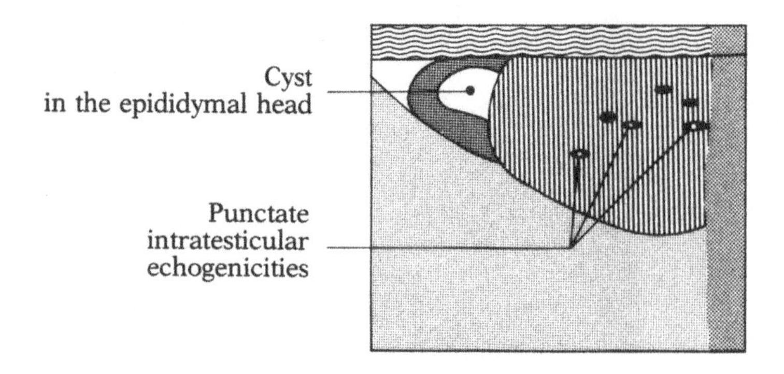

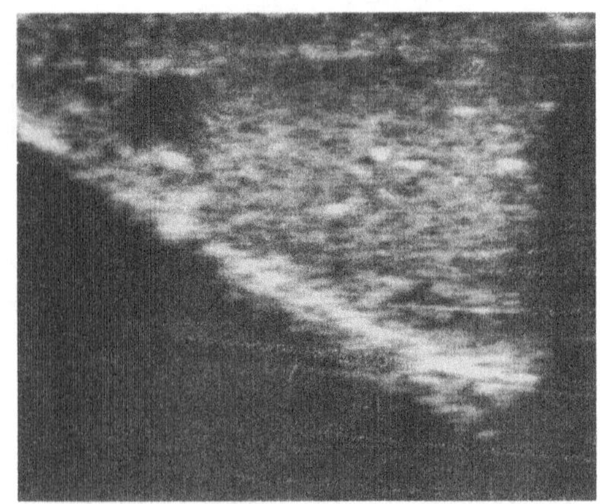

Fig. 35. ***Testicular abnormalities. Echopattern.*** A 34 year old sterile patient. At ultrasound, large bilateral varicoceles with other abnormalities. Sagittal section of the right testis. Normal size epididymal head containing a solitary large cyst. Multiple micro-echogenic punctate areas are seen mainly in the centre of the testis. Different appearance to the larger echogenic structures seen in Case 35. Uncertain patho-physiology: ?phleboliths of the superficial veins of the testis

Abnormalities of the pelvic genital organs

Prostate

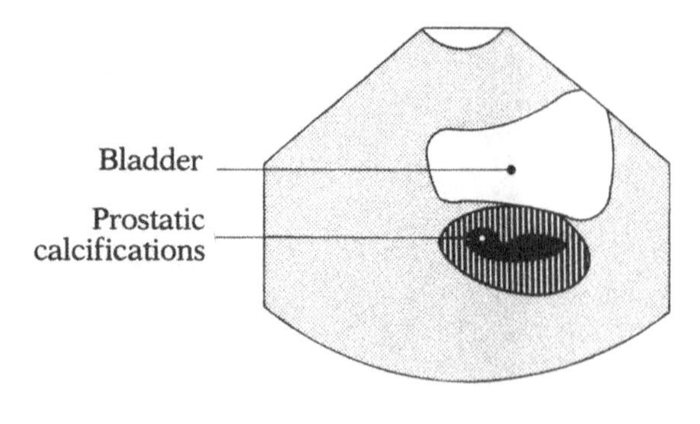

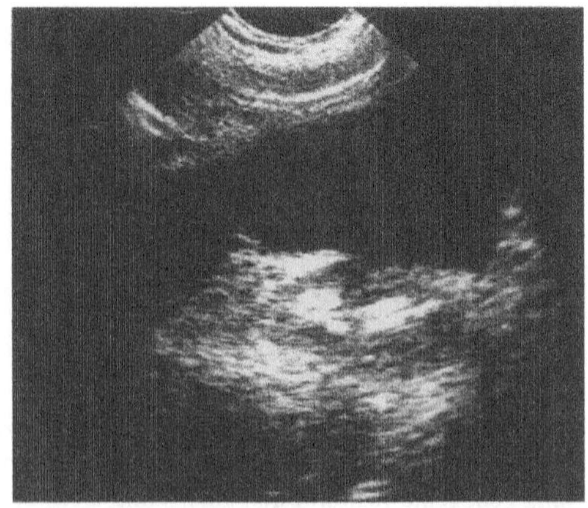

Fig. 36. ***Prostatic calcifications.*** Primary sterility. Transverse suprapubic scan. Symmetrical clumps of calcification lying centrally in the prostate. Very slightly attenuating

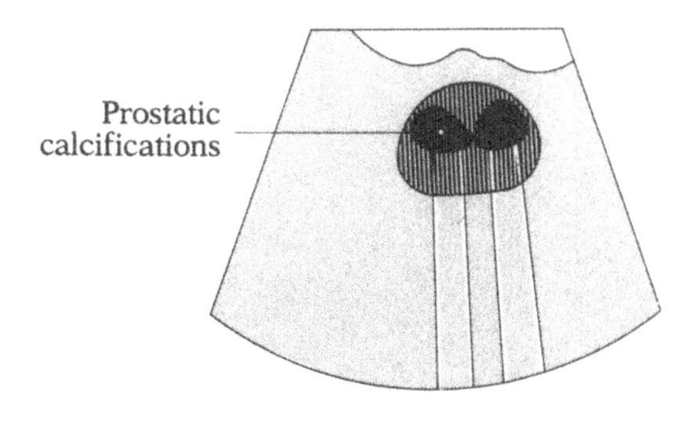

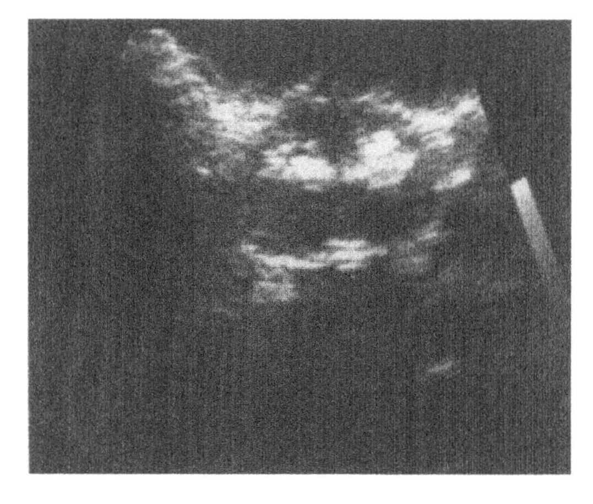

Fig. 37. ***Prostatic calcification***. Severe oligoasthenospermia in a 30 year old man. Same level of section. Same distribution and morphology of the calcifications but with more marked posterior attenuation

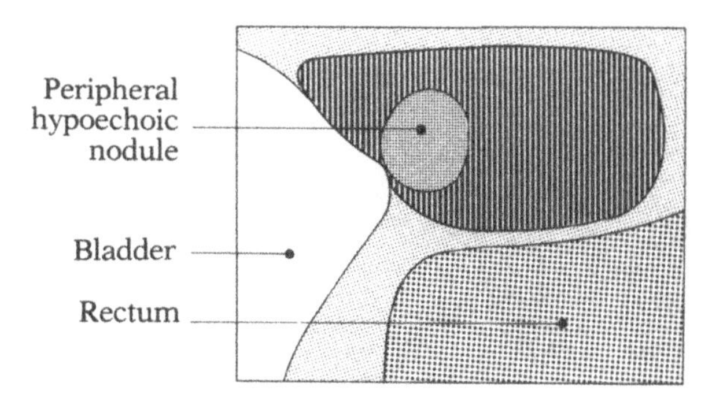

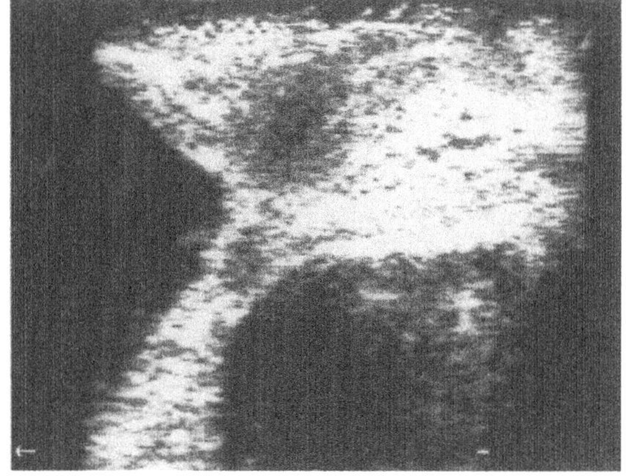

Fig. 38. ***Prostatitis.*** Primary sterility. Bacteria isolated in replated sperm cultures. Endorectal scan (linear array). Peripheral hypoechoic nodule indicating a focus of prostatitis, given the clinical context

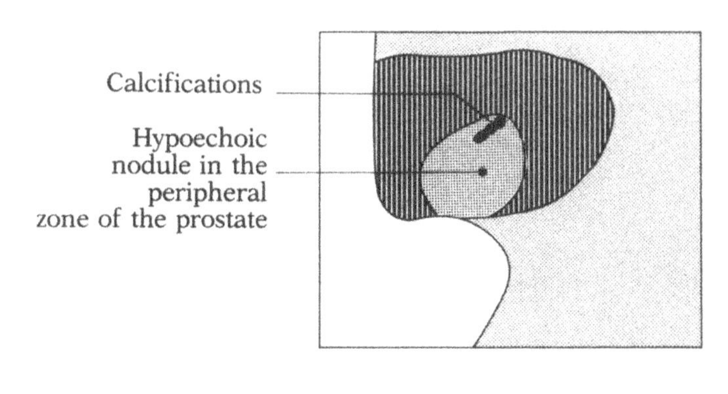

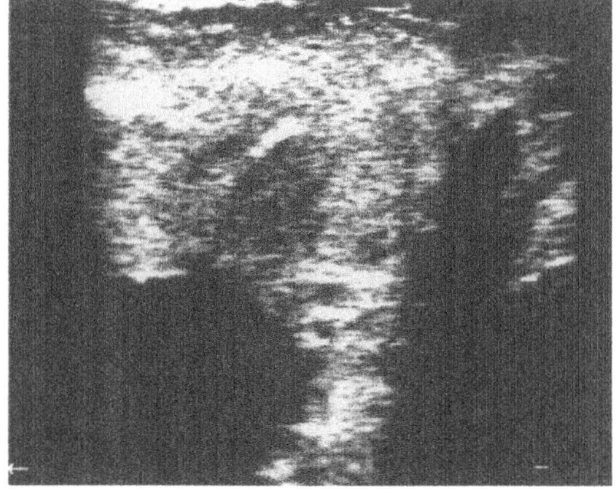

Fig. 39. ***Prostatitis.*** Identical clinical picture and scan technique. Large rounded peripheral hypoechoic zone containing small flecks of calcification in a chain: chronic prostatitis with lithiasis

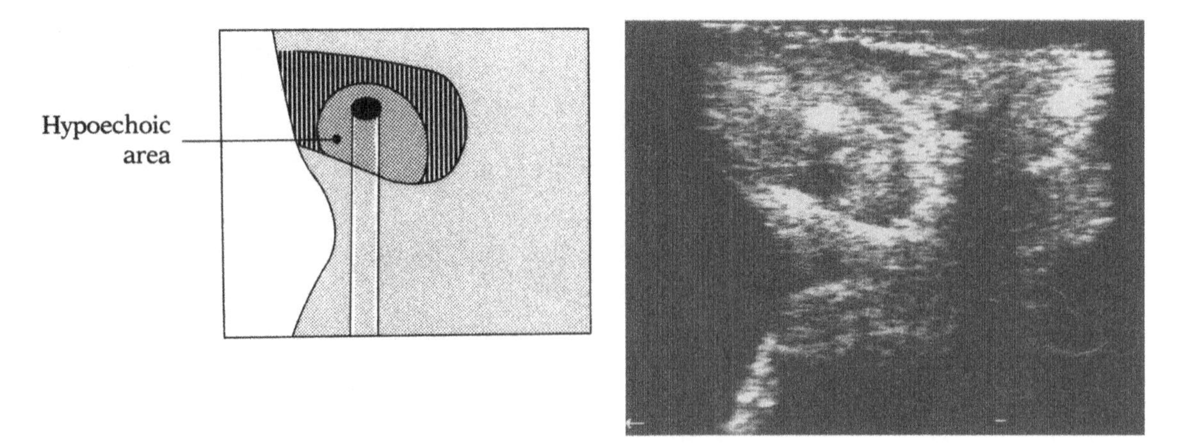

Fig. 40. ***Prostatitis.*** Same context. Peripheral hypoechoic area with less well-defind boundaries, containing a highly attenuating calcified nodule: chronic prostatitis

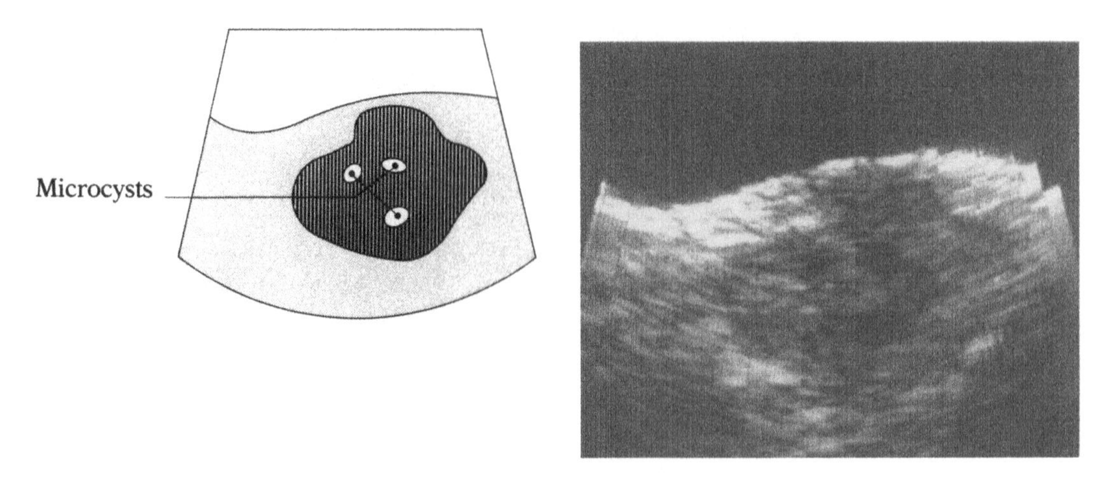

Fig. 41. ***Intra-prostatic cysts.*** A 45 year old patient with secondary sterility. Transverse suprapubic scan. There are 3 cysts (of about 1 mm) lying centrally within the prostate. Given the age of the patient and their central position, the appearances are almost certainly due to microcyst formation in benign adenomatous hyperplasia

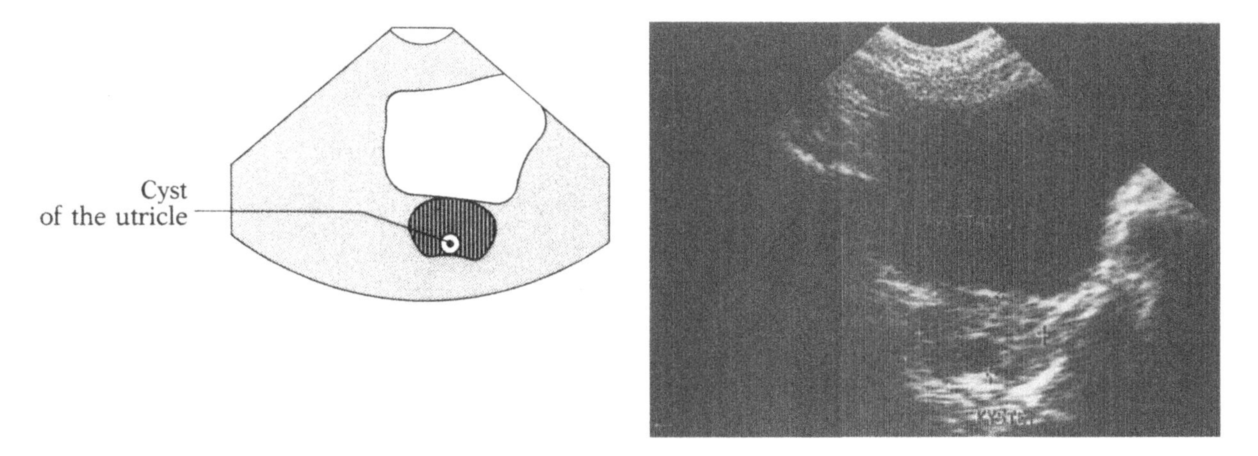

Fig. 42. ***Cyst of the prostatic utricle.*** A 30 year old patient. Primary sterility. Transverse suprapubic scan: incidental finding of a small cyst of the utricle: anechoic nodule within the prostate in a posterior and median position

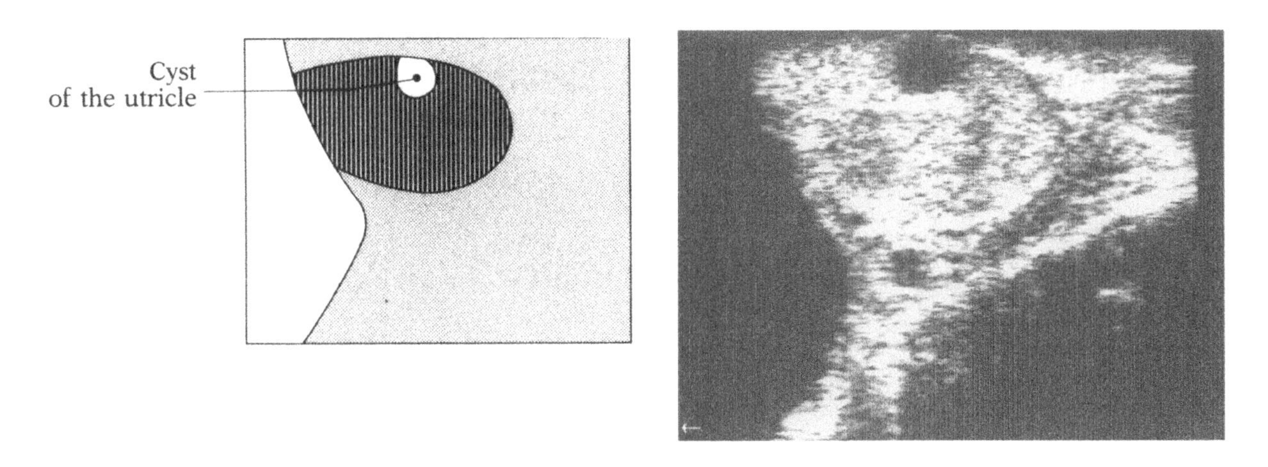

Fig. 43. ***Cyst of the prostatic utricle.*** Same context. Endorectal scan (linear array). Intra-prostatic postero-median cyst of almost 1 cm: small uncomplicated cyst of the utricle. This makes the possibility of obstruction to the ejaculatory canals less likely but, in this clinical context, must be taken in conjunction with the levels of the markers of the seminal vesicles (fructose) and prostate (zinc) in the semen

Seminal vesicles

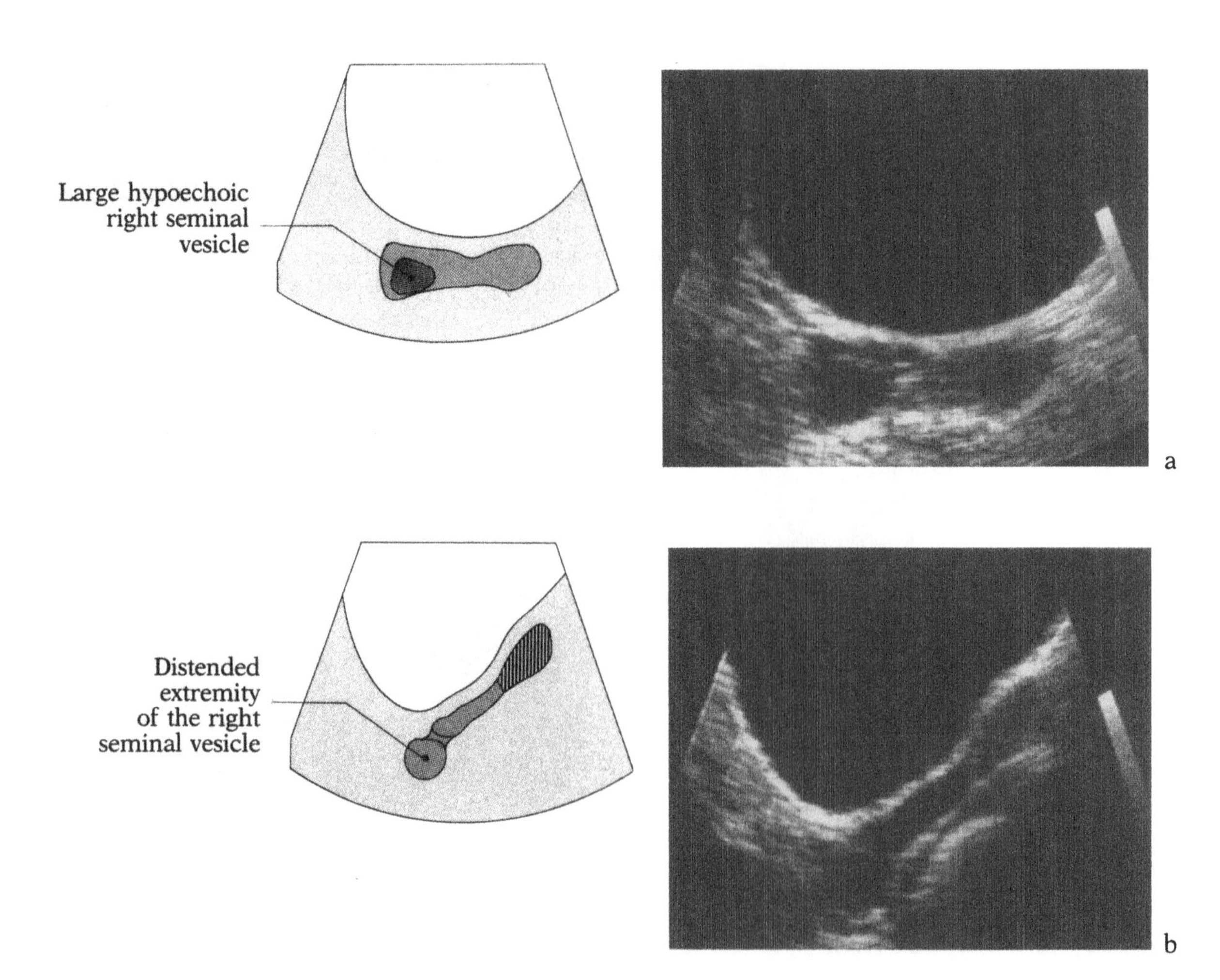

Fig. 44a, b. ***Asymmetry of the seminal vesicles*** A 35 year old patient. Primary sterility. Suprapubic examination. **a** Transverse section of the seminal vesicles at the level of the base: frank asymmetry as shown by the more hypoechoic and swollen right seminal vesicle. **b** Right para-sagittal section: visualisation of the whole of the right seminal vesicle, very hypoechoic due to distension. In this context, the presence of this degree of asymmetry should raise the possibility of stenosis of the homolateral ejaculatory duct

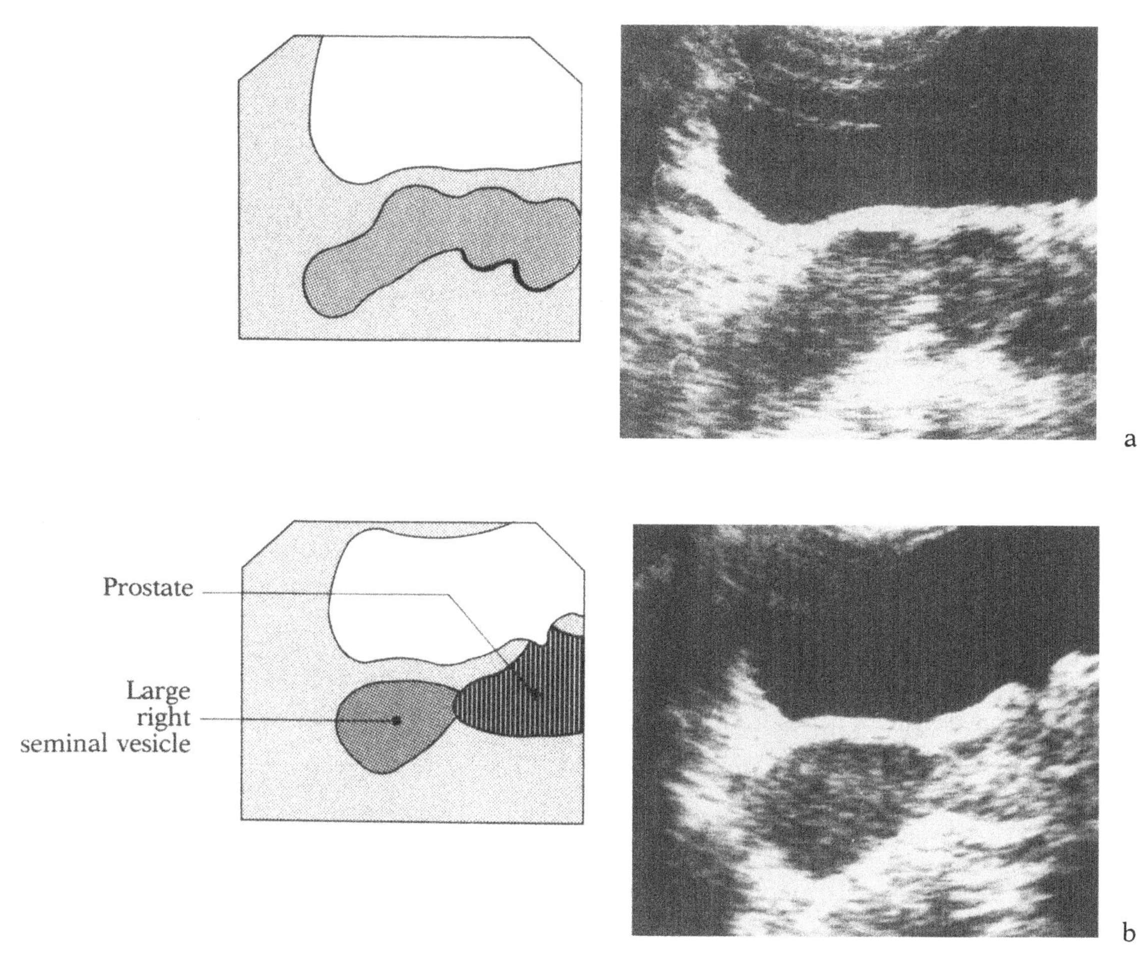

Fig. 45a, b. ***Enlarged seminal vesicles.*** Primary sterility. Last ejacul...on *48 hours* previously. Suprapubic examination. **a** Transverse section through the extremities of the seminal vesicles. Symmetrical enlargement of both organs: their distension accentuates the physiological bulging. **b** Para-sagittal section through the body of the seminal vesicle. This confirms the pathological enlargement (greater than 2 cm width). Uniform hypoechogenicity. In conclusion: the appearances suggest a bilateral obstruction, most likely an obliteration of the ejaculatory ducts

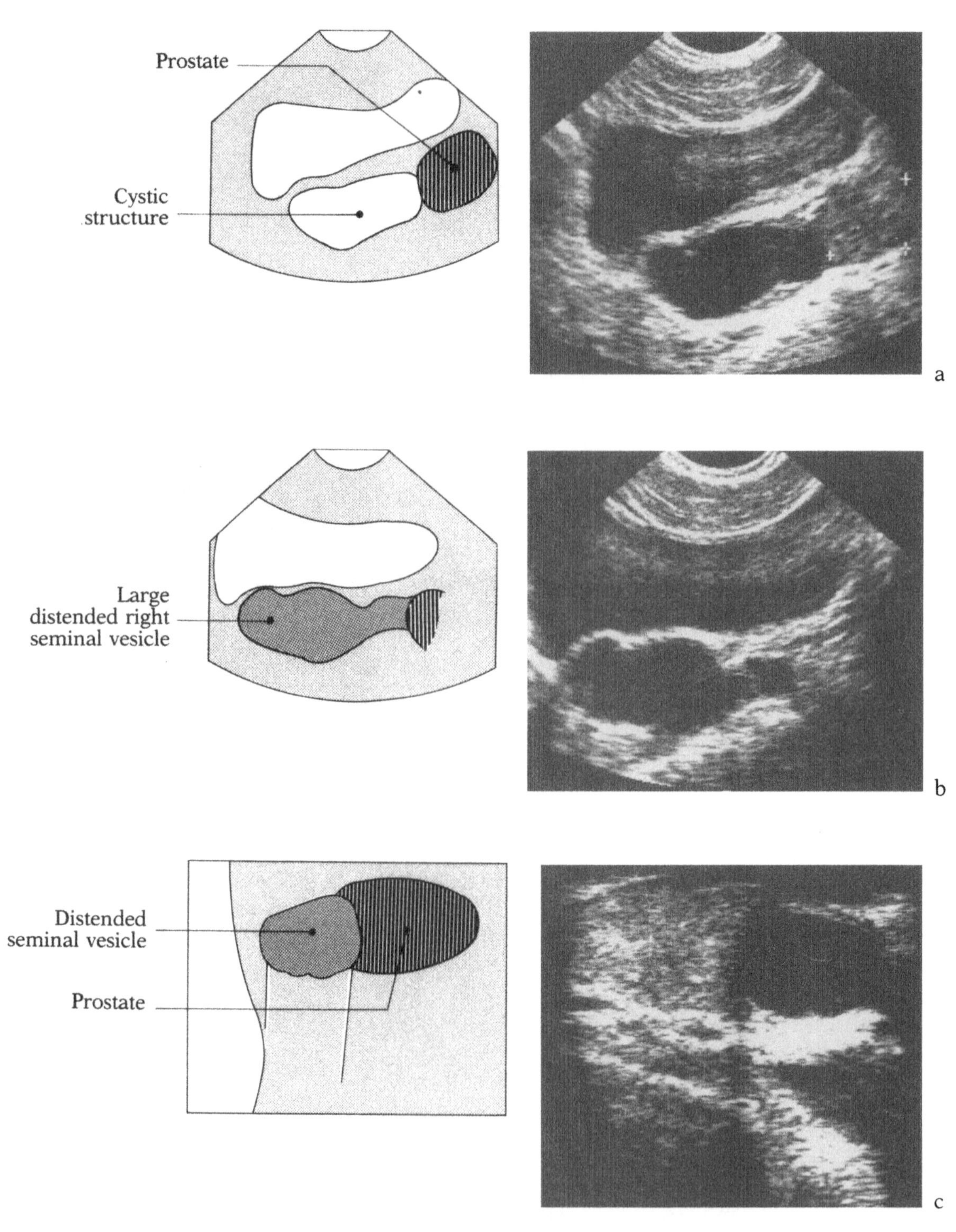

Fig. 46a-c. ***Cystic distension of a seminal vesicle.*** A 38 year old patient. Hypofertility with a right epididymal nodule, left varicocele and anti-spermatozoal antibodies. No signs of pelvic pathology. **a** Suprapubic scan, right para-sagittal section. Large cystic structure (2.5 x 4 cms) in the right lateral aspect of the prostate. **b** Section along the length of the mass: the appearances confirm that this structure is a grossly distended right seminal vesicle with bulging contours and maximum distension in its extremity. **c** Endorectal scan. This confirms the absence of sediment or an internal fluid level. No evidence of thickening of the wall of the seminal vesicle. A distal obstruction, namely a stenosis of the right ejaculatory duct should be excluded. However, given the clinical context, there are likely to be multiple factors accounting for the sterility in this patient

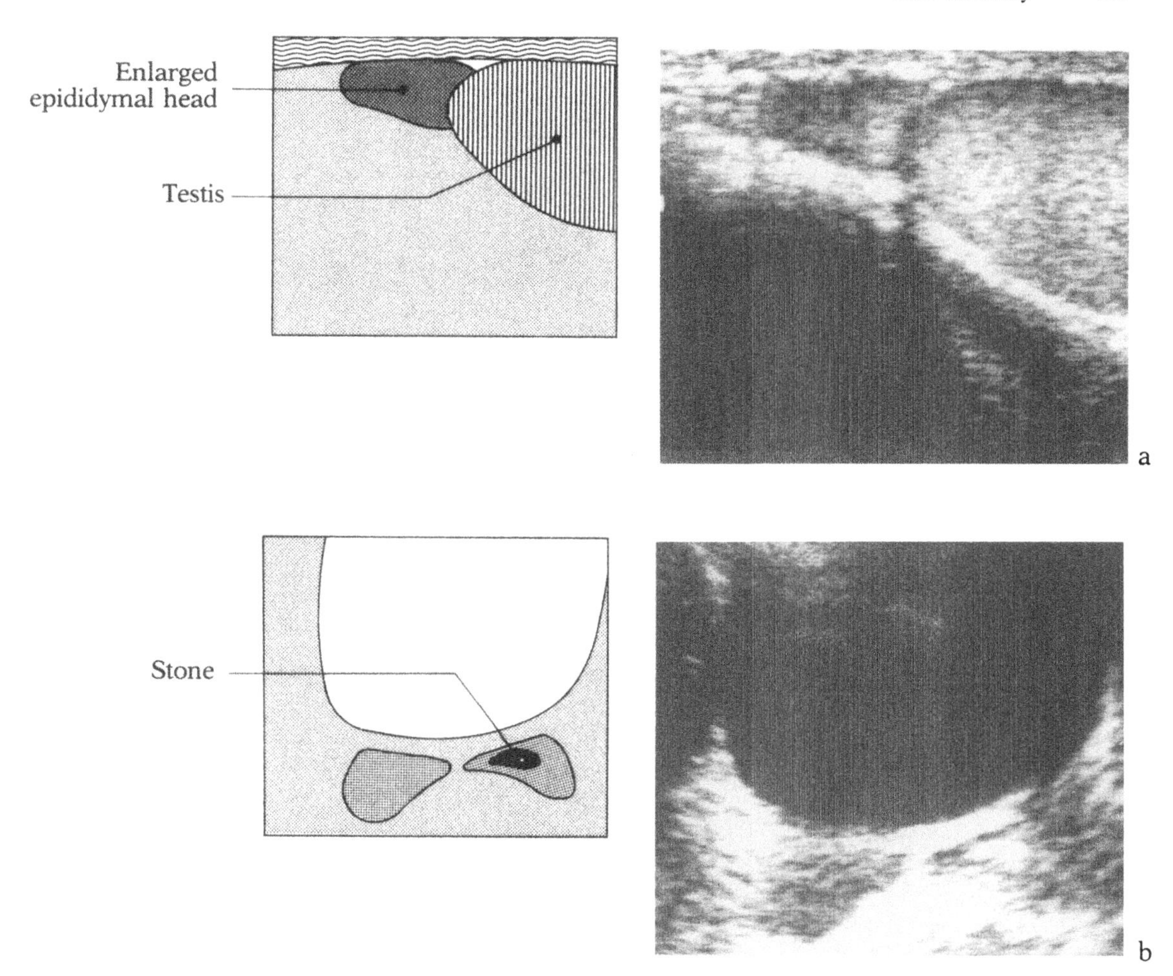

Fig. 47a, b. ***Seminal lithiasis.*** A 26 year old patient. Azoospermia. **a** Sagittal section of the superior pole of a testis (first part of the genital ultrasound examination). The epididymal head is too prominent due to enlargement and appears relatively hypoechoic. Same appearances on the opposite side. **b** Transverse section of the seminal vesicles through their base (second part of the genital ultrasound), suprapubic scan. Regular homogenous echogenicity in the base of the left seminal vesicle due to a calculus which , in association with the enlargement of both epididymal heads , suggests a bilateral obstruction (obliteration of the ejaculatory ducts)

Post-surgery scrotal sac

Scrotal ultrasound may be indicated in three different periods following surgery:

- In the immediate post-operative stage
Ultrasound is requested by the Clinician who suspects a complication has occurred in the scrotum or neighbouring structures following surgery: haemorrhage, infection or ischaemia.

- In the medium- to long- term
Ultrasound is useful for follow -up:

• *often in cases of malignant disease*: Initially an annual follow-up scan of the single remaining testis following orchidectomy for a malignant testicular tumour. In fact,the risk of cancer developing in the remaining testis is 60 times greater than in the normal population. This risk is even greater if it involves a testis of cryptorchidism which has been lowered and/or is atrophic;

• *much rarer* is to objectively observe the development of a testis (by measurements, in particular the thickness and volume, and also the echopattern) in cases of late correction of an ectopic testis or following the treatment of an idiopathic varicocele;

• finally, the examination of surgically corrected ectopic testes associated with male infertility is considered separately (see Chapter "Male infertility").

In all these cases it is vital to know the nature of the previous surgery in order to adapt the examination and give a clear interpretation of the ultrasonic abnormalities.

Surgery of the testis

Orchidectomy

This is the surgical removal of the whole of the testis and epididymis, always performed via the inguinal approach with high ligation of the spermatic cord.

- Technical points

• Often accompanied either at the same time or secondarily by insertion of a silicon testicular prosthesis attached to the inferior surface of the scrotum (young subject; contra-indicated in cases of infection or immunosupression).

• The exception is *pulpectomy* : bilateral subcapsular orchidectomy leaving behind the testicular appendages and the tunica albuginea of the testes.

- Indications

• Principal indications (tumours):
- tumours of the testis. If bilateral, castration necessary;
- the exception is cancer of the prostate (pulpectomy).

• Other indications:
- severe trauma;
- necrotising infection of the testis;
- ischaemic necrosis (neglected or unrecognized torsion).

-Ultrasound appearances

• Orchidectomy or pulpectomy: a sheet of variable echogenicity is seen in place of the normal scrotal contents.

• Prosthesis: structure and morphology similar to that of the testis, uniformally hypoechoic.

- Complications

• Haemorrhagic: haematoma;

• infectious (rare);

• specific for the prosthesis: rejection, very rare (biocompatibility of the materials used). Late complication, periprosthetic fibrous capsule which is painful and unacceptable cosmetically. Ultrasound is of value to detect the predisposing signs (indentations, localised deformity) which would result in early treatment with anti-inflammatory agents.

Table 1. ***Principal operations of the scrotal structures***

Organ (s) concerned / **Usual indications**	**Testis**	**Epididymis**	**Cord**		**Tunica vaginalis**
			Vas deferens	**Spermatic Plexus**	
	←----------	**Orchidectomy**	----------→		
		- Tumour (++) - Purulent liquefaction - Ischaemic necrosis			
	• **Pulpectomy** - Prostatic cancer • **Lowering of ectopic testis(es)** • **Orchidopexy** - Torsion • **Tumourectomy** • **Biopsy** - Infertility	• **Epididymectomy** - Abscess - Trauma • **Epididymotomy** - Risk of ischaemic necrosis of the testis by severe epididymitis • **Epididymo-deferential anastomoses** (homolateral or crossed) - Infertility due to obstruction • **Neospermatocele**	• **Vasectomy** - Contraception	• **Varicocelectomy**	• **Needle aspiration** - Hydrocele • **Plication** - Recurrent hydrocele • **Vaginalectomy** - Infected hydrocele - Tumours

Orchidopexy

This is the fixation of the epididymo-testicular complex to the posterior wall of the scrotum or to the median raphe.

- Indications

• Principal indications; torsion of the spermatic cord. This requires a bilateral orchidopexy (the contralateral testis may also be lying abnormally in the scrotal sac and is therefore operated on prophylactically);

• recommended: solitary testis either congenital or acquired in an adolescent (failure of correction or removal of a contralateral ectopic testis).

- Ultrasound appearances

• Often indistinguishable from a non-operated testis;

• sometimes, slightly horizontal position of the hilum.

- Complications

• Haemorrhagic: haematocele;

• inflammatory: hydrocele; granuloma.

Lowering of ectopic testes

This concerns the fixation of a testis into the scrotum from a persistently abnormal position (along the path of migration: cryptorchidism, or outside the path of migration: ectopic testis).

- Technical points

The surgery is specialized, delicate and usually performed on a small child. It is preceded by examination under general anaesthetic if the testis cannot be localised pre-operatively. This is being replaced by laparoscopy.

The surgical approach is initially inguinal. The degree of difficulty and the type of surgery depend essentially on the length of the spermatic cord and any abnormalities of the epididymo-testicular junction.

The fixation of the testis requires the creation of a neo-pouch between the fibrous capsule and the scrotum.

- Indications

•The sole indication is the lowering of abnormally situated testes which, if left in an abnormal position, have twice the risk of cancer formation (10-40 times greater than the risk for a normally situated testis) and sterility.

- Ultrasound appearances
These are variable depending on the results of the surgery.

For the testis the appearances are essentially:

• size , which may be normal, slightly reduced (hypotrophy) or very reduced (atrophy);

• the echopattern is sometimes echogenic in cases of atrophy. The examination should be meticulous to detect a focal lesion within the at-risk testis;

• a slightly piriform shape when the testis is of reasonable size and a little deformed by a small capacity, surgically fashioned sac;

• the hilum is occasionally aligned horizontally following fixation.

In the funiculo-scrotal position there is often an echogenic band, too wide to be a normal spermatic cord, due to surgical elongation of the cord.

- Complications

• Haemorrhage,
• infections,
• vascular.

If any of these occur, they generally lead to atrophy of the lowered testis. However, they are rare if this surgery is performed, as it should be, by a specialized surgical team.

Tumourectomy

This is the enucleation of a tumour.

-Technnical points
Initially the approach is scrotal in order to visualise the lesion. If the lesion is not visible or difficult to palpate clinically, ultrasound guidance can be useful.

- Indications
Only performed in exceptional circumstances although it depends on the surgical team.

- Ultrasound appearances

• In the early post-operative period, the resection cavity appears hypoechoic.

• Later it fills up with more echogenic fibrous tissue, although it still appears non-expansive, this distinguishing it from a possible recurrent tumour.

Surgery of the testicular appendages

Tunica vaginalis

Surgery on this structure is almost exclusively concerned with curative surgery for a symptomatic hydrocele. Its performance depends on the state of the patient (physiological age), the severity of the pachyvaginalitis and the possibility of the hydrocele becoming septated.

- Needle puncture: aspiration
This is a minor procedure reserved for a simple hydrocele in an elderly subject.

- Plication of the tunica vaginalis
This consists of incision and plication of the tunica vaginalis (apposition of the two layers) and aims to prevent recurrence of the hydrocele.

- Vaginalectomy
This is the surgical excision of the tunica vaginalis, very rarely indicated (progressive tuberculosis and tumour).

- Technical points
Surgical approach is always scrotal.

- Ultrasound appearances
Plication of the tunica vaginalis results in an extra structure seen as a band of variable echogenicity deep to the inferior surface of the investing layers.

- Complications

• Haemorrhagic: haematocele. This can occur following a needle puncture which damages an anterior epididymis. This can be avoided by a pre-aspiration ultrasound;

• infectious: epididymo- orchitis.

Epididymis

Selective surgery of the epididymis is rare.

- Epididymectomy
Total or less commonly, partial removal of the epididymis.

- Epididymotomy
This is conservative surgery making an opening in the length of the epididymis.

- *Indications*

• Trauma: tear of the epididymis;

• inflammation; abscess:

- in this situation, urgent epididymotomy can have a role to prevent ischaemic necrosis of the testis due to compression of the vascular pedicle by a grossly enlarged epididymis;

- cystectomy (excision of a cystic mass, usually a spermatocele) has been virtually abandoned due to the risk of secondary sterility by a ligature or accidental transection of the epididymis.

- *Ultrasound appearances*
This can be summarised as the non-visualisation of the epididymis.

- *Complications*

• Essentially vascular, due to damage to the testicular branch of the spermatic atery resulting in a partial ischaemia of the testis and often a segmental atrophy;

• infectious, secondary to the initial ischaemia;

• haemorrhagic: rare.

Vas deferens

If one excludes the surgery for sterility, which is dealt with later, surgery of the vas is restricted to bilateral division or vasectomy.

- *Indications*
An irreversible method of male contraception. This is not frequently performed except in the countries of Anglo-Saxon origin .

- *Technical points*
Inguinal approach.

- *Ultrasound appearances*
No specific features in the absence of complications.

- *Complications*

• Frequent, hence the operation is rarely performed in certain countries;

• in the immediate post-operative period: vascular complications due to damage to the deferential artery, ischaemic necrosis of the inferior pole of the testis. .In the medium- to long- term: pseudo cystic distension, usually bilateral, of the epididymo-testicular canalicular system.

Surgery for infertility

The surgical lowering of ectopic testes has already been considered.

Varicocelectomy

Ligation of the varicocele in the cord by an inguinal approach.

Epididymo-deferential anastomosis

This is in the field of microsurgery and is restricted to a few Specialists. Two patent sections are anastomosed in order to by pass the non-functioning occluded segment. The anastomosis usually involves the body or tail of the epididymis and is often a side-to-side anastomosis. It is sometimes bilateral or even crossed. Testicular biopsy is performed routinely pre-operatively.

Neo-spermatocele

An epididymal fistula is fashioned, from which the secretions are collected by means of a pouch of the tunica vaginalis. Needle aspiration is performed secondarily for medically assisted fertilisation.

- *Ultrasound appearances*
These are restricted to those of the neo-spermatocele which is a pseudocystic structure.

- *Complications*

• Following varicocelectomy: a simple procedure, virtually non-existent;

• following anastomoses on the other hand, these may leak or become stenosed giving the appearance of a collection adjacent to the anastomosis or cystic dilatation distally;

• complications are rare following neo-spermatocele (mainly infection) because it is aspirated so rapidly.

The post-surgery scrotal sac

Surgery of the ectopic testes

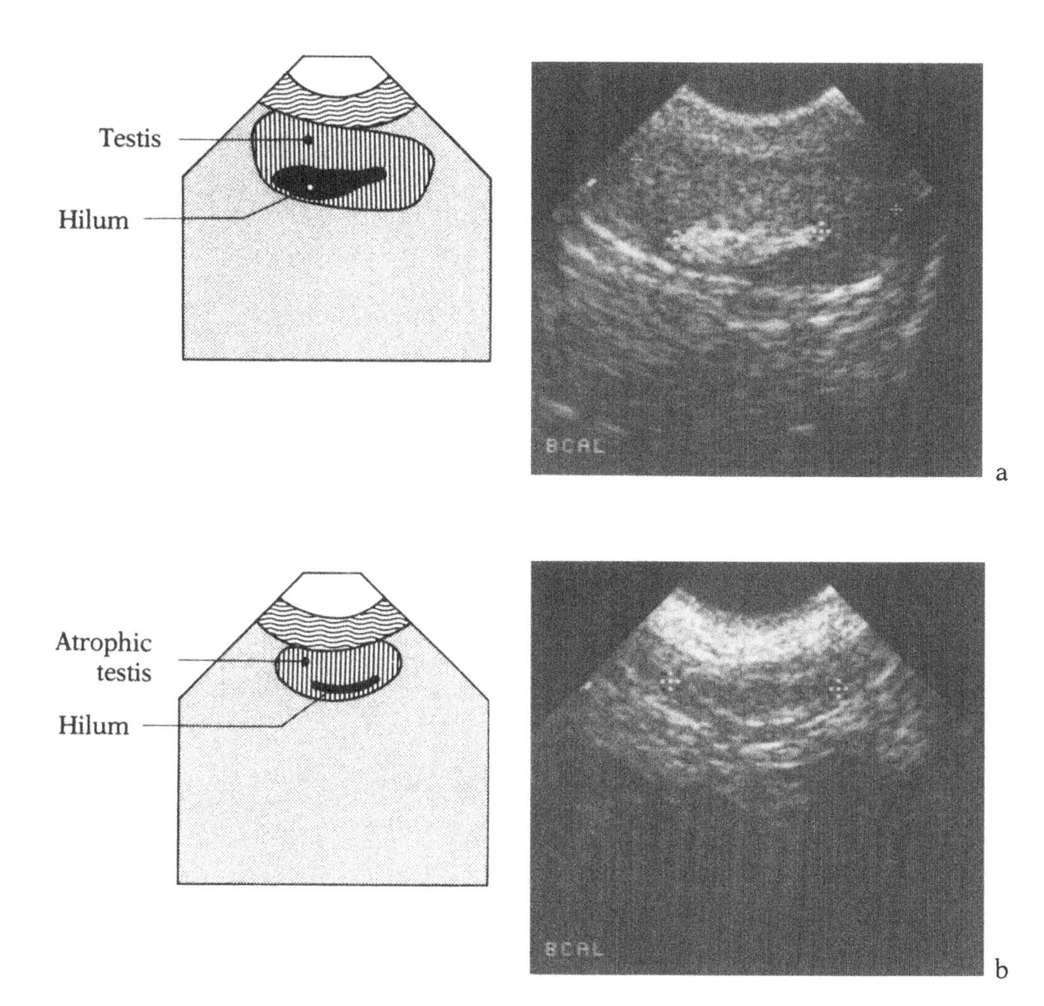

Fig. 1a, b. ***Post-operative appearance.*** A young boy of 13. Bilateral ectopic testes operated on as a small child. **a** Sagittal section of the right testis. The testis is in place and of normal size (almost 3 cm) with a normal echo pattern for the age of the patient. The hilum is particularly well seen, without doubt due to its horizontal position as a result of the orchidopexy. **b** Sagittal section of the left testis: the testis is also in place and is recognized by the linear echogenicity of the hilum. In comparison to the opposite side it appears atrophic. Conclusion: Failure of the corrective surgery on the left; good result, at least with respect to testicular volume, on the right

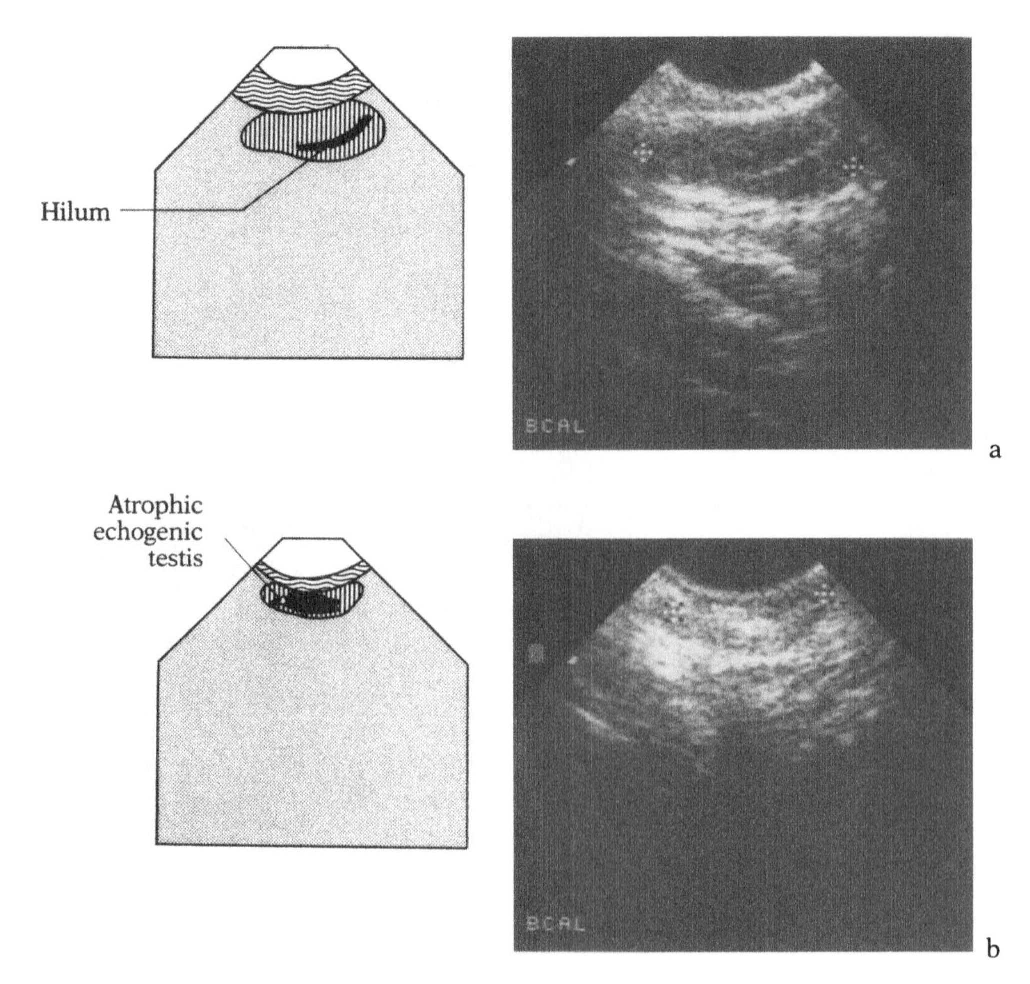

Fig. 2a, b. ***Post-operative appearance.*** A 6 year old child. Surgery at the age of 2 for bilateral ectopic testes. **a** Sagittal section of the left testis: the size and echopattern of the testis are normal for the age of the patient. The hilum is visible. **b** Sagittal section of the right testis: small abnormally echogenic testis. Fibrous atrophy

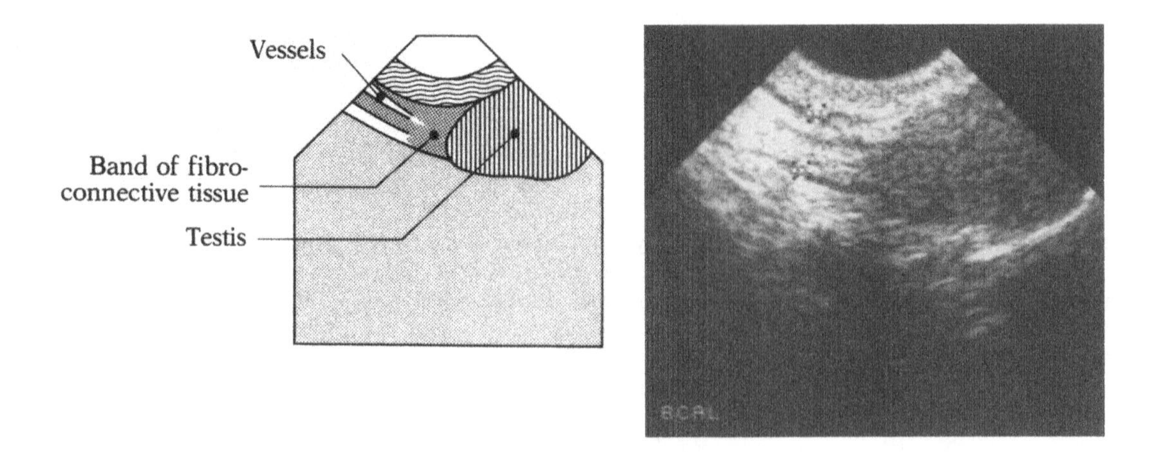

Fig. 3. ***Post-operative appearance.*** Sagittal section: normal volume and echogenicity of the testis for a 10 year old child. The echogenic band in the region of the spermatic pedicle is related to the technique of lowering the testis and corresponds to the detachment of the fibro-connective tissue

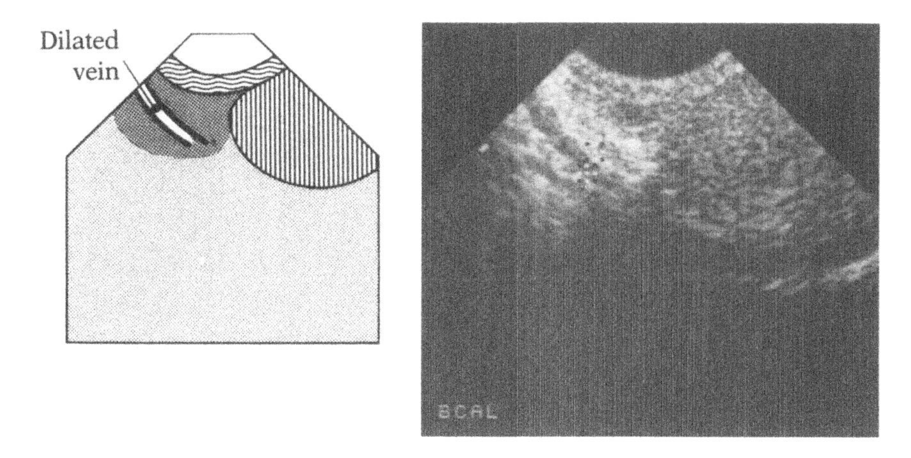

Fig. 4. ***Post-operative appearance.*** Sagittal sections of the superior pole: same appearance of the echogenic band in the spermatic pedicle but,in this case,it is associated with narrow tubular and transonic structures of a few millimetres due to an associated varicocele

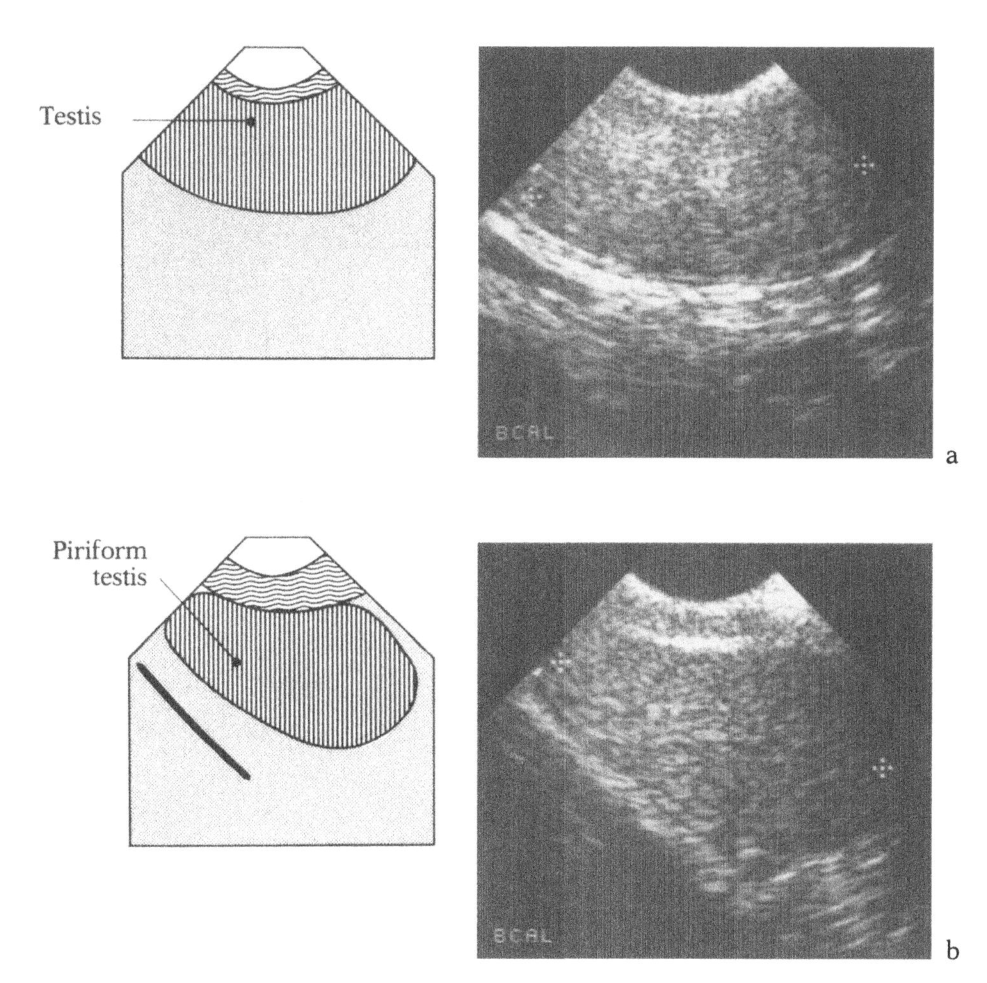

Fig. 5a, b. ***Post-operative appearance.*** **a** Sagittal section of the non-operated testis with a normal morphology. **b** Sagittal section of the lowered testis: its pear-shape is related to the small capacity of the newly fashioned sac

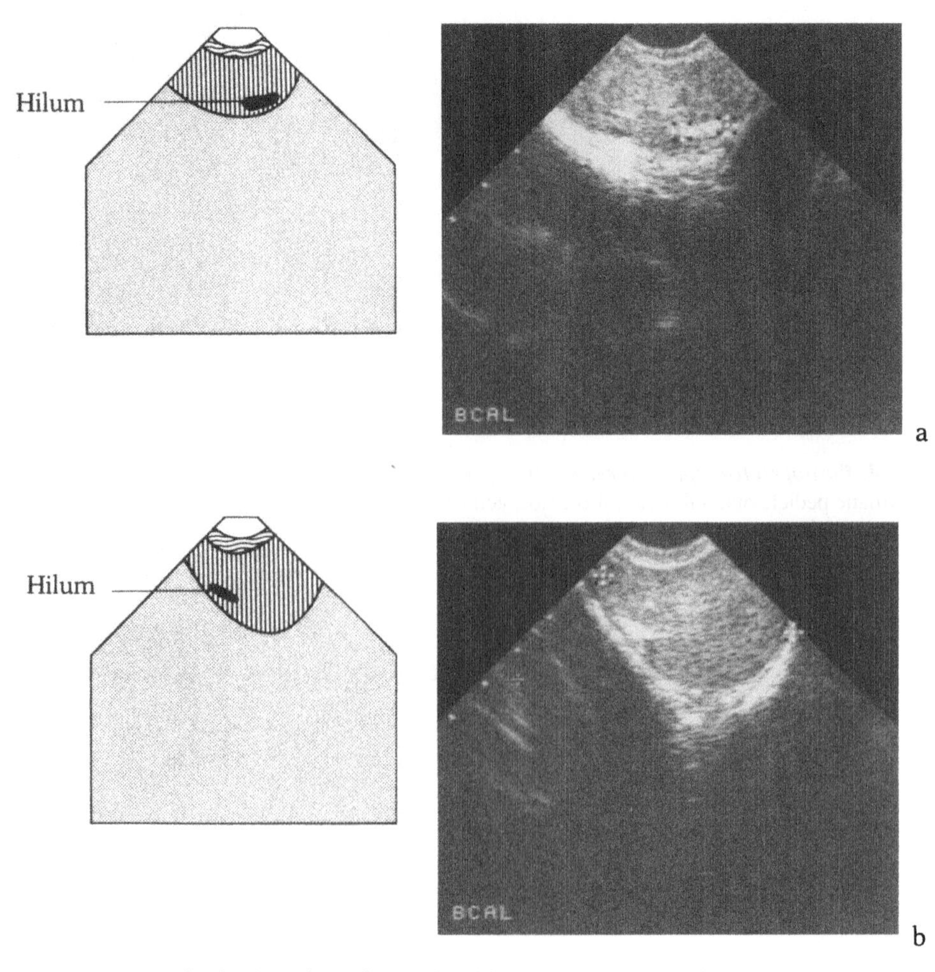

Fig. 6a, b. ***Post-operative appearance.*** **a** Sagittal section of a testis which has been lowered due to cryptorchidism: normal size and echopattern, but the position of the hilum is modified by the surgical fixation: postero-inferior rather than the normal postero-superior position. **b** Sagittal section of the contralateral testis which has been within the scrotum since birth: the testis is slightly larger with the hilum in a normal position

Orchidectomy

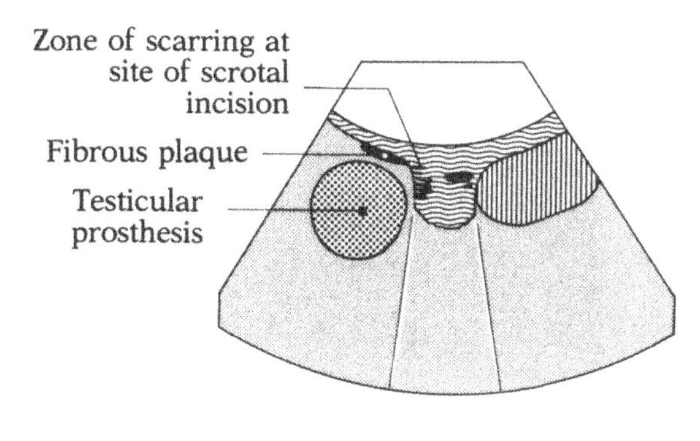

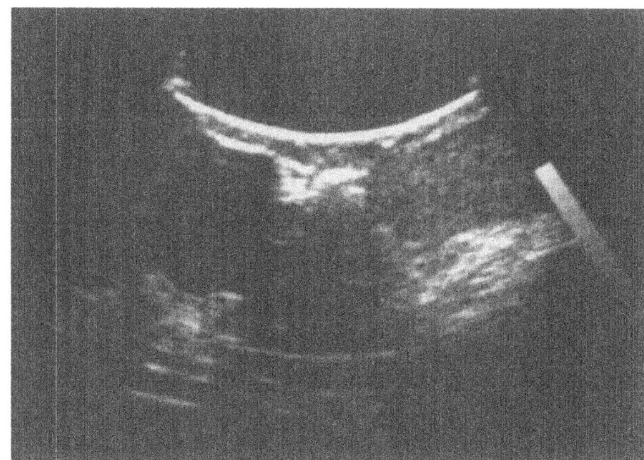

Fig. 7. ***Testicular prosthesis.*** A 32 year old patient. Orchidectomy for a tumour (seminoma) with insertion of a prosthesis at the same time. Transverse section of both testes: the silicon prosthesis appears as a regular rounded echo-free area with no posterior enhancement. No peri-prosthetic abnormality; the small fibrous reaction of the investing layer in the form of an anterior echogenic line is normal. Similarly, the echogenic areas in the median raphe are due to scar tissue secondary to the median scrotal incision

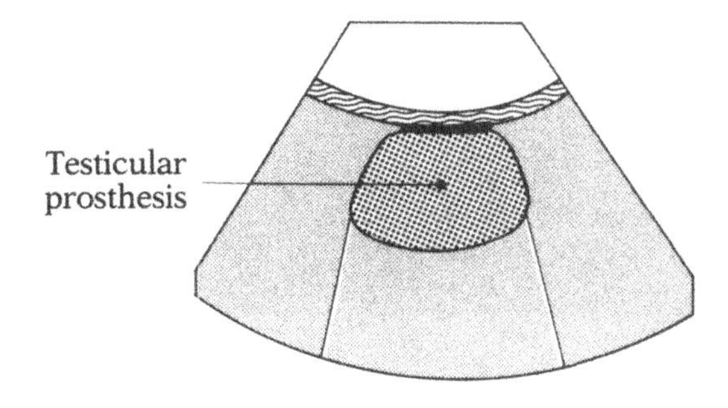

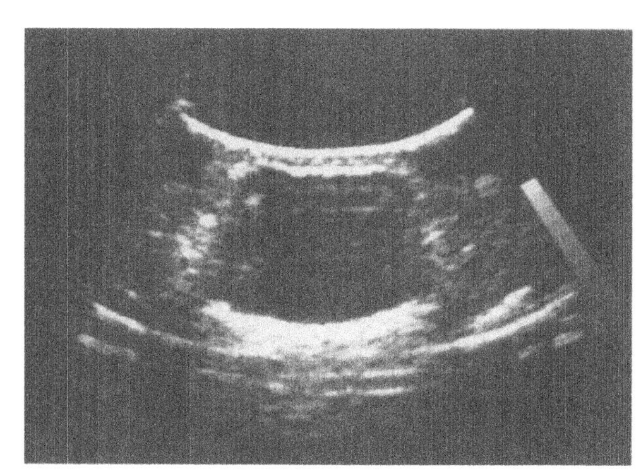

Fig. 8. ***Testicular prosthesis.*** Sagittal section of a silicon testicular prosthesis: in this case the prosthesis does not appear purely transonic and this is due to the gain setting which is on maximum and does not indicate an abnormality of the prosthesis

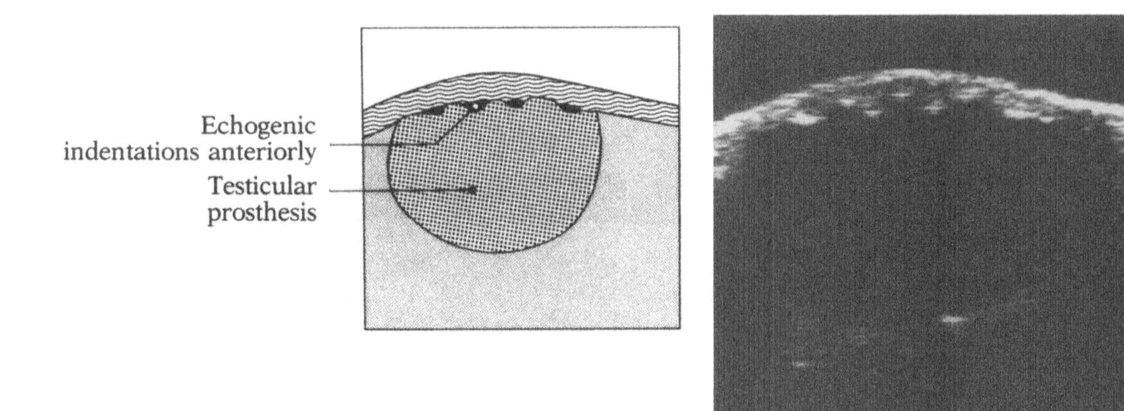

Fig. 9. ***Testicular prosthesis.*** Orchidectomy with secondary insertion of a prosthesis in a patient with a large Leydig cell tumour. The scrotum remains sensitive after several months. Sagittal section: the anterior surface of the silicon prosthesis has lost its regularity and there are several echogenic indentations present: peri-prosthetic fibrosis which has reached the stage where the use of anti-inflammatory agents to prevent the formation of a painful fibrous capsule is justified

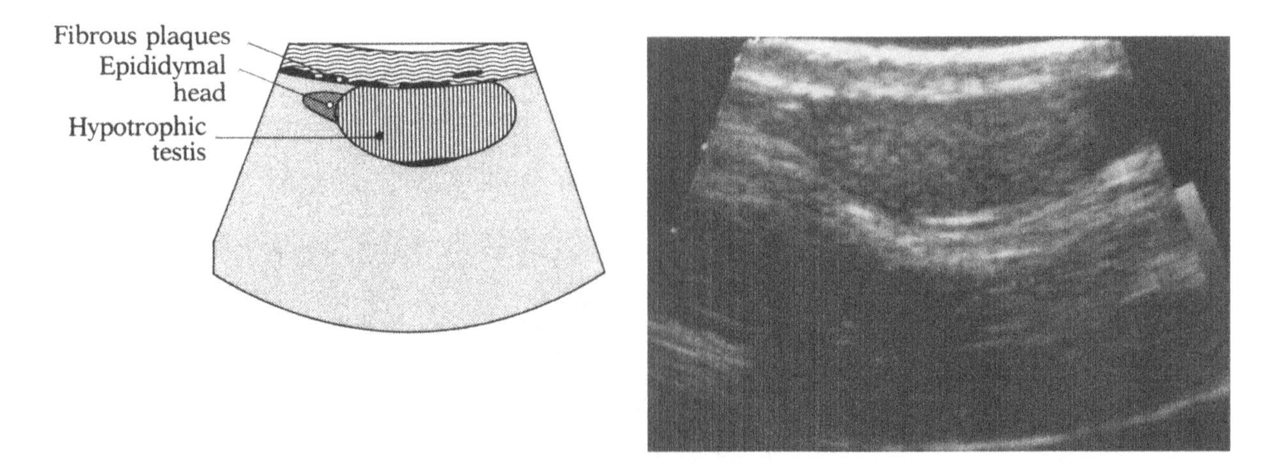

Fig. 10. ***The remaining testis.*** A 30 year old patient treated for a mixed germinal tumour by orchidectomy followed by chemotherapy. Ultrasound follow-up of the remaining testis. Sagittal section: no focal abnormality to suggest a parenchymal secondary. However, there is a certain degree of atrophy (thickeness barely greater than 10 mm) and fibrous plaques are seen on the deep surface of the investing layers; these are frequently seen after chemotherapy

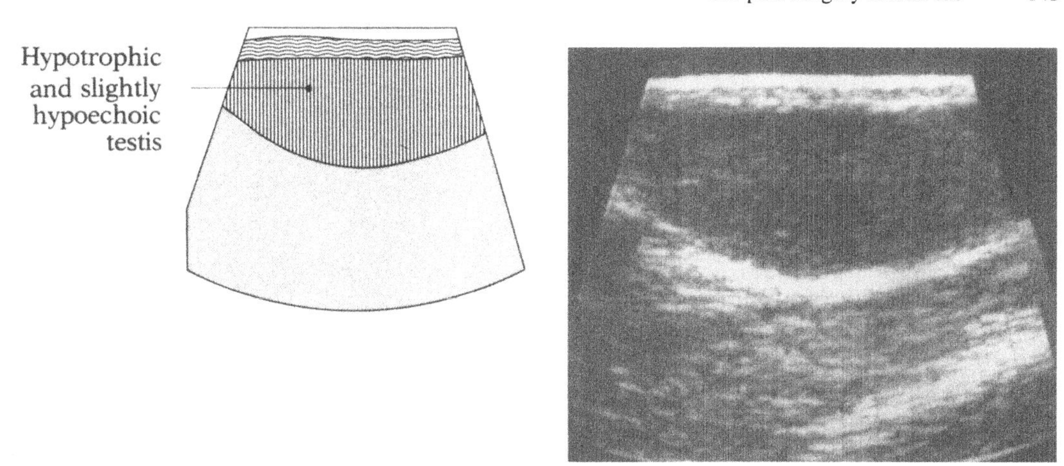

Fig. 11. ***The remaining testis.*** Same context. Sagittal section of the solitary testis: reduced thickness of the testis, slightly hypoechoic: post-chemotherapy atrophy

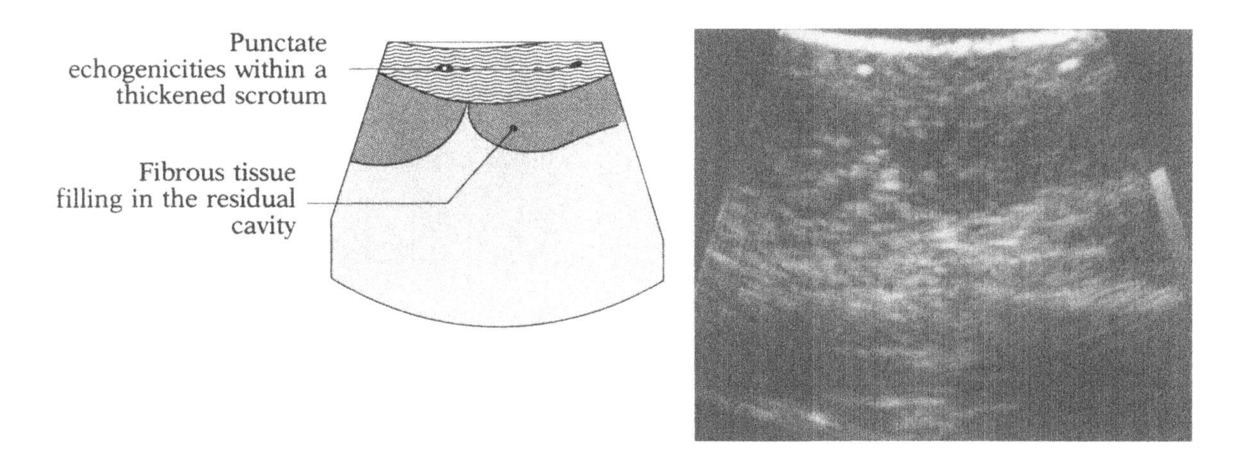

Fig. 12. ***Post-operative appearance.*** Removal of the testis for acute necrotizing infection. One week later, persistent fever. Collection ? Sagittal section: thickened investing layers containing small echoes due to residual air bubbles. Normal hypoechoic filling in of the residual cavity. No evidence of a collection

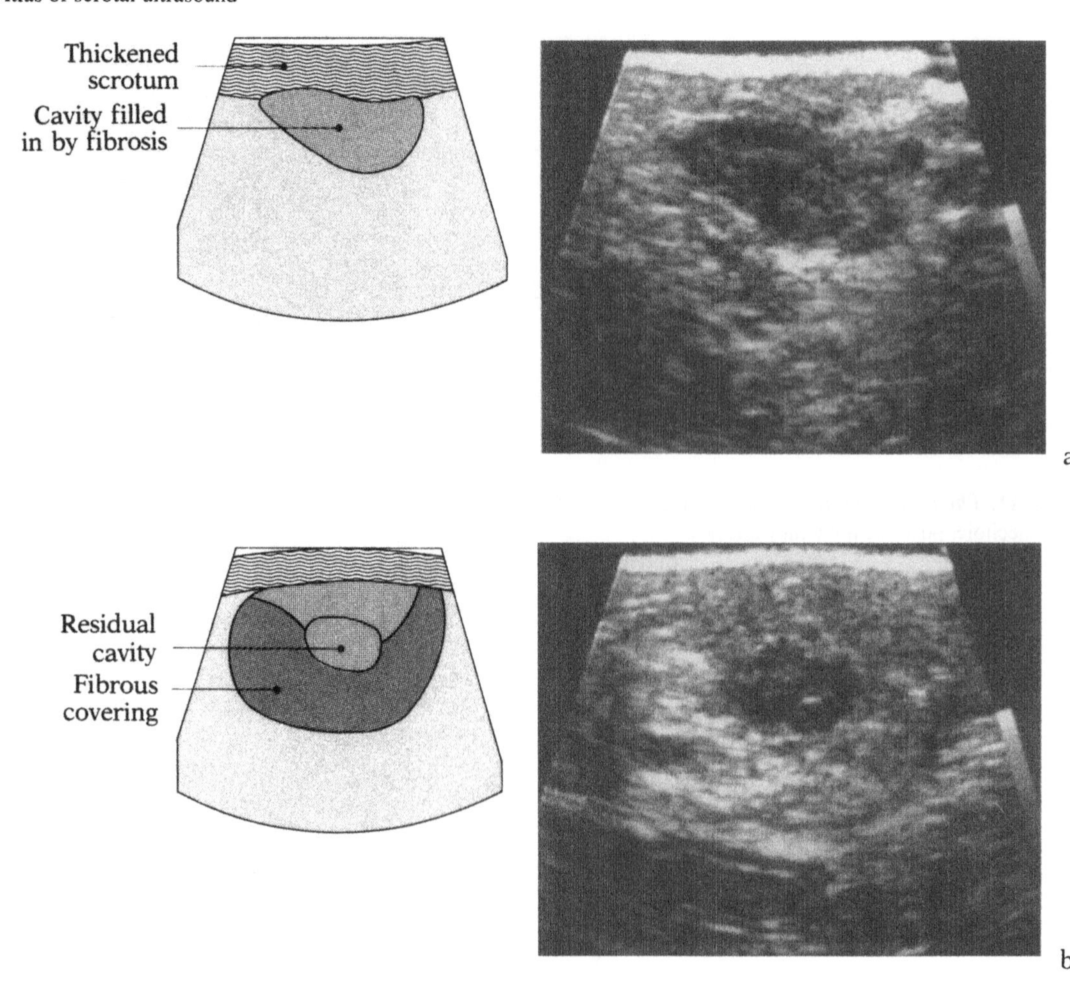

Fig. 13a, b. ***Pulpectomy. Post-operative appearance. Complication.*** Bilateral pulpectomy for cancer of the prostate. Three months later, the left testis is indurated and painful. **a** Sagittal section of the right scrotal sac: the gland is replaced by fibrous tissue which appears as a fairly homogenous, slightly echogenic area: normal post-pulpectomy appearances. **b** Sagittal section of the left scrotal sac: the residual cavity is surrounded by a thickened echogenic ring: a fibrous capsule without doubt secondary to a surgical complication, probably a haematoma

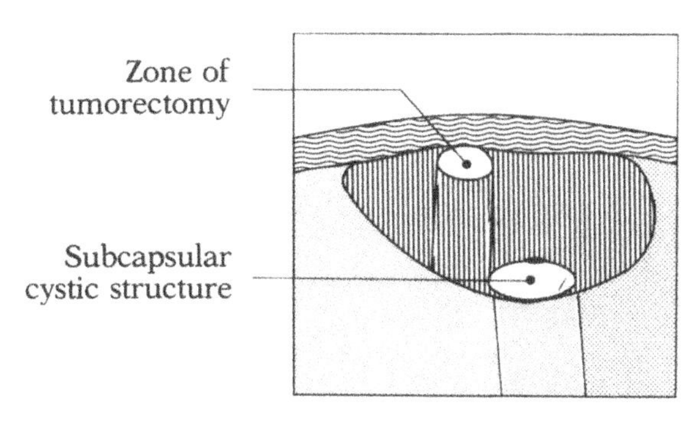

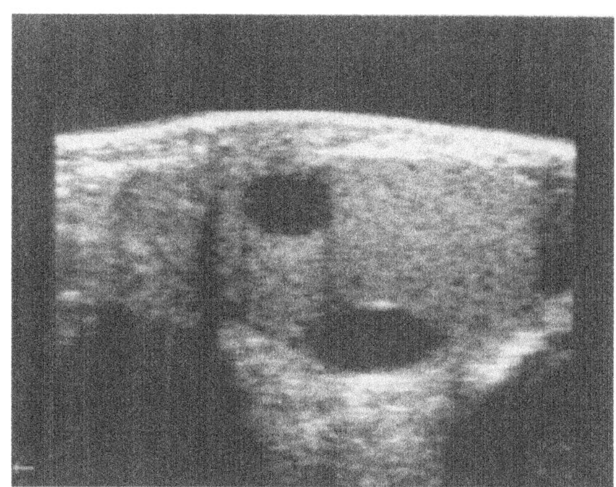

a

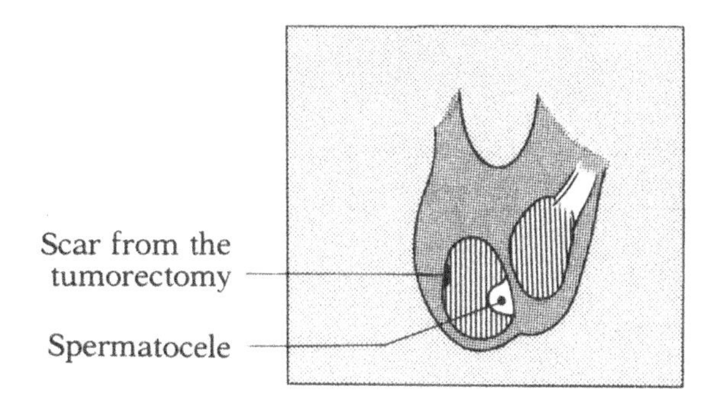

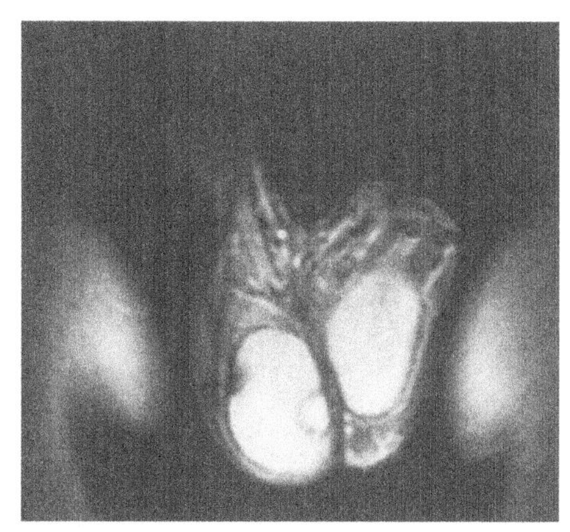

b

Fig.14a, b. ***Tumourectomy . Post-operative appearances.*** Appearance of a sensitive solid nodule in the testis, one month after a tumourectomy for benign fibroma of the tunica albuginea (see Fig. 10 in chapter "Impalpable testicular tumours within a clinically normal scrotum"). **a** Sagittal section (Image courtesy of Dr. Tordjman): two apparent abnormalities. One is a hypoechoic area, without posterior enhancement, filling the tumourectomy cavity. The appearances are those of a normal fibrotic replacement of the residual cavity and not a collection. The other abnormality is an oblong structure, more transonic with definite posterior enhancement: a small fluid collection in the rete testis without doubt secondary to a small parenchymal injury and is therefore a spermatocele. The subcapsular position of this spermatocele is causing some stretching of the tunica albuginea and may explain the patient's pains. **b** Frontal section of the scrotum by Magnetic Resonance Imaging (T2-weighted Spin Echo sequence): scar from the tumourectomy is hypointense since it is composed of fibrous tissue. In contrast, the fluid nature of the second abnormality is confirmed, as is its non-haemorrhagic character, by the appearances on several sequences. Spontaneous resolution is likely and the patient should be simply reassured

Surgery of the neighbouring structures

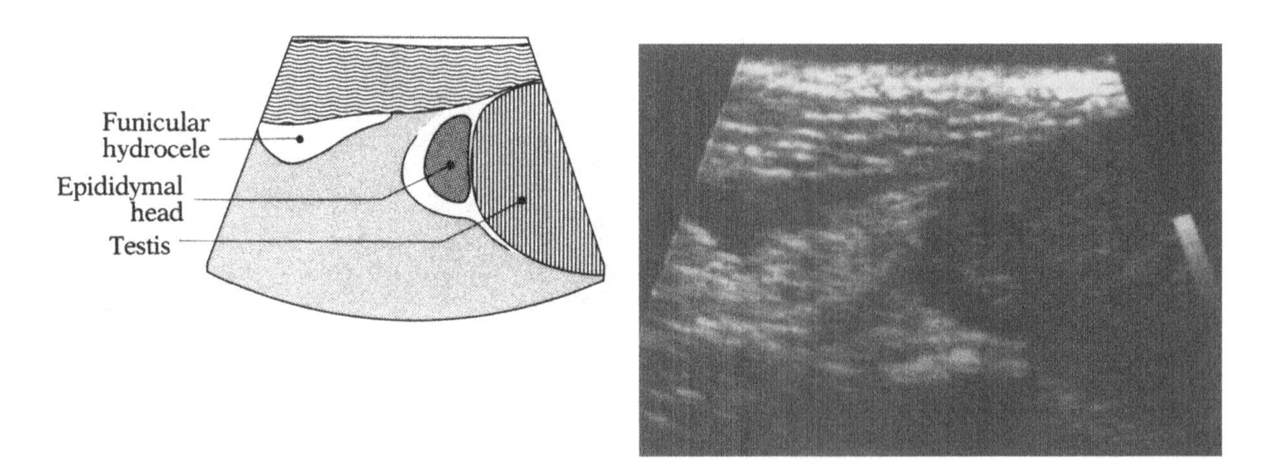

Fig. 15. ***Complication. Inflammation.*** Enlarged testis *three months* after bilateral inguinal hernia repair . Sagittal section of the inguino-scrotal region. Enlarged testis and hypoechoic epididymis: funicular fluid collection with oedematous infiltration of the investing facia: epididymo orchitis

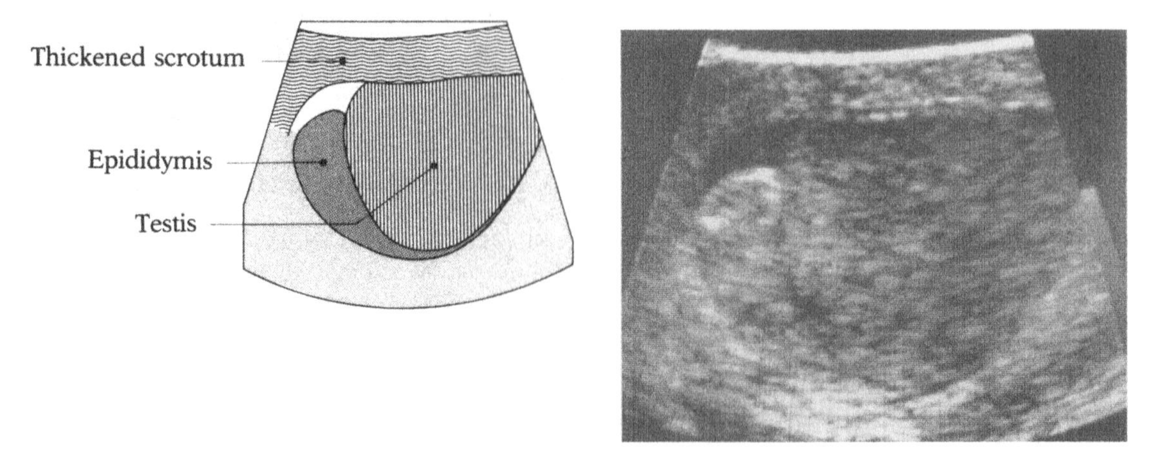

Fig. 16. ***Complication. Inflammation.*** Enlarged testis *three days* following repair of an ipsilateral inguinal hernia. Transverse section. Acute epididymo-orchitis: enlarged testis and epididymis with reduced echogenicity: thickened scrotum

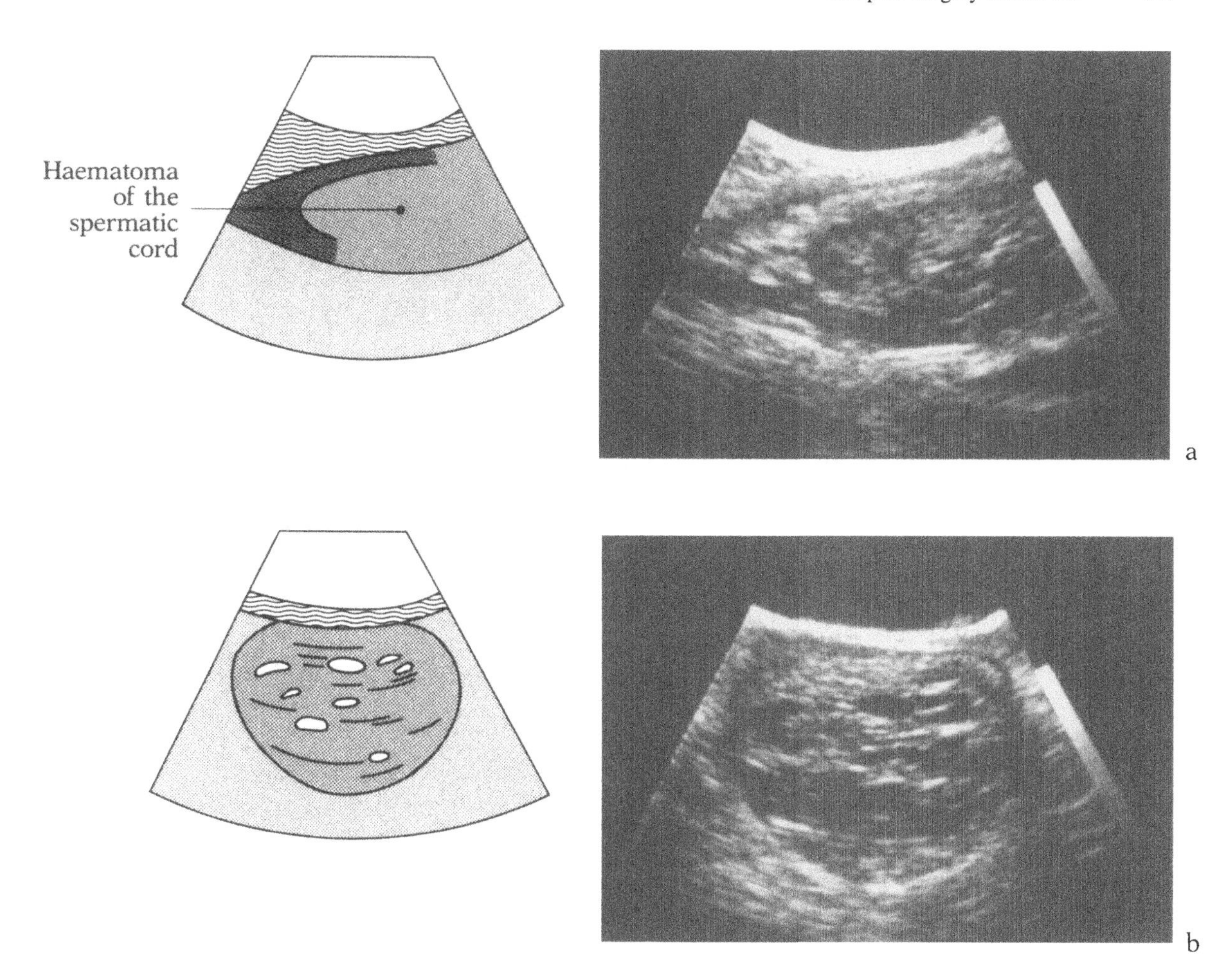

Fig. 17a, b. ***Complication. Haematoma.*** Indurated and painful spermatic cord, *one month* following an ipsilateral herniorraphy. **a** Sagittal section of the inguinal region. Heterogenous oblong mass along the line of the spermatic cord. **b** Transverse section. In the context of recent surgery, the structure containing alternating echogenic and transonic areas is typical of a haematoma of the cord in the process of organisation

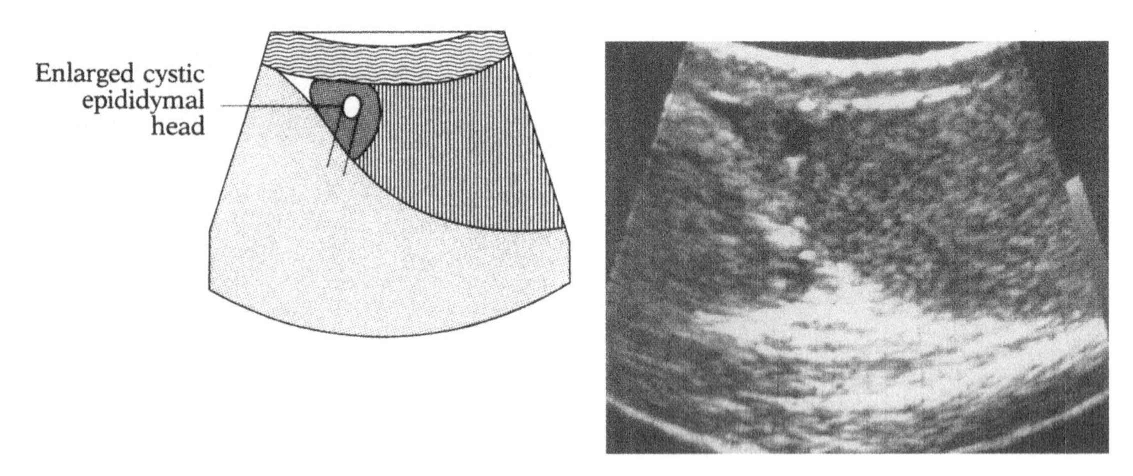

Fig. 18. ***Late complication.*** A 28 year old patient, surgical exploration for an excretory sterility (azoospermia with anti-spermatozoal antibodies), history of previous operation for a right inguinal hernia repair in childhood. Right sagittal section: normal testis. However the epididymis is enlarged and cystic due to distal obstruction from accidental ligation of the vas deferens

Surgery of the scrotum

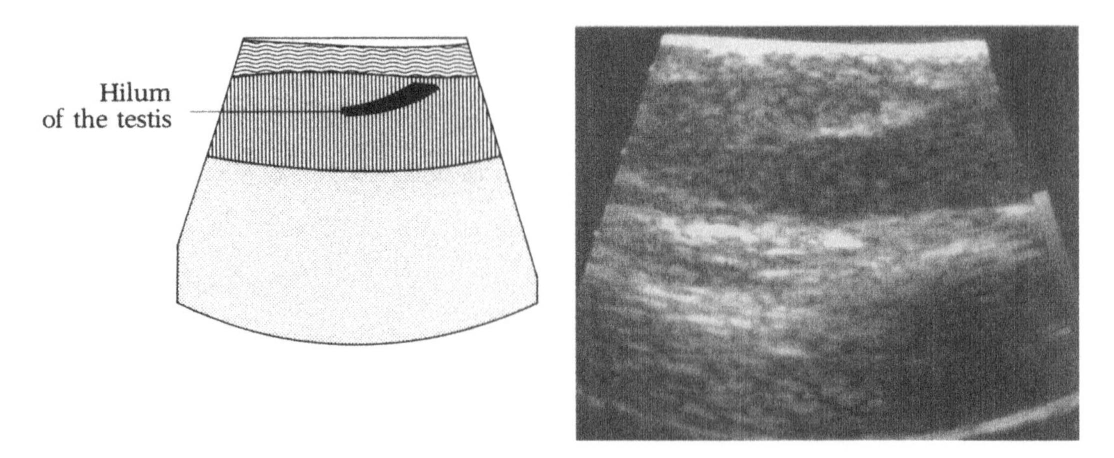

Fig. 19. ***Orchidopexy.*** Orchidopexy following correction of torsion of the spermatic cord. Sagittal section: change in the position of the hilum which is now postero-inferior due to the fixation of the epididymo testicular junction to an anchorage point in the inferior part of the scrotum

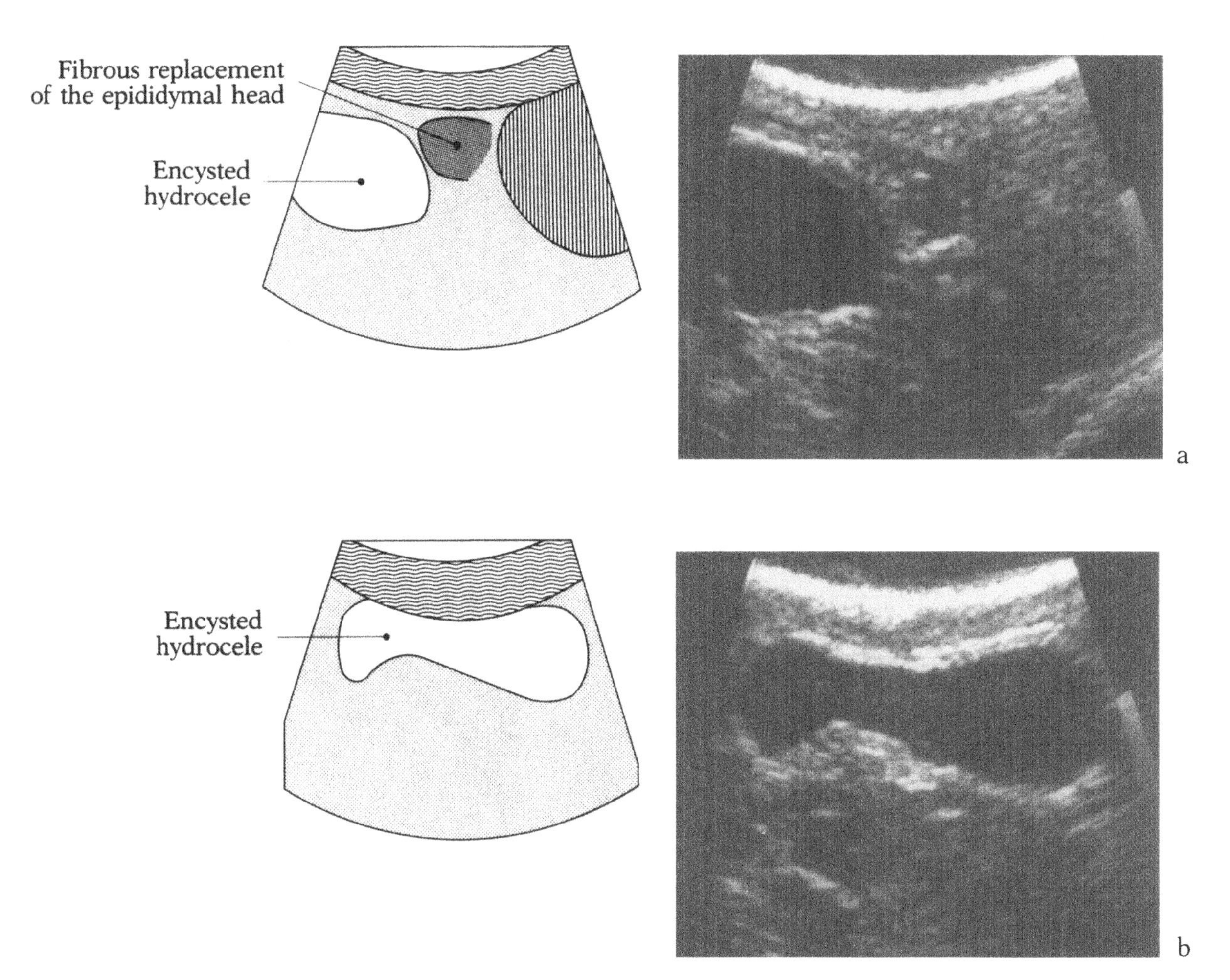

Fig. 20a, b. ***Epididymectomy. Sequellae.*** Epididymectomy for an abscess of the epididymal head. *Three months* later, palpable mass in the superior pole of the testis. **a** Sagittal section. Normal superior pole of the testis. Replacement of the epididymal head by an area of mixed echogenicity due to scar tissue. Superior to this is a transonic collection. **b** High oblique section: purely fluid "hour-glass" shaped collection: encysted hydrocele of the superior pole secondary to surgery

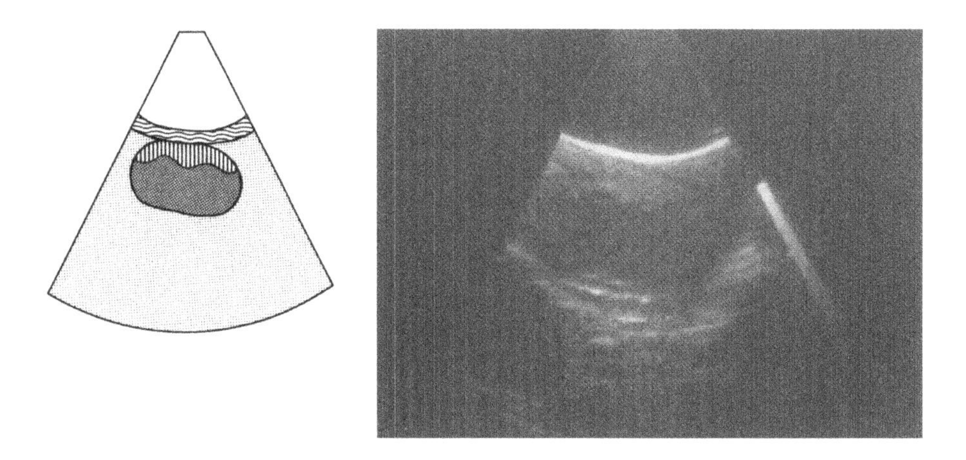

Fig. 21. ***Epididymectomy. Complication.*** Same indication for the epididymectomy. *One month* later, palpable softening of the testis. Transverse section. The testis is unequally divided into geometrically limited zones with different echopatterns. The anterior band has a normal appearance. However, the posterior 2/3 of the gland is hypoechoic. The appearance is characteristic of a vascular territory: testicular ischaemia secondary to ligation of the spermatic artery, causing non-vascularisation of the territory supplied by the testicular branch

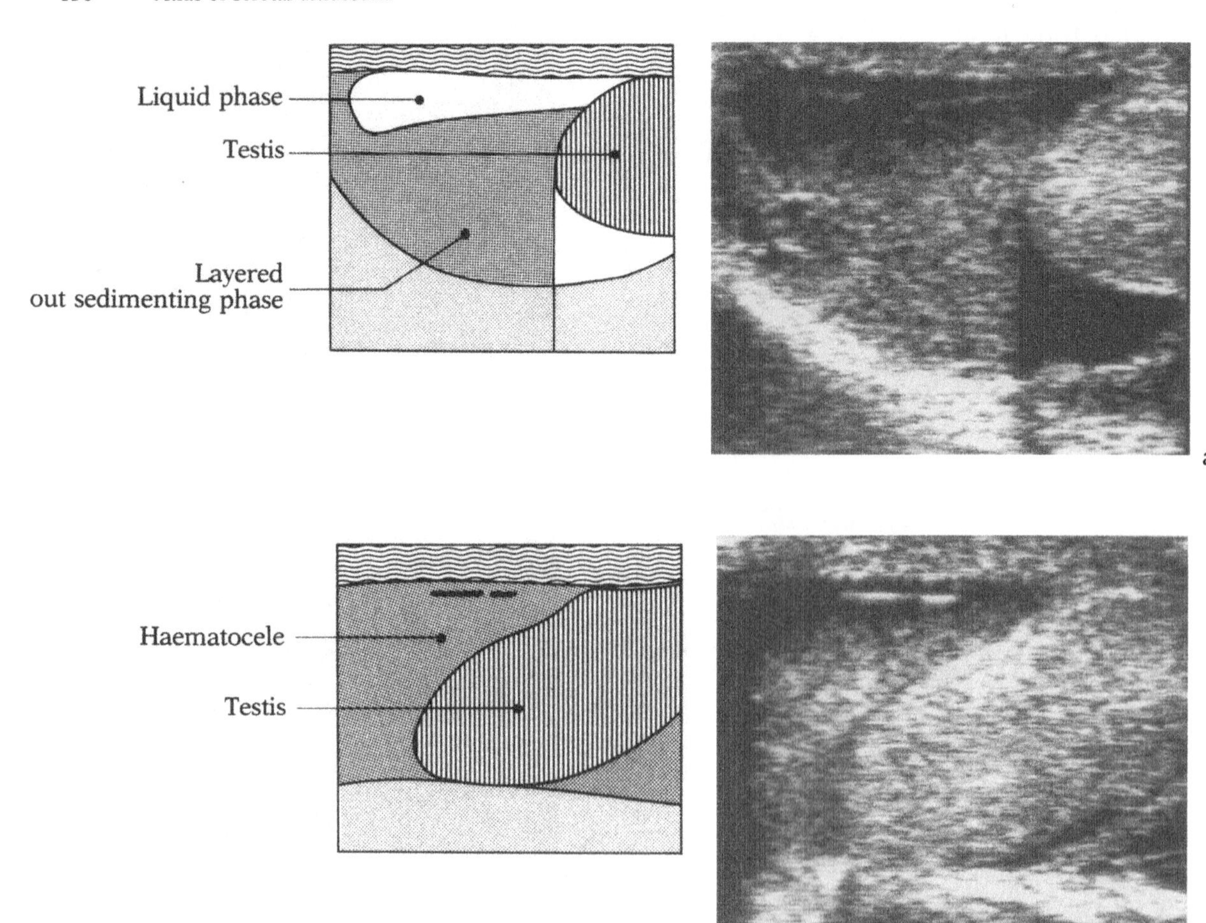

Fig. 22a, b. ***Scrotal excision. Complication.*** Scrotal excision for a chronic abscess with fistula to the skin. *Two weeks* later, large sensitive testis. **a** Sagittal section of the superior pole: large effusion in the tunica vaginalis with two components, one is purely liquid, the other is an echogenic sheet. **b** Sagittal section of the inferior pole: the normal testis is displaced inferiorly by the effusion which contains sediment: typical appearances of a hydro-haematocele, secondary to post operative vascular injury

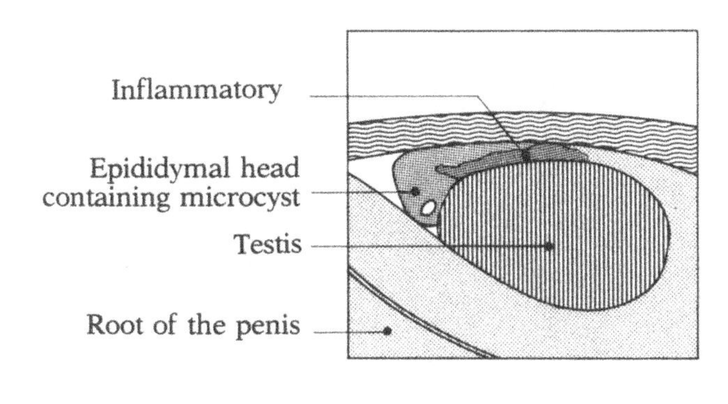

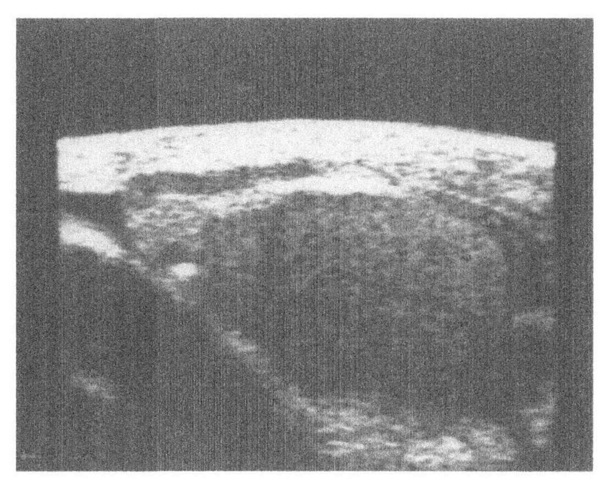

Fig. 23. ***Post-curative treatment of a traumatic haematocele.*** Very inflamed testis *five days* later. Sagittal section: sheet of tissue, partially echogenic, covering the superior part of the testis and epididymis: the testis is attached to the deep surface of the investing layers by inflammatory adhesions, no other underlying abnormality

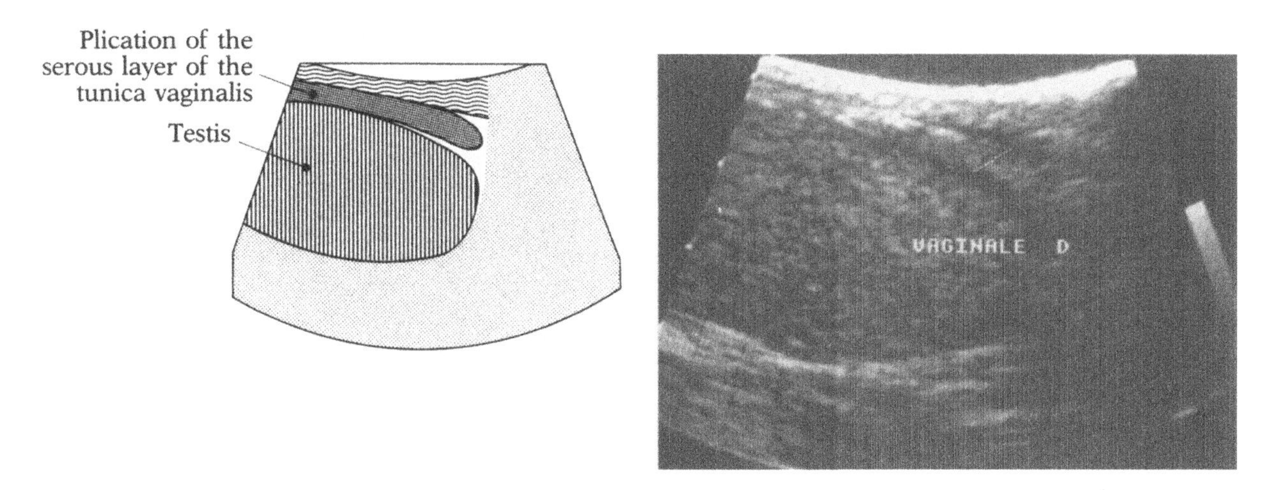

Fig. 24. ***Post-curative treatment of a hydrocele.*** Inferior sagittal section: no recurrence of the fluid collection. There is surgical adhesion of the two layers of the tunica vaginalis to the inferior pole of the testis shown as a regular band of tissue a few millimetres thick

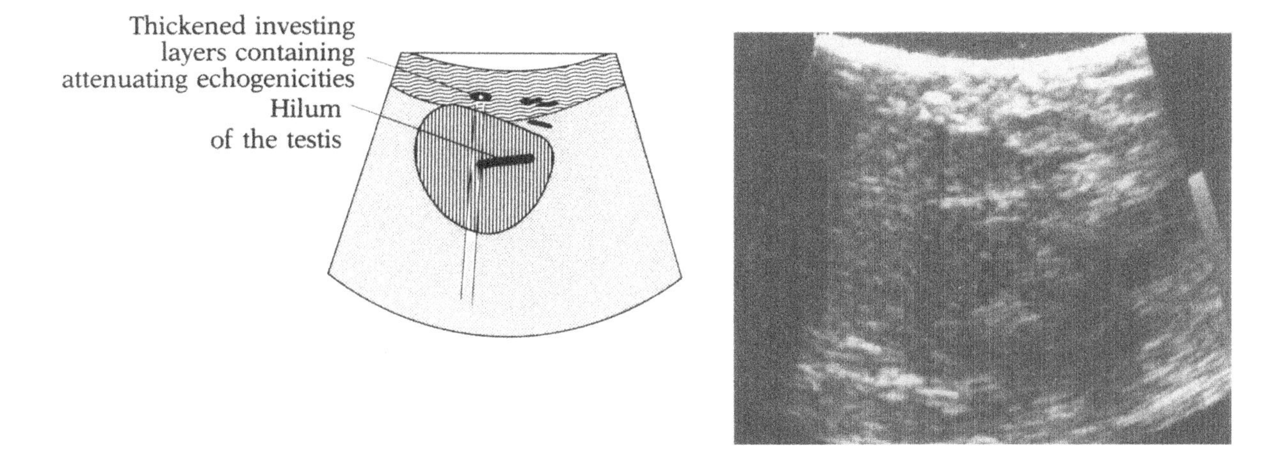

Fig. 25. ***Needle aspiration of a hydrocele. Inflammatory complication.*** Inflamed and sensitive testis *three weeks* following aspiration of a hydrocele. Transverse section: normal testis, well visualised due to the fine echogenicity of the hilum. Inflammatory reaction in the thickened investing layers which appear abnormally echogenic

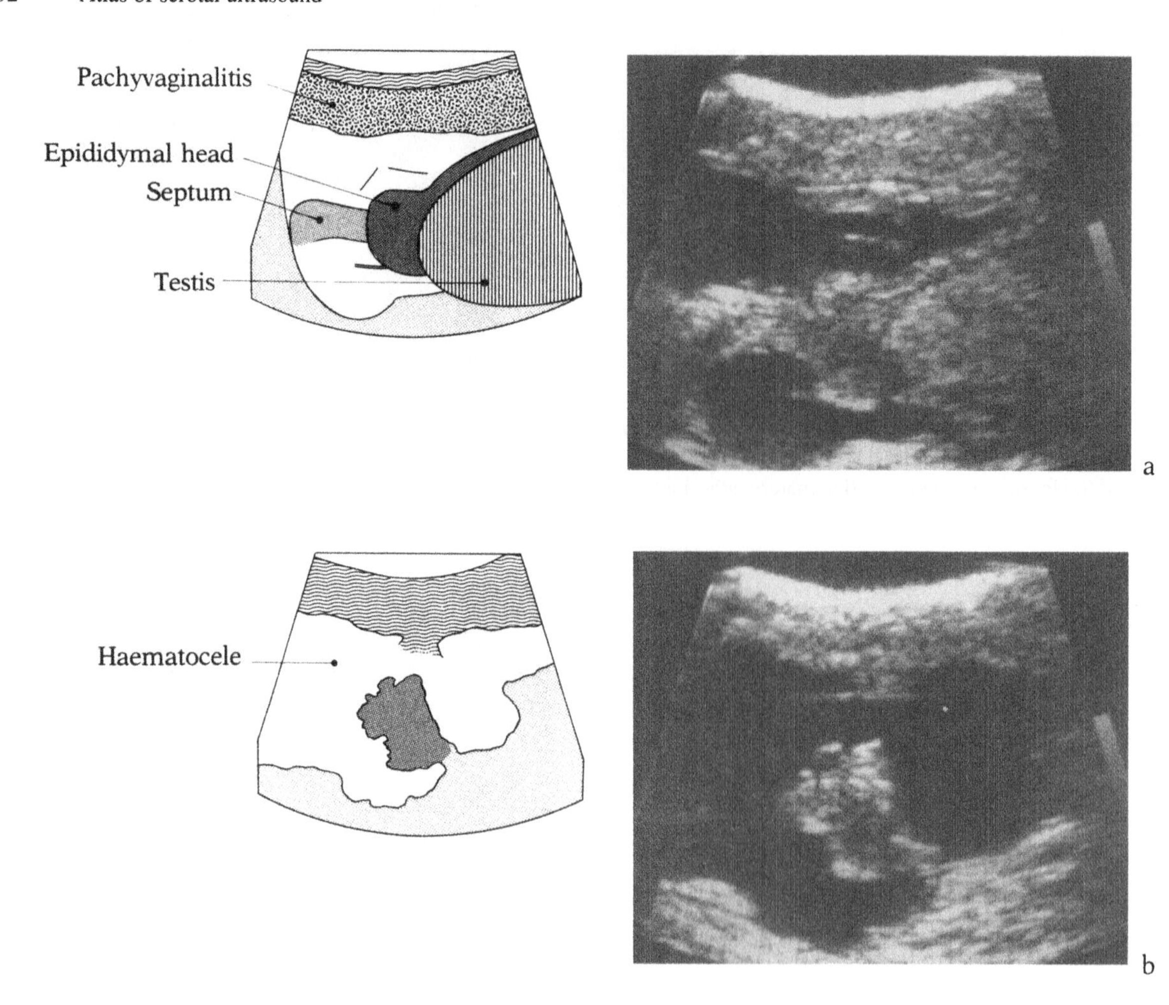

Fig. 26a, b. ***Needle aspiration of a hydrocele. Haemorrhagic complication.*** Progressive enlargement of the testis *one week* after a haemorrhagic aspiration of a hydrocele. **a** Sagittal section. Marked thickening of the investing layers involving mainly the parietal layer of the tunica vaginalis. Large septated effusion which is displacing the normal testis against the postero-inferior surface of the scrotum. The magma (paste-like material) covering the testis corresponds to a sediment of fibrin and blood-clot. The epididymis is definitely lying anteriorly and injury of this structure following needle puncture is the commonest cause of post-aspiration haematoceles. **b** Transverse section: debris of fibrin and blood-clot are floating in a recent haematocele which is predominantly still liquid

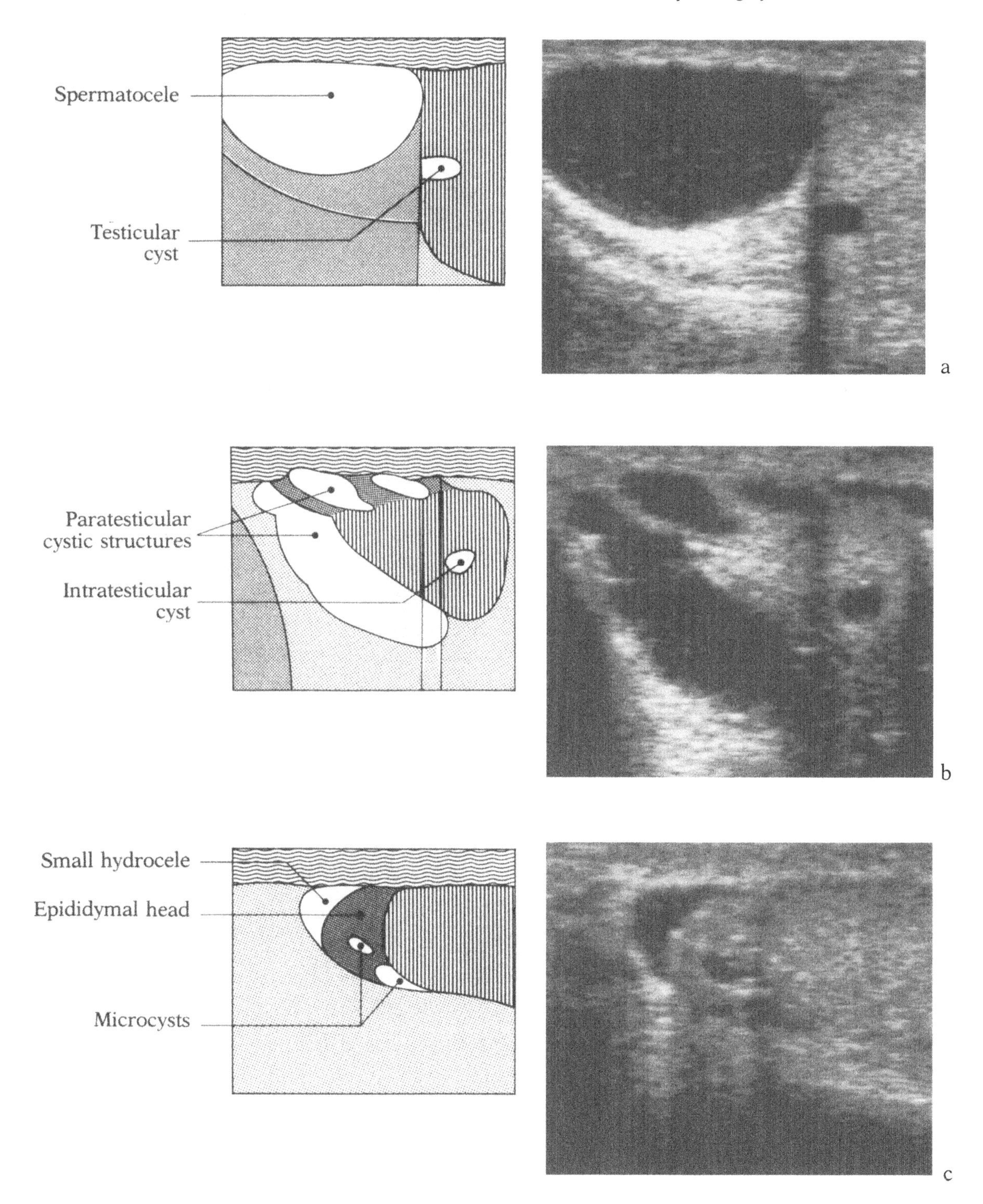

Fig. 27a-c. ***Vasectomy. Complication.*** Bilateral vasectomy *ten years* ago. Enlarged sensitive right testis. **a** Oblique section of the right testis. A large spermatocele (which represents a retention cyst) lying above the testis. **b** Transverse section of the same testis: multiple para testicular cysts. **c** Sagittal section of the contra lateral testis. Enlarged epididymal head with cystic dilatation leading to the region of the efferent canals. Conclusion: pseudo cystic distension of the internal excretory passages predominantly on the right, secondary to the vasectomy

Surgery for sterility

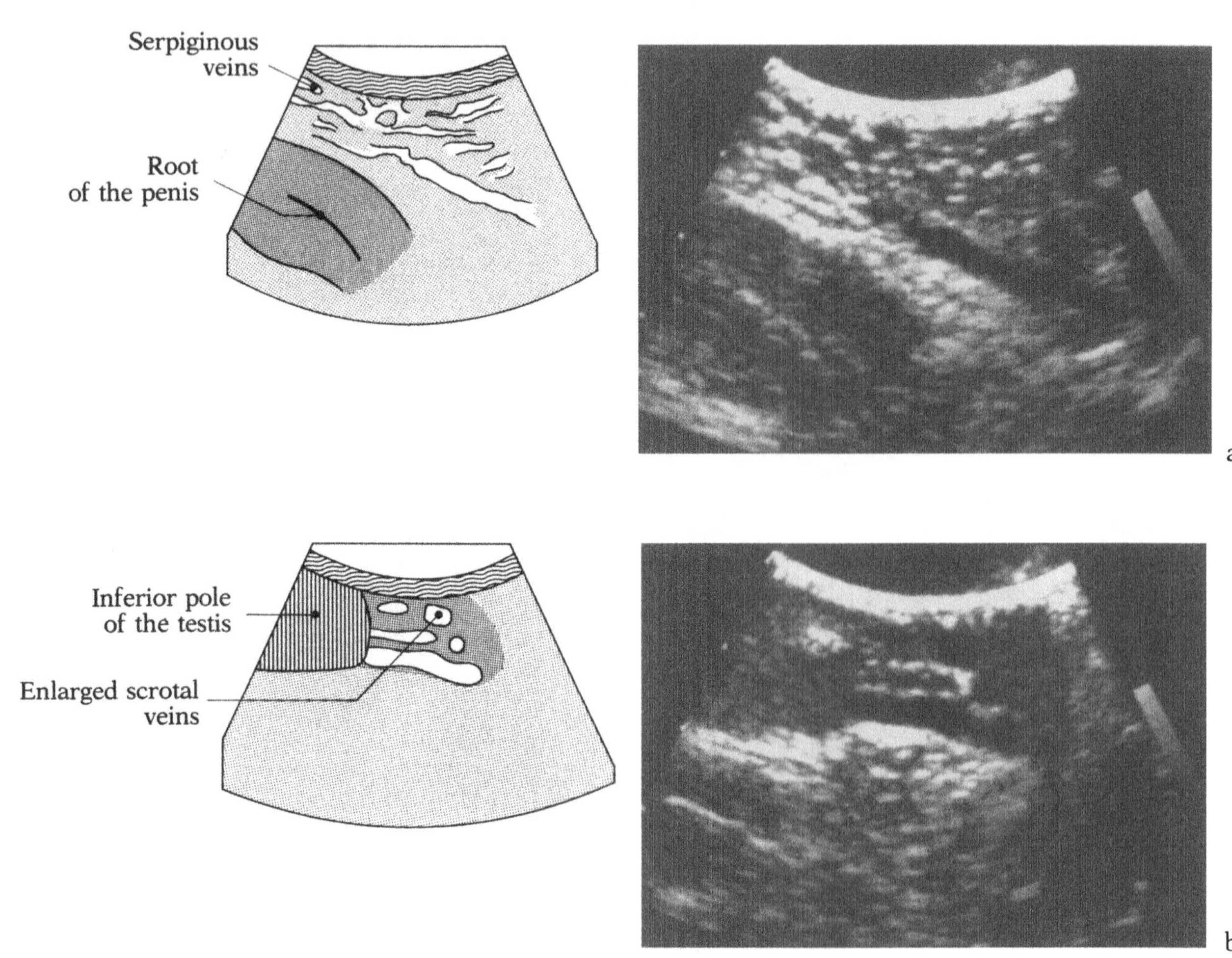

Fig. 28a, b *Varicocelectomy.* *Several months* post-surgery for a left varicocele, no improvement either in the sperm count or in the feeling of heaviness in the testis. **a** Sagittal section of the superior pole. Network of small transonic structures along the cord, with a principal draining vein. **b** Sagittal section of the inferior pole. Inferior to the testis there are dilated scrotal veins giving a mesh-like appearance. Conclusion: recurrence of a global varicocele involving the pampiniform and cremasteric plexi

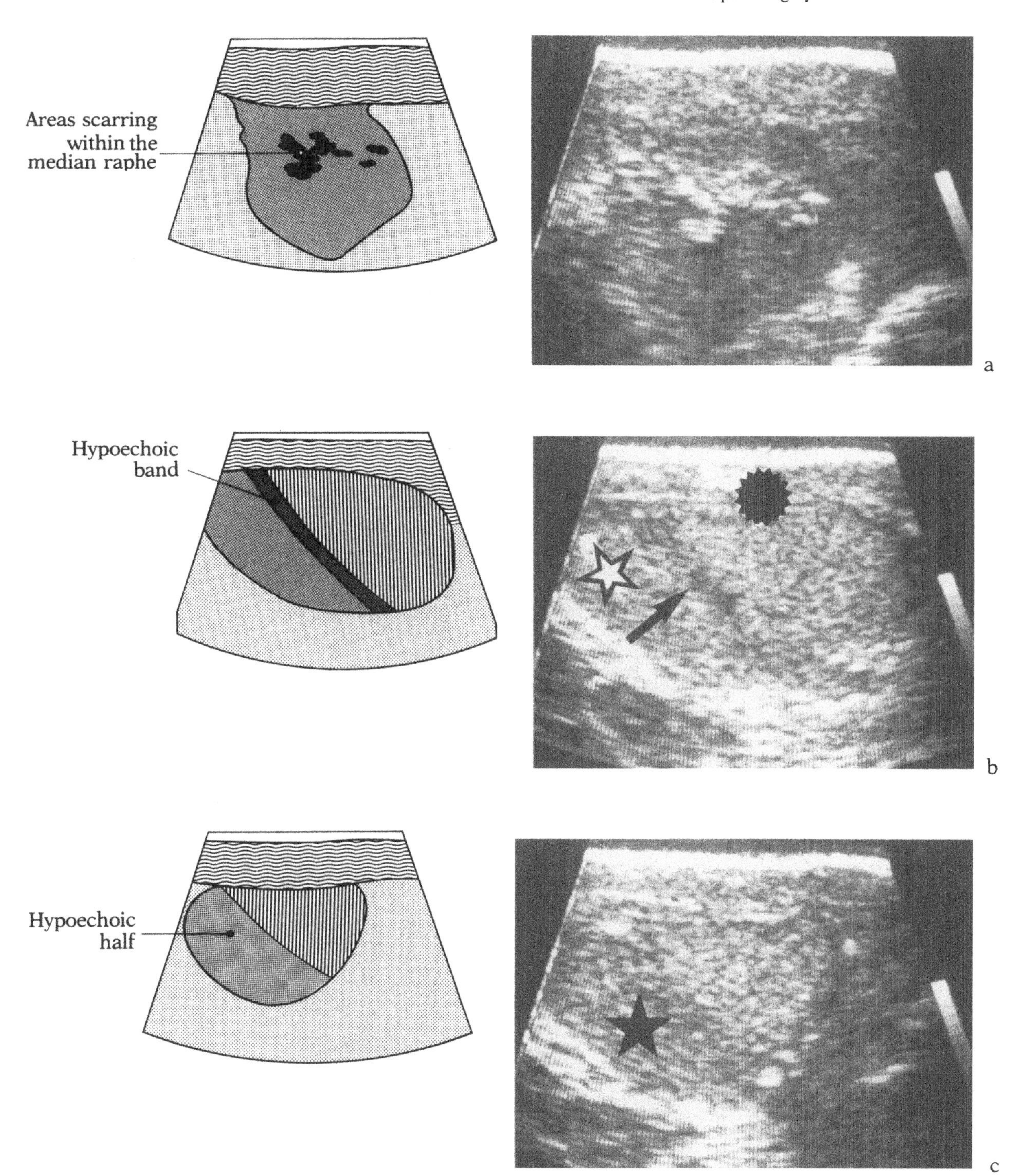

Fig. 29a-c. ***Testicular biopsy. Complication.*** Bilateral testicular biopsy for the investigation of azoospermia. *One month* later the right testis remains abnormally sensitive. **a** Transverse section of the median raphe. Usual changes following scrototomy: thickening of the median raphe punctuated by several echogenicities due to fibrotic plaques of scar tissue. **b** Sagittal section. The right testis is crossed by a hypoechoic band. The echo pattern of one part of the testis appears different to the other. **c** Transverse section. The comparison of the orthogonal scans confirms the difference in echogenicity of the two halves of the testis, the superior part is abnormally hypoechoic due to ischaemia following damage to a branch of the testicular artery sustained at the time of biopsy

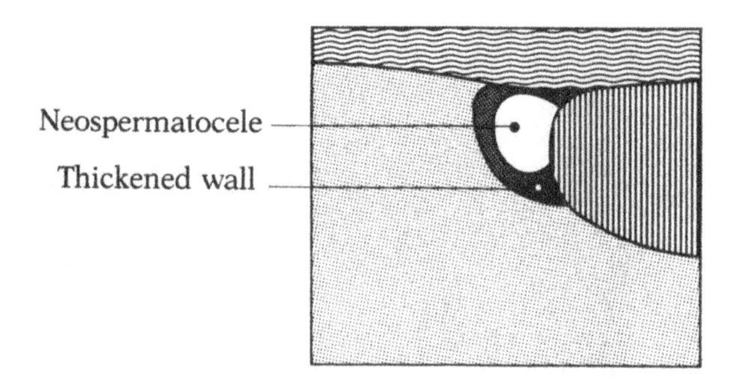

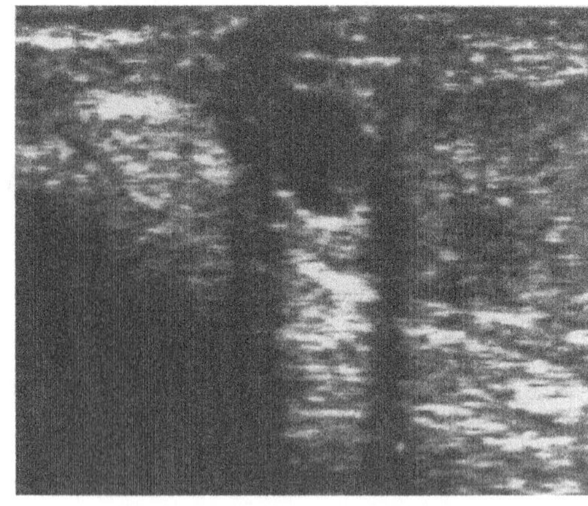

Fig. 30. ***Neo-spermatocele.*** Bilateral agenesis of the vas deferentia. Creation of a spermatocele,essentially a reservoir for the spermatozoa formed from a pouch of the tunica vaginalis. Control scan on the *eighth day* to measure the volume in order to decide the time for aspiration . Sagittal section. The neo-spermatocele is a fairly thick-walled spherical structure, 1 cm in diameter. No adjacent effusion

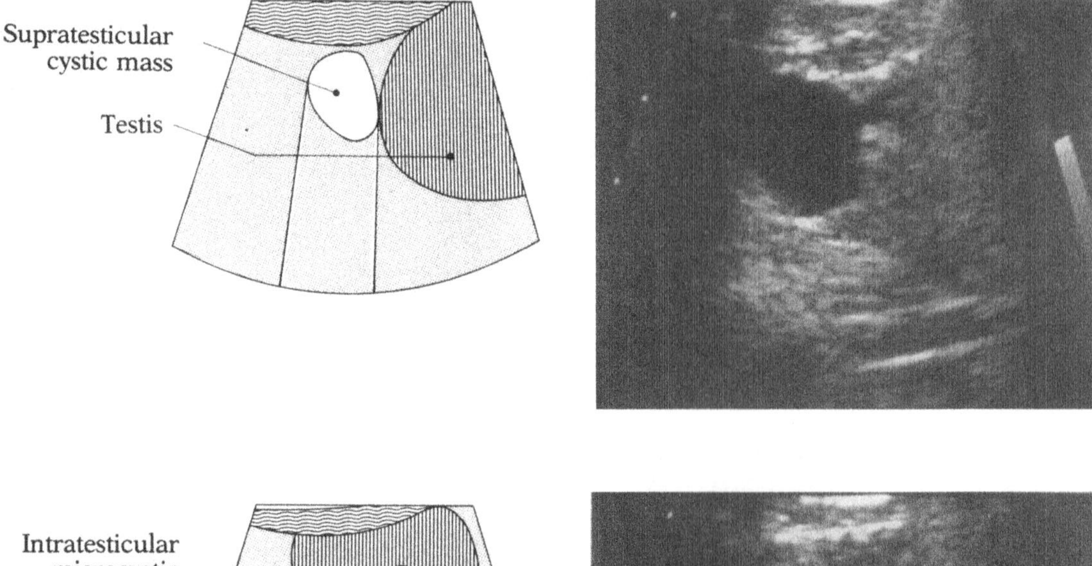

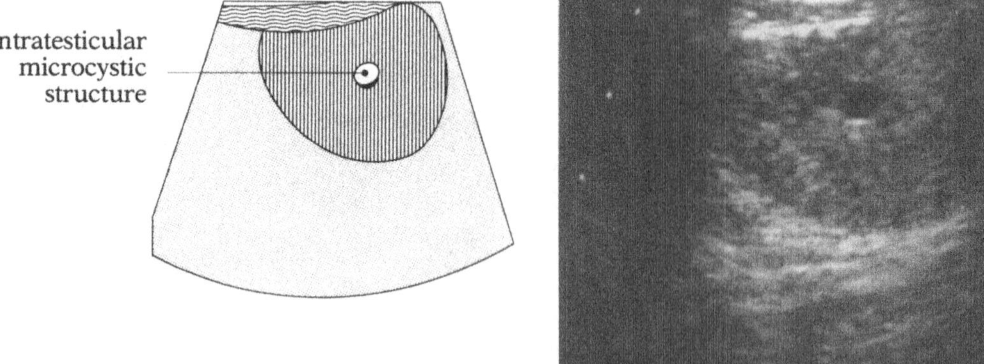

Fig. 31a, b. ***Crossed epididymo-deferential anastomosis.*** Agenesis of the left vas deferens. At testicular biopsy: on the left spermatozoa were present; on the right absence of spermatozoa. Formation of an anastomosis between the right vas deferens and the left epididymal head. One week later, nodule in the superior aspect of the right scrotal sac. **a** Oblique scan of the right superior pole. Cystic formation overlying the testis: leak at the sight of the anastomosis. **b** Sagittal section on the left. Appearance of microcysts in the testis: ectasia of the straight tubes indicating that the anastomosis is not functioning resulting in dilated tubules proximally

Calcifications of structures within the scrotum and the periscrotal region

These are not unusual and are generally secondary to previous infection within the scrotum (Table1). The mechanism of formation is by a secondary calcification of a fibrous scar. Occasionally, other rarer aetiologies should be considered, particularly the possibility of an underlying neoplasm containing calcification within a normal size or even small testis.

The diagnosis by ultrasound is made in three stages:

- *Nature of the calcification:* calcification of a structure is recognized by a definite fairly homogenous hyperechogenicity with variable posterior acoustic shadowing (depending both on the degree of fibrosis relative to the amount of calcification in the structure and the nature of the surrounding tissue through which the ultrasound beam passes) The acoustic shadowing is not a constant feature and its absence does not preclude a diagnosis of calcification. Once this has been established, the characteristics of the calcification must be noted: number, size and form.

- *Site of the calcification:* this is a key feature in reaching a differential diagnosis. It should be possible to determine whether the calcification is within one of the structures in the scrotum or in one of the neighbouring structures. It is of vital importance to establish whether the calcification is intra- or extra-testicular. As a rule, any calcification outside the testis is benign. By contrast, intra testicular calcification is suggestive of a neoplastic aetiology, particularly in certain clinical contexts.

- *Consideration of the differential diagnosis.* This is ultimately determined by the clinical picture, including the age, ethnic background and previous medical history of the patient.

List I : Gamut of the causes of calcifications of the testicular appendages in relation to their localisation

Tunica vaginalis

- *Chronic or previous inflammation* (frequent):
  - common organisms,
  - tuberculosis (++; necrosis; caseation),
  - syphilis (gumma).
- *Traumatism* (sequellae).
- *Tumours* (rare):
  - fibrous pseudotumour

Tunica albuginea of the testis

- *Inflammation .*
- *Torsion .*

Sessile hydatids

- *Inflammation .*
- *Torsion .*

Epididymis

- *Inflammation :*
  - common organisms,
  - tuberculosis(++),
  - gonococcus

- syphilis,
- hydatidosis,
- exceptionally sarcoidosis.
- *Previous torsion*

Cord

- *Parasites*
  - filariasis.
- *Traumatism* .
- *Tumours and pseudotumours*
  - rhabdomyosarcoma,
  - leiomyosarcoma,
  - lymphangioma.
- Post treatment
  - embolisation.

Investing layers of the testis (scrotum)

- *Inflammation* .
- *Parasites: cysticercosis.*
- *Traumatism* .
- *Tumours and pseudotumours* (rare)
  - rhabdomyosarcoma,
  - leiomyosarcoma,
  - angiokeratoma,
  - lymphangiomatosis.

List II : Gamut of the causes of calcification within the testis

- *Tumours* (++).
- *Torsion* (ischaemic necrosis).
- *Traumatism.*
- *Inflammation and pseudotumours*
  - granulomatous orchitis,
  - malacoplakia.
- *Idiopathic*
  - phleboliths (varicocele)

List III : Gamut of the causes of calcification of the penis

- *Peyronie's disease.*
- *Traumatism.*
- *Blood disorders.*
  - haemoglobinopathies (sickle cell disease)
  - storage disorders (lipoidoses, Gaucher's disease),
  - excess of glucocorticoids (Cushing's syndrome).
- *Iatrogenic* (injection of Papaverin).
- *Tumours* (rare).
- *Urethral lithiasis.*

List IV : Principal types and characteristics of calcified lesions of the testicular appendages

Tunica vaginalis

- *Calculi*
  - Calcified concretions or sludge, layering, mobile++ (move the patient; orthostatic), generally associated with chronic hydrocele.
- *Granuloma*
  - Fixed on one of the layers, solitary; en plaque or granular.
- *Pachyvaginalitis*
  - Septations with usually an associated hydrocele.
- *Fibrous haematocele*
  - Localised (inferior or superior pole) or surrounding the testis (risk of ischaemic necrosis of the testis)

Tunica albuginea of the testis

- *Granuloma*
  - Fixed to the testis and solid to palpation;
  - single;
  - multiple grains: rounded and about 1 mm in size.

Epididymis

- *Fibrous nodule from a previous chronic epidiymitis*
  - Rounded, not uncommonly bipolar;
  - rarely affects the body.
- *Spermatic granuloma*
  - Resulting from the presence of abnormal spermatozoa in the epididymal stroma (trauma, loosening of a suture following vasectomy),
  - usually occurs in the epididymal head.
- *Complicated spermatocele*
  - Occurs in the head,
  - haemorrhage or superadded infection.
- *Hydatid cyst*
  - Calcified wall,
  - indistinguishable from a complicated spermatocele -> Serology.

Spermatic cord

- *Calcified filarial larvae*
  - Multiple, arcuate, often bilateral. Situated in the lymphatic vessels,
  - organised in a chain (plain x-ray radiograph with soft tissue exposure).

- *Calcified haematoma*

Regular, oblong and homogenous

- *Malignant tumour*
  - Haemorrhagic or necrotic remnants,
  - heterogenous disorganised calcifications associated with a solid expansive process.

Investing layers

- *Granuloma*
  - Isolated, mobile relative to the testis,
  - fixed.

- *Calcified larvae of cysticerci*
  - Generally bilateral,
  - regular, aligned, tapering to the extremities (seen on plain radiographs with soft tissue exposure).

- *Tumour*
  - Haemorrhagic or necrotic zones,
  - scattered microcalcifications within a mass.

Calcifications of structures within the scrotum and of periscrotal region

Calcifications of the testicular appendages

Tunica vaginalis

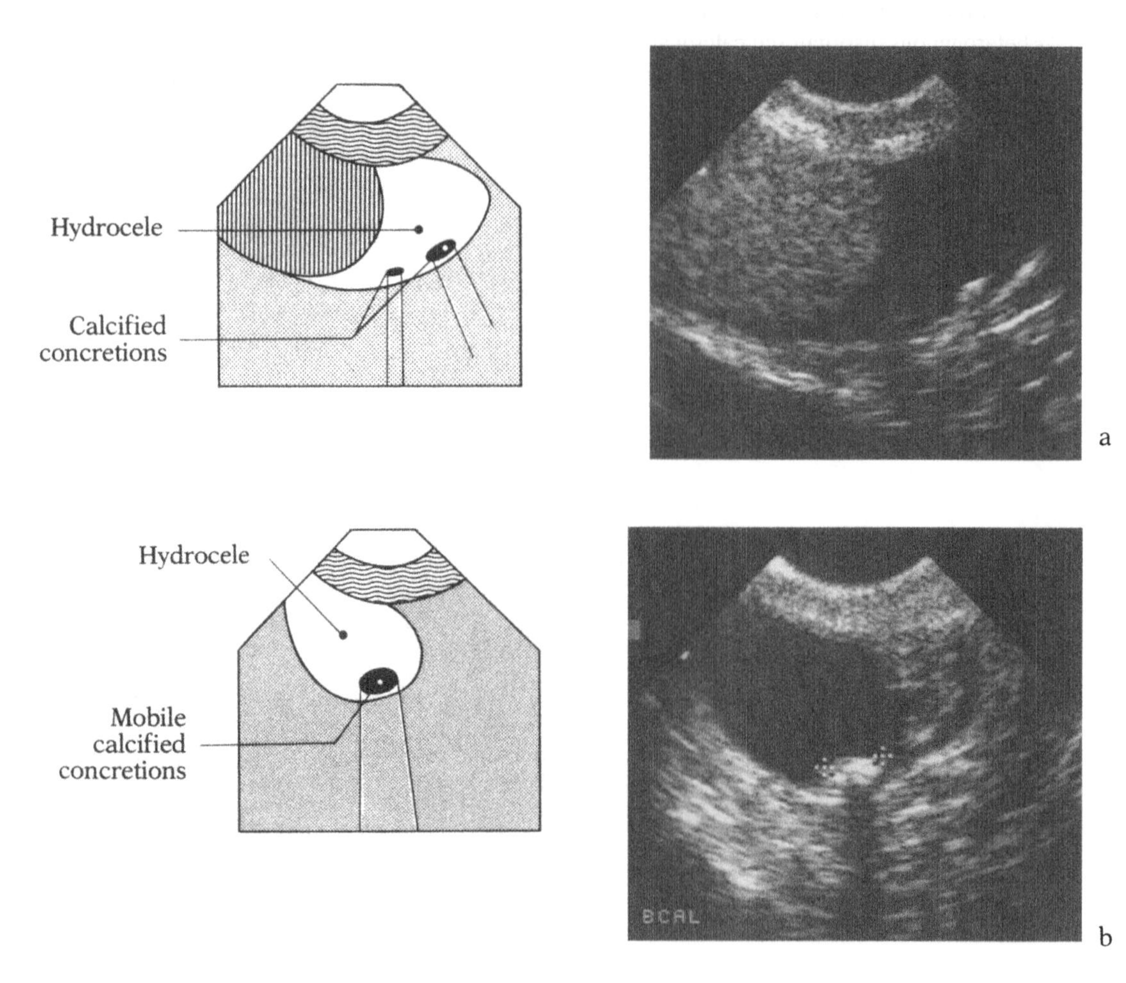

Fig. 1a, b. ***Calcific concretions.*** **a** Sagittal section of the inferior pole. Normal testis. Simple medium sized hydrocele containing a small rounded structure of a few millimetres which is very echogenic and attenuating. Another similar smaller structure is also seen mainly recognized by its acoustic shadowing. **b** Transverse section of the inferior pole, patient standing up. Mobility and sedimentation of the two structures which have now settled together against the parietal layer of the tunica vaginalis: calcified concretions, often seen in old hydroceles or detached hydatids, floating within the tunica vaginalis and secondarily calcified

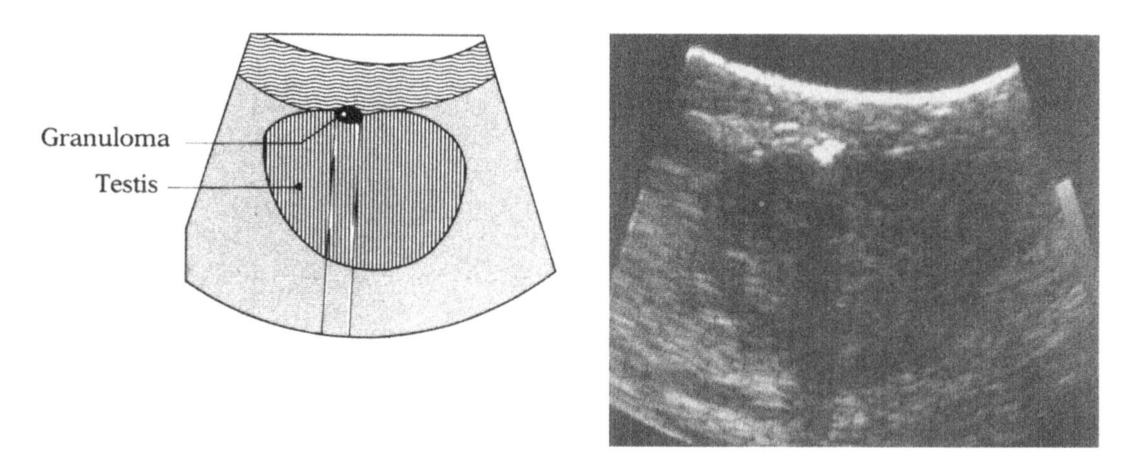

Fig. 2. ***Granuloma.*** Transverse section: enlarged hypoechoic testis , due to acute orchitis, across which runs the posterior acoustic shadowing from a calcified granuloma of the parietal layer of the tunica vaginalis

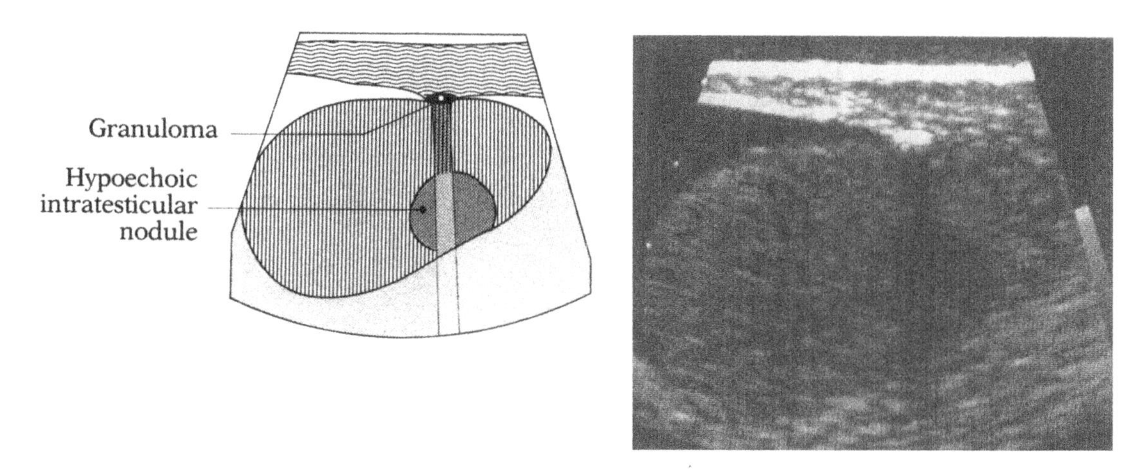

Fig. 3. ***Granuloma.*** Sagittal section. Same appearance of a calcified granuloma of the tunica vaginalis, associated with a hydrocele. It is essential not to miss the intra-testicular hypoechoic nodule which turned out to be a secondary tumour, partially obscured by the posterior acoustic shadowing

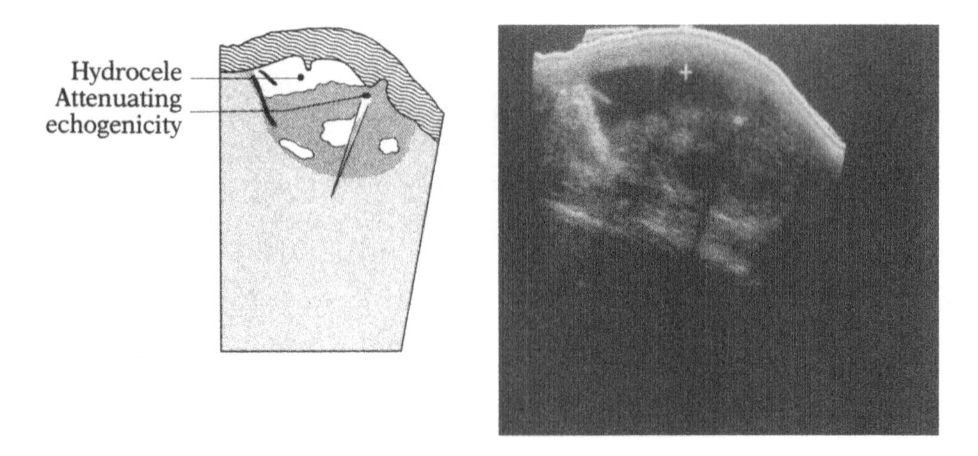

Fig. 4. *Tuberculosis.* Progressively enlarging and indurated testis in an elderly man. Oblique scan: pachyvaginalitis with thickened walls punctuated with attenuating echogenicities lining the hydrocele: granulomatous lesions with caseation due to subacute tuberculosis shown on histopathological examination

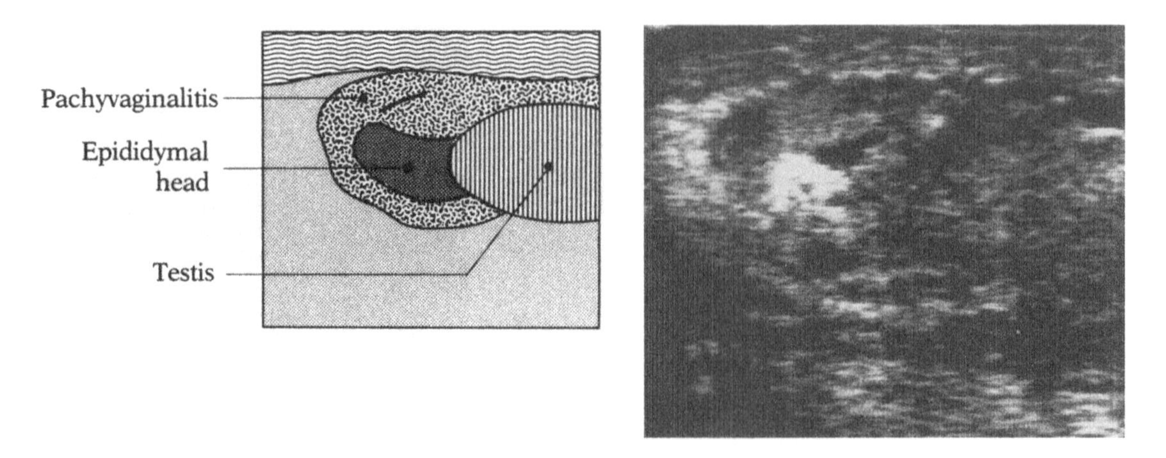

Fig. 5. *Atypical inflammation.* Epididymo-orchitis. No improvement on medical treatment. Oblique section: numerous adhesions between the testis, epididymis and the two layers of the tunica vaginalis with highly echogenic areas, of variable attenuation, with an absence of or only a small hydrocele: the appearances are suggestive of tuberculosis

Tunica albuginea of the testis

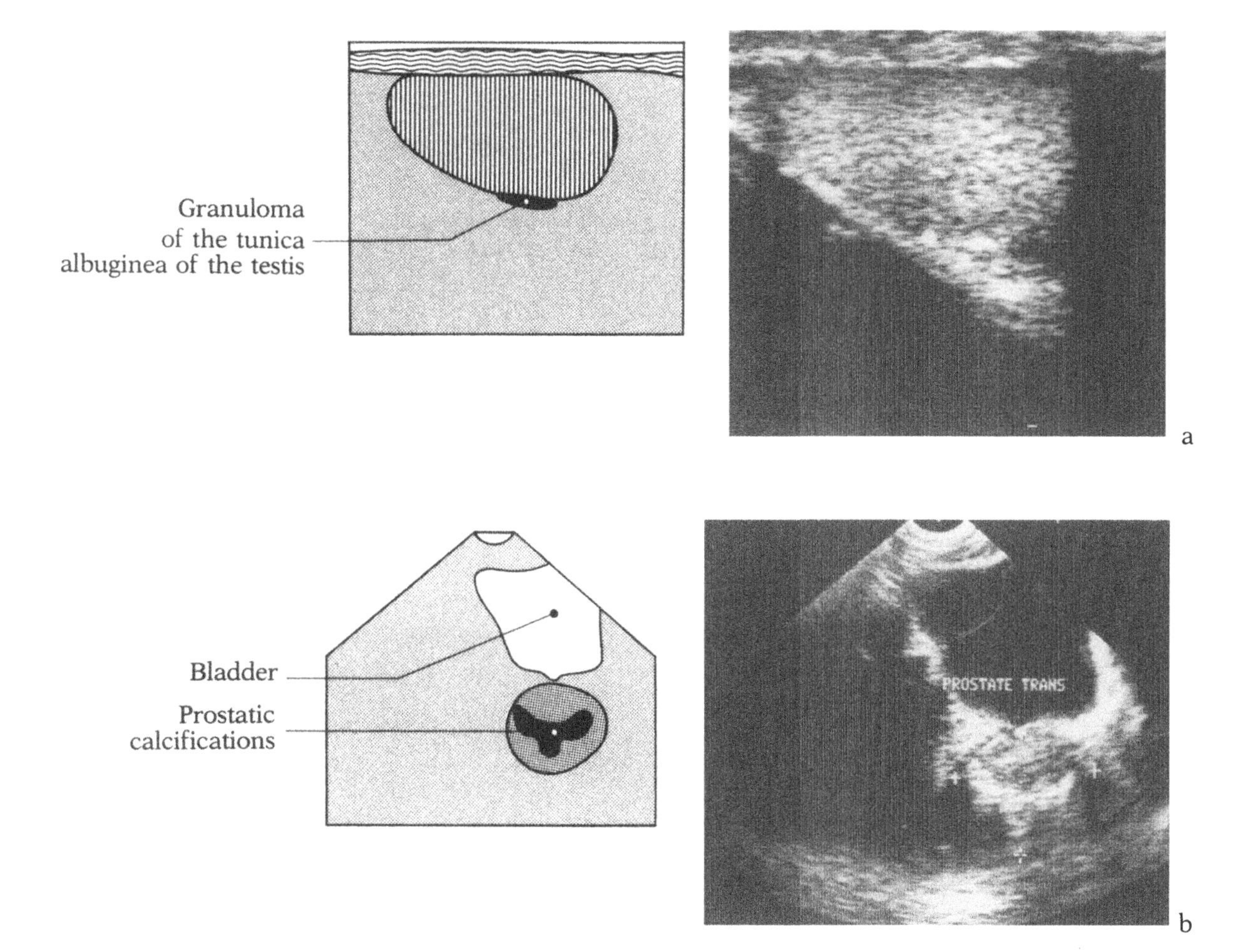

Fig. 6a, b. ***Granuloma.*** Investigation of hypofertility in a 34 year old man: genital ultrasound. **a** Sagittal section of the right testis: incidental finding of an echogenic, slightly attenuating plaque in the periphery of the testis: benign granuloma, absence of or minimal calcification of the tunica albuginea. **b** Transverse section of the prostate (supra-pubic scan). Large symetrical echogenicities in the intermediate zone: clumps of calcification, no specific features. Their association with the granuloma of the tunica albuginea indicates a definite previous infection

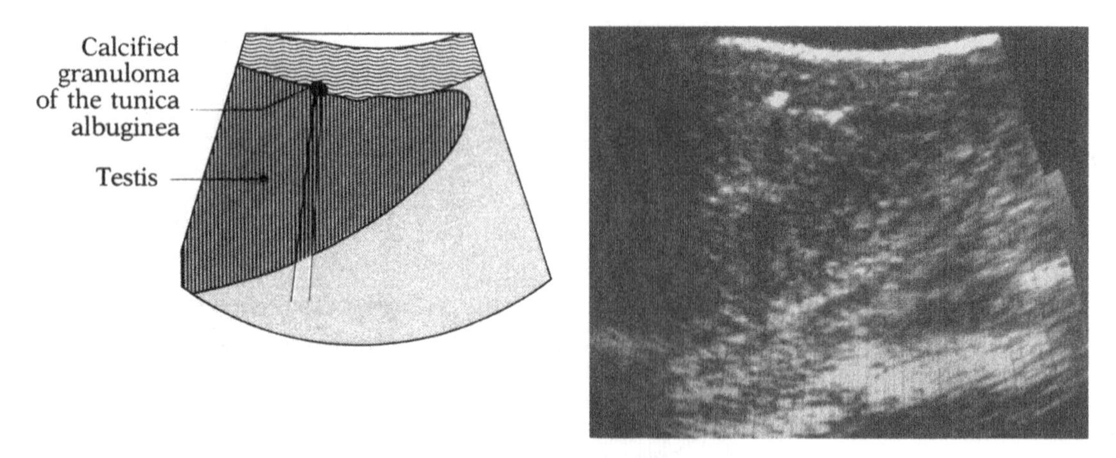

Fig. 7. ***Granuloma.*** Acutely enlarged testis containing a palpable small solitary nodule in a 30 year old man : tumour presenting acutely ? Sagittal section of the inferior pole: large globally hypoechoic testis suggestive of inflammation with a calcified granuloma explaining the palpable nodule

Epididymis and hydatid

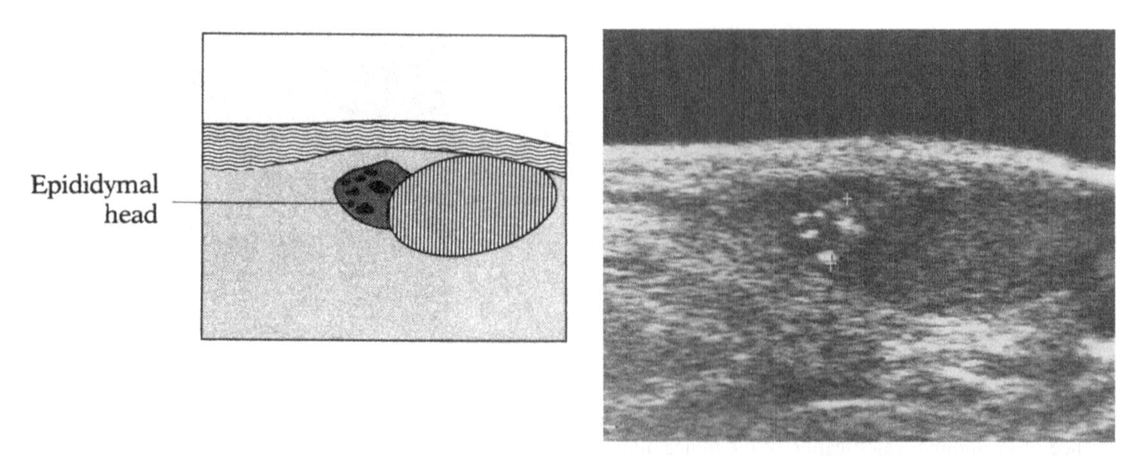

Fig. 8. ***Sequellae of tuberculosis.*** Investigation of sterility in a 35 year old man with a previous history of tuberculosis. Sagittal section. Homogenous but hypotrophic testis. The head of the epididymis is of normal size but contains several echogenicities: fibro-caseous lesions which have become secondarily calcified due to tuberculosis of the epididymal head

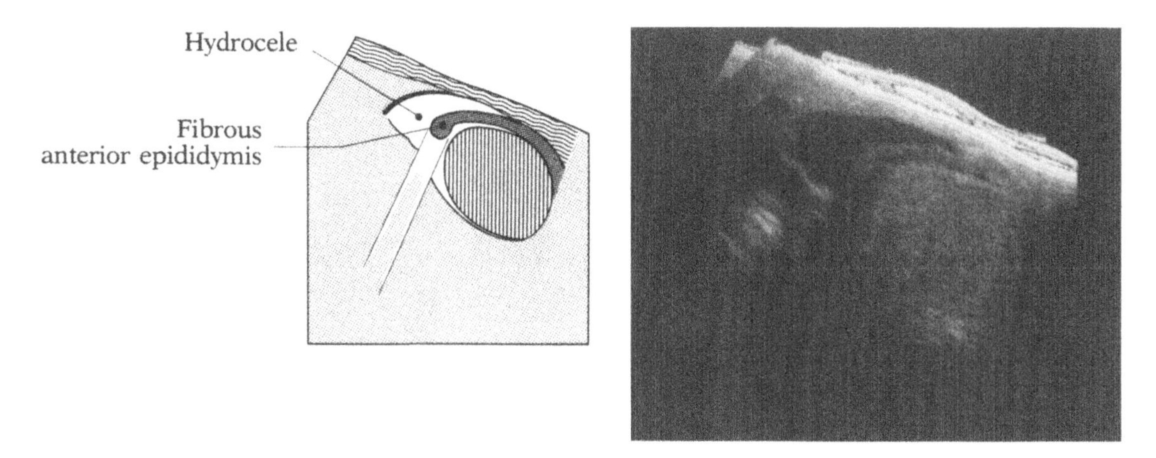

Fig. 9. ***Calcified fibrosis of the epididymal head.*** Investigation of azoospermia. Sagittal section. Normal testis. Anteriorly placed epididymis (seen in 10% of cases) giving a "cobra head" appearance. Complete attenuation of the beam behind the head indicating fibrotic calcified epididymitis compatible with previous tuberculosis or syphilis which must be confirmed to be inactive

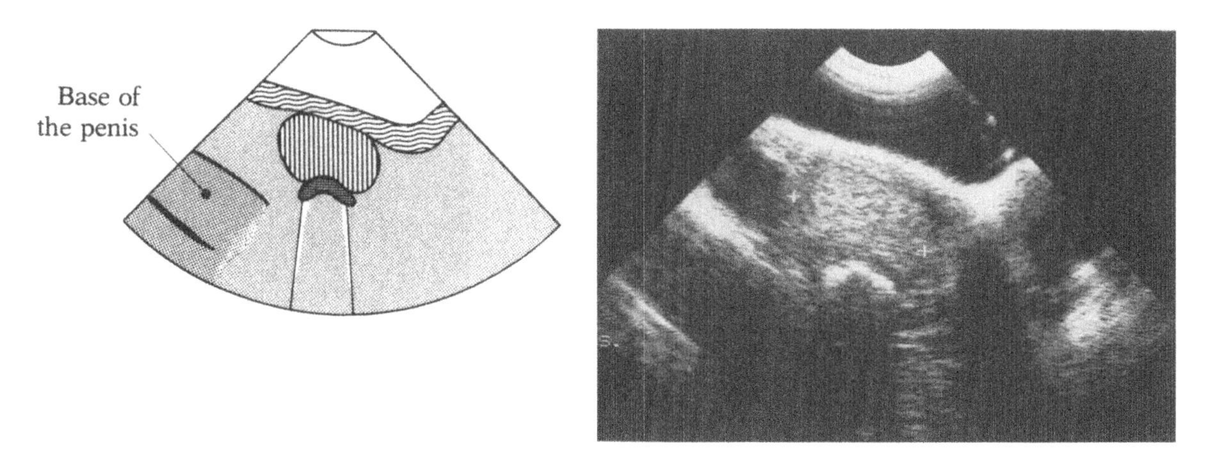

Fig. 10. ***Misleading image.*** Sagittal section. The attenuating hyperechogenicity in an arc posterior to the testis is not a calcified body of the epididymis but simply the finger of the operator which is immobilising the testis!

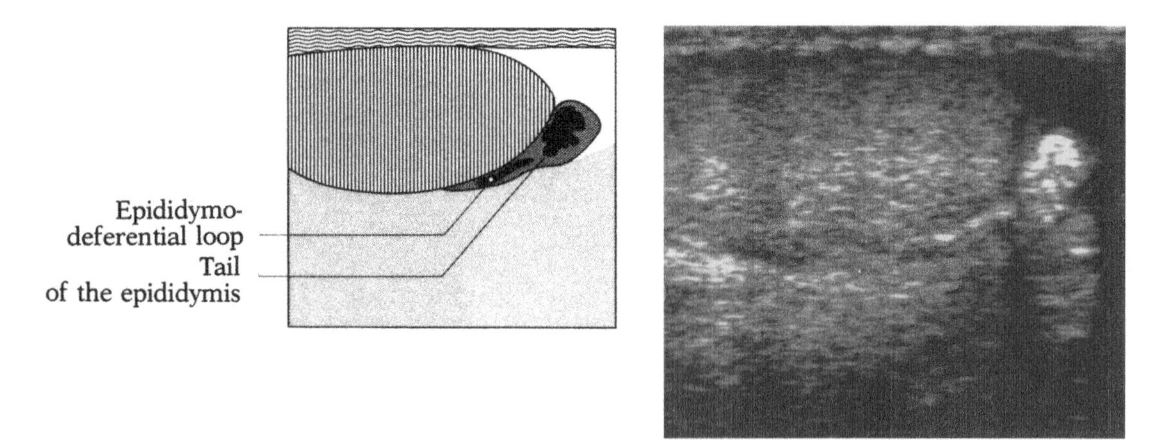

Fig. 11. ***Calcified fibrosis of the epididymal tail.*** Hard painless nodule in the scrotum. Sagittal section of the inferior pole. Normal testis. Inferiorly, the epididymal tail is very enlarged and completely echogenic extending up as a linear structure, also echogenic: calcified fibrous lesions of the epididymal tail and vas deferens

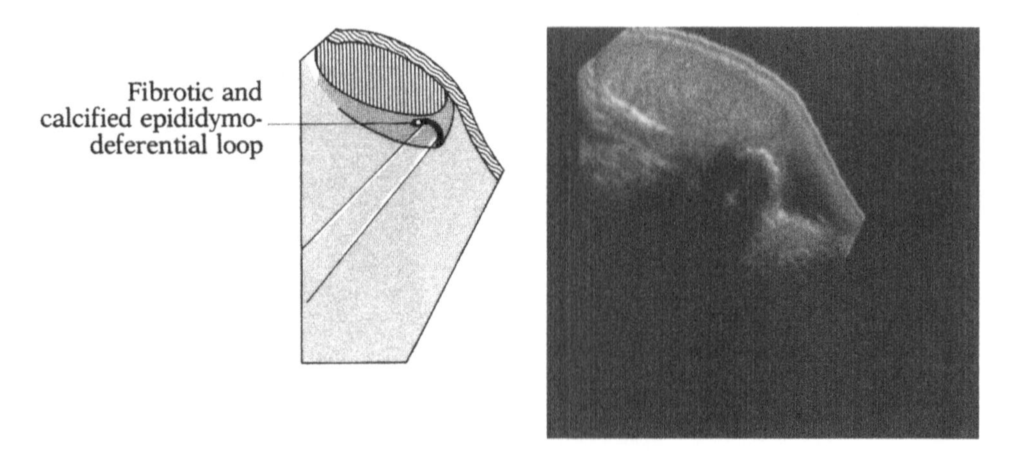

Fig. 12. ***Sequellae of tuberculosis.*** Elderly patient. Previous tuberculosis. Sagittal section. Enlarged epididymo-deferential loop with a completely attenuating echogenic arc: old calcified tuberculous lesions

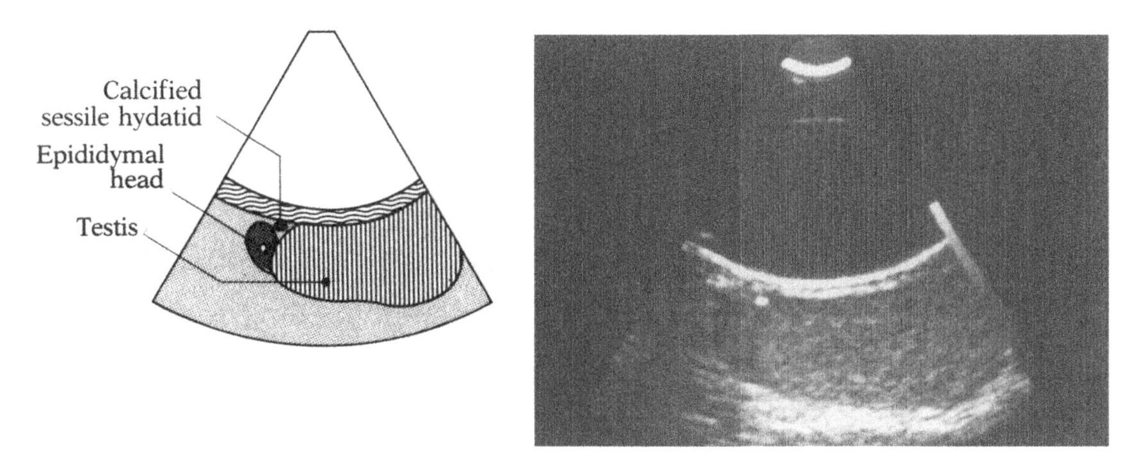

Fig. 13. ***Sessile hydatid.*** Sagittal section. Highly echogenic and attenuating micronodule at the anterior junction of the testis and epididymis: calcified sessile hydatid

The vessels

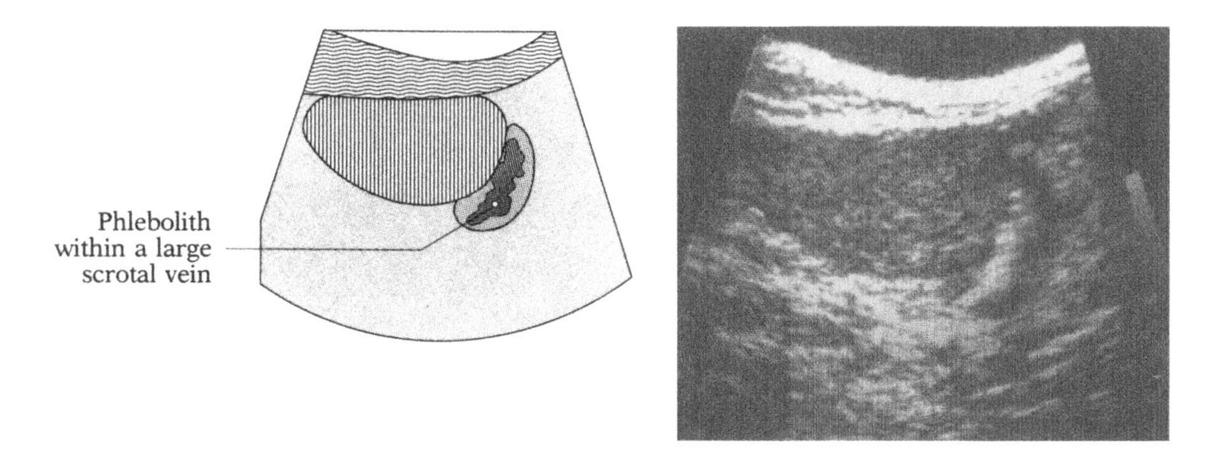

Fig. 14. ***Phleboliths.*** A 73 year old diabetic patient. Sagittal section of the inferior pole. Beneath the testis is an echogenic curvilinear structure within a similar but hypoechoic structure which increases in size following the Valsalva manoeuvre and after standing up. Phleboliths in enlarged scrotal veins

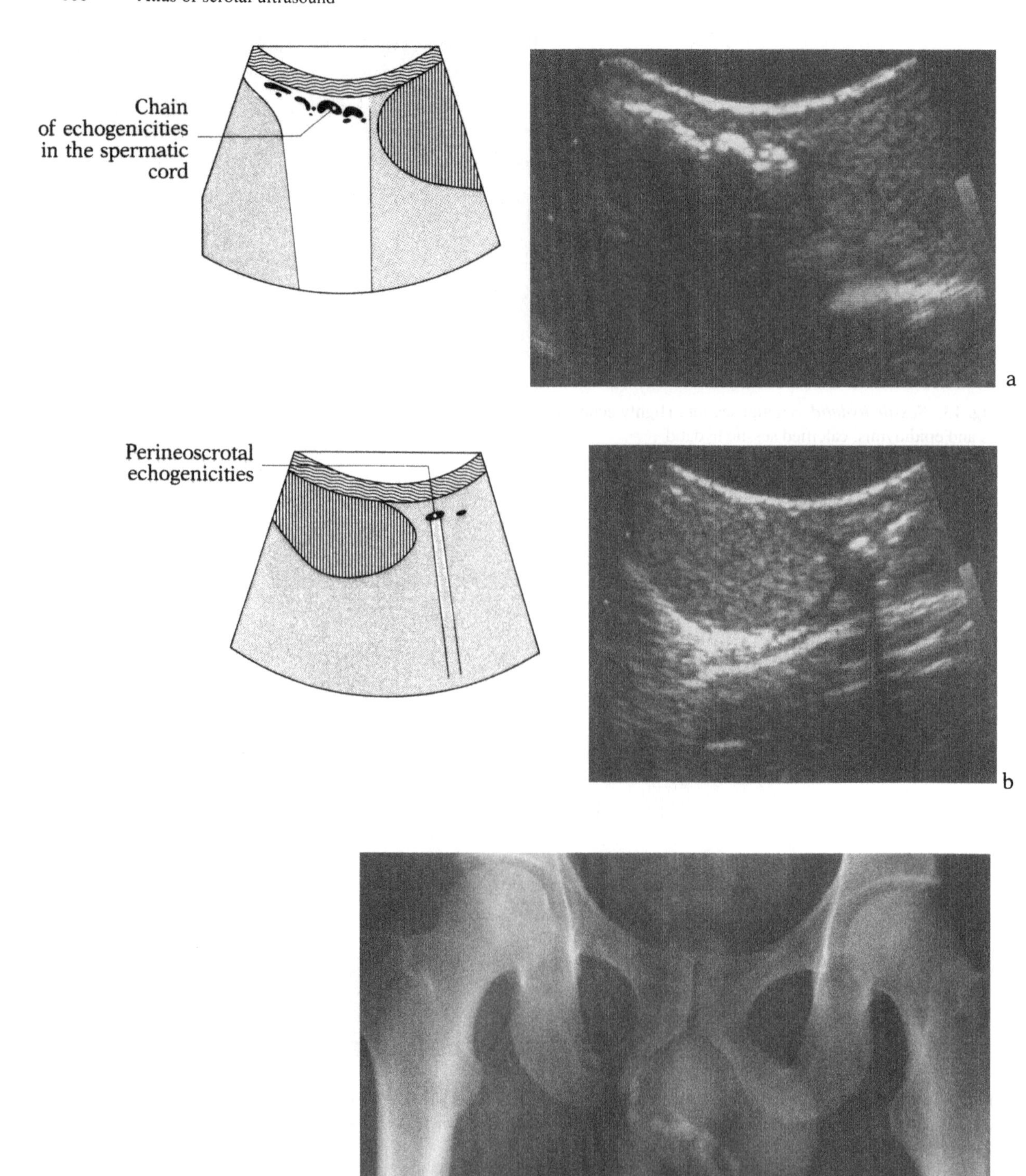

Fig. 15a-c. ***Calcified filaria.*** A young man of 28 from Mali. Induration of the right spermatic cord. **a** Sagittal section high in the right scrotum. Overlying the testis, in the spermatic cord is a chain of attenuating echogenic lesions. **b** Sagittal section low in the left scrotum, beneath the testis and epididymis in the peno-scrotal region, same type of attenuating echogenicities. **c** View centred on the inguino-scrotal region during an intravenous urogram (IVU). Regular linear calcifications throughout the scrotum and right spermatic cord. Conclusion: typical appearances of calcified microfilaria in the line of the lymphatic vessels, particularly those in the right spermatic cord. Note the absence of any associated hydrocele which would suggest impaired lymphatic drainage

Calcification of the penis

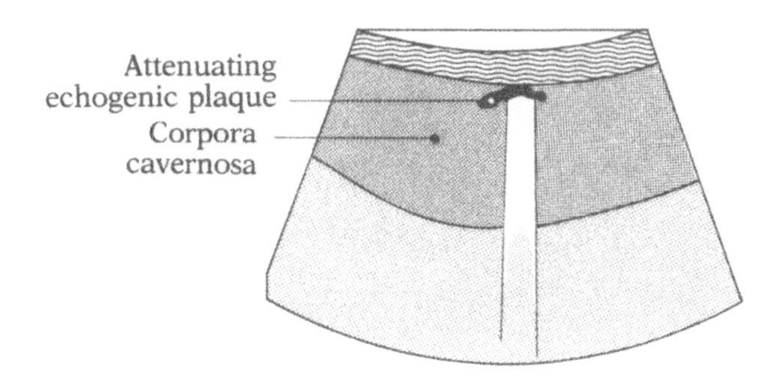

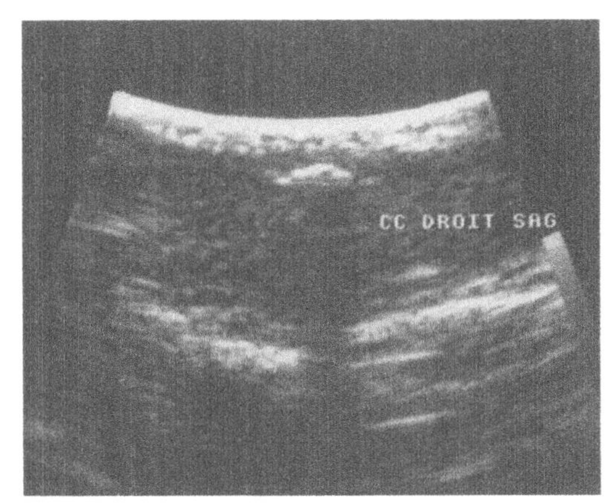

a

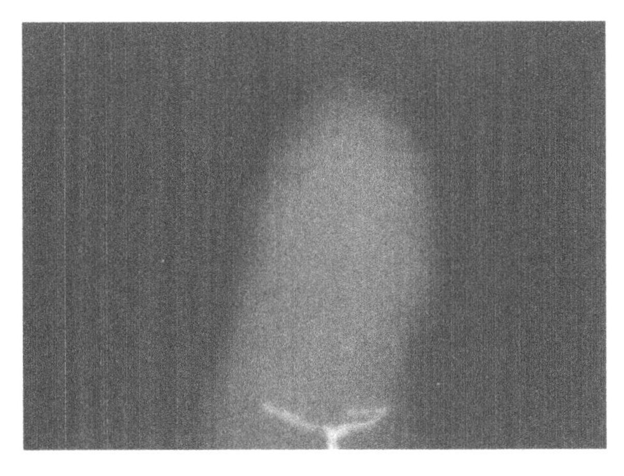

b

Fig. 16a, b. ***Peyronie's disease.*** A 46 year old patient. Deformity of the root of the penis for several months during erections. **a** Sagittal right paramedian section of the penis. In its proximal third there is an echogenic attenuating linear structure of almost 1 cm at the periphery of the corpus cavernosum. Same abnormality on the left. **b** Soft tissue exposure centred on the penis. T-shaped calcification at the base of the penis corresponding to the ultrasound images, namely calcified fibrous plaques due to Peyronie's disease

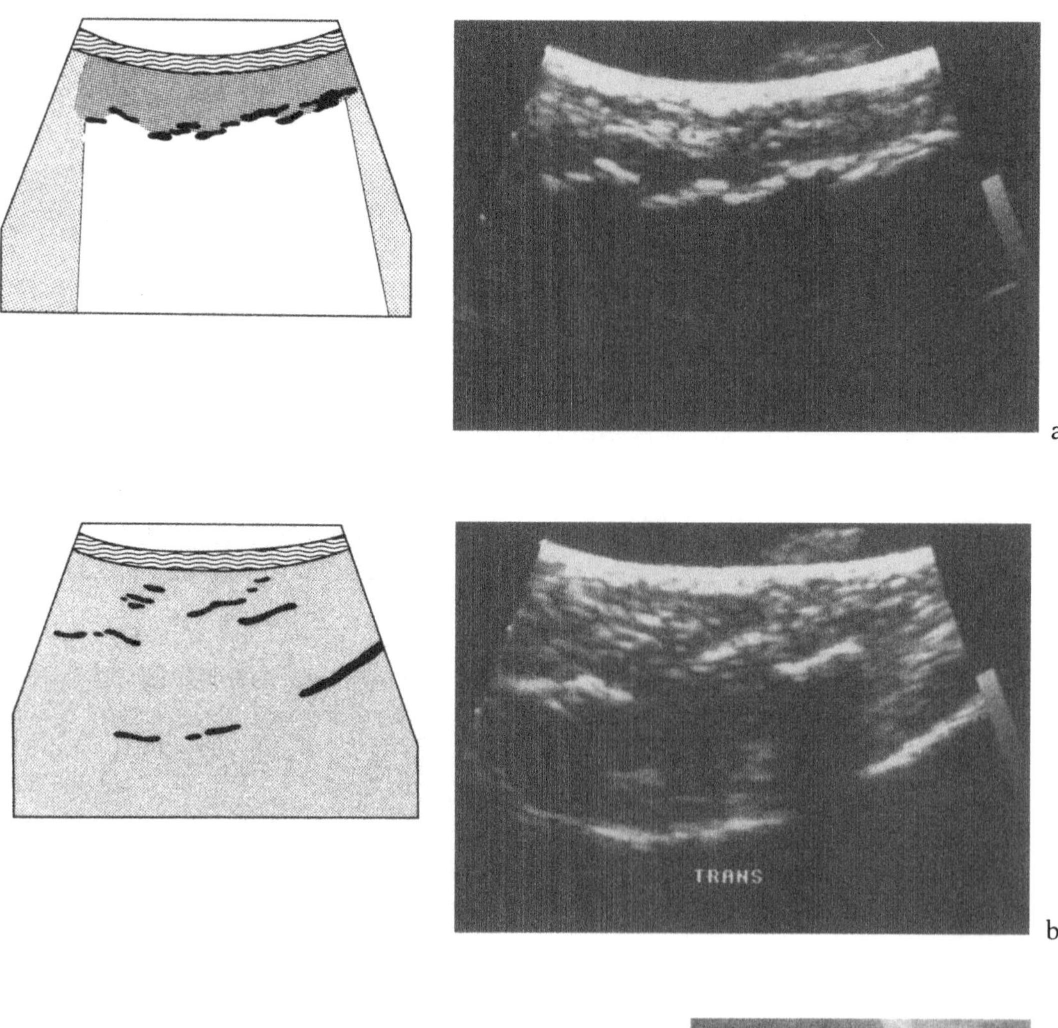

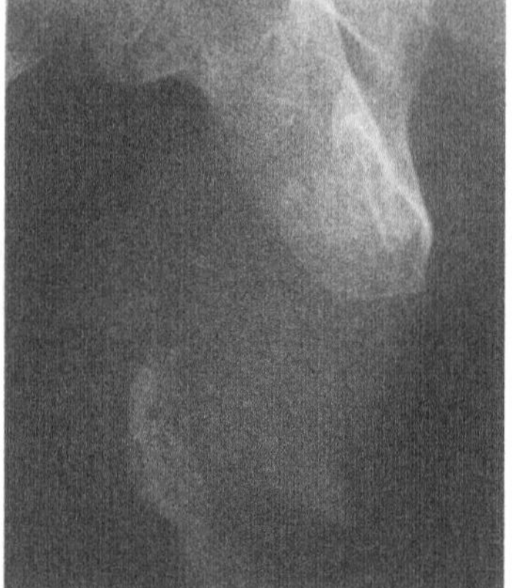

Fig. 17a-c. ***Complication of acute thrombosis in sickle cell disease.*** A 42 year old patient from the Congo, homozygous for sickle cell disease SS. Following a crisis episode of priapism for five days. **a** Sagittal right paramedian section of the penis: large echogenic lesions arranged in chains giving a total acoustic void posteriorly and situated more centrally in the corpus cavernosum. **b** Transverse left paramedian section. Same abnormalities, fairly central in the left corpus cavernosum. **c** Left anterior oblique view during an IVU. Large central bulging calcifications situated right along the two corpora cavernosa: calcified thrombii of the corpora cavernosa secondary to an acute thrombotic episode during a sickle cell crisis

Calcifications of the testis

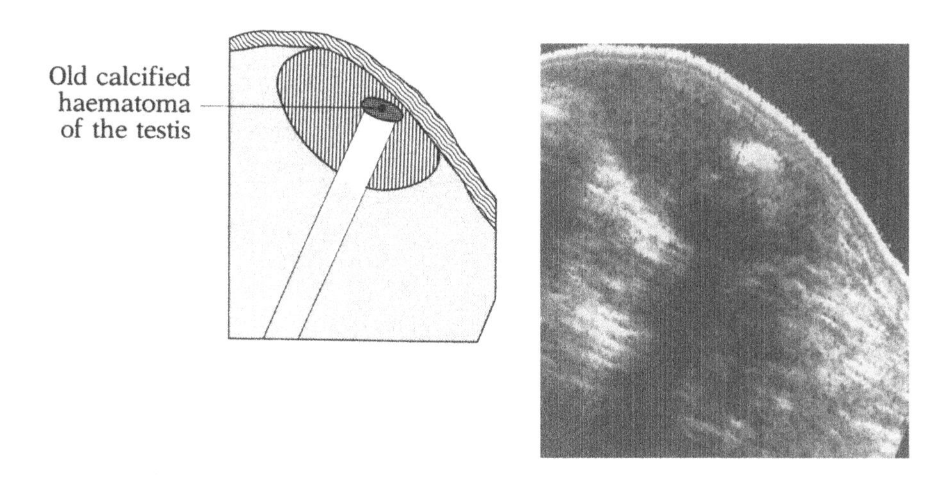

Fig. 18. ***Trauma.*** A 25 year old patient. Trauma to the left testis two months earlier, now painless induration. Sagittal section. Large oval echogenicity, very attenuating, lying in the periphery of the parenchyma in the inferior half of the testis. Subcapsular haematoma, secondarily calcified

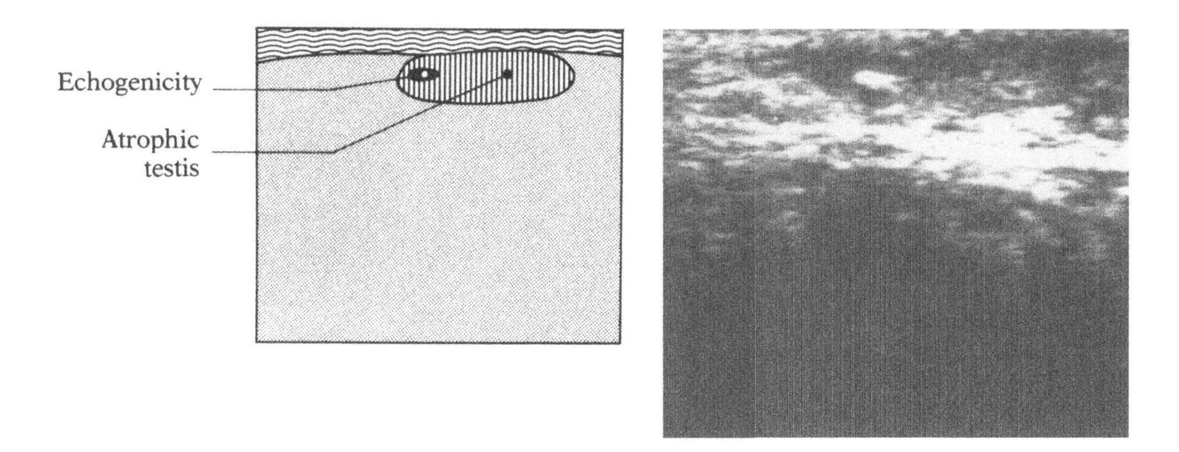

Fig. 19. ***Inflammation.*** Severe epididymo-orchitis six months previously. Secondary shrinkage of the testis with a hard palpable nodule. Sagittal section. Marked testicular atrophy with an echogenic nodule at the superior pole due to a calcified fibrous scar probably from an area of purulent necrosis

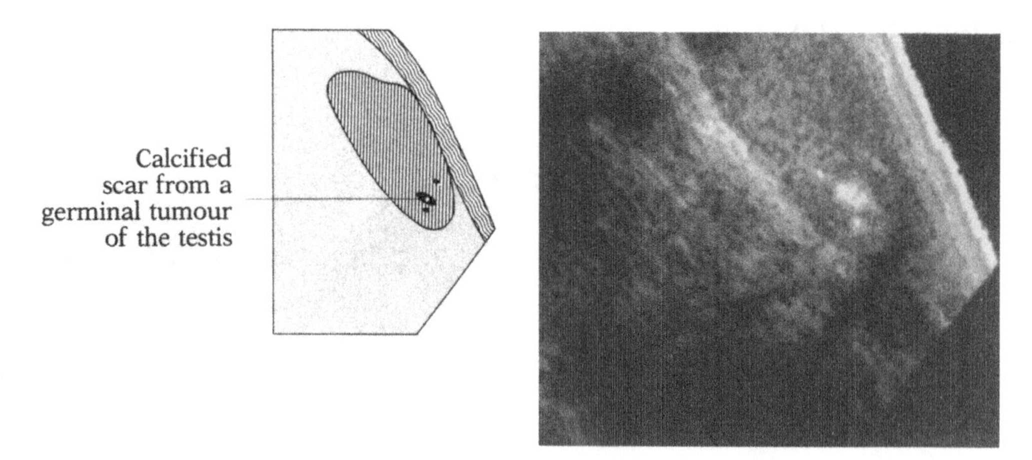

Fig. 20. ***Tumours.*** Investigation of retroperitoneal lymphadenopathy in a young man. Normal testes clinically. Sagittal section. At the inferior pole of a slightly hypotrophic testis is a mass of several echogenicities, the largest is situated centrally, surrounded by identical lesions of about 1 mm with no posterior acoustic attenuation. In this context, the appearances are typical of calcified fibrous scarring in a germinal tumour, confirmed by histopathological examination of the orchidectomy specimen

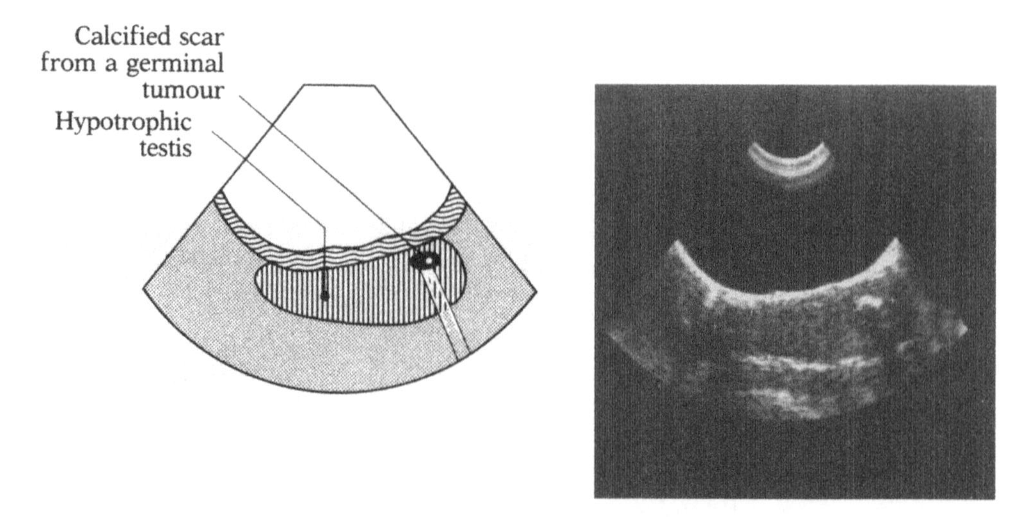

Fig. 21. ***Tumours.*** Same clinical picture. Sagittal section. Hypotrophic testis (reduced thickness) with a clump of very attenuating echogenic material of about 1 cm at the inferior pole: calcified scar of a proven mixed germinal tumour (seminoma and embryonic carcinoma)

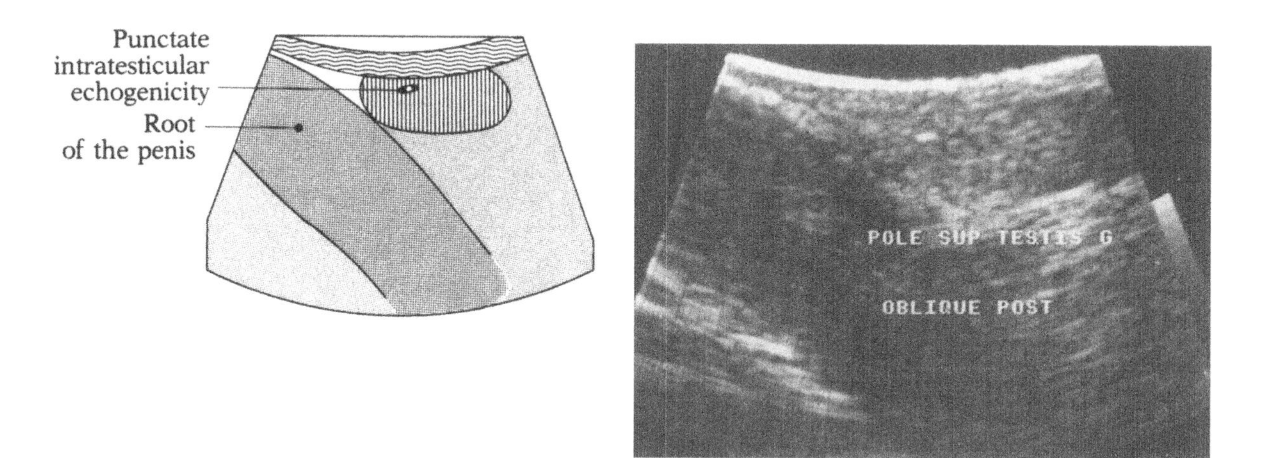

Fig. 22. ***Tumours; differential diagnosis.*** A 35 year old patient operated on for a seminomatous mass in the mediastinum. Search for a primitive subclinical testicular tumour. Sagittal section of the left testis. Small homogenous testis apart from a solitary echogenicity of a few millimetres in the superior half. Despite its smallness, in this context, the possibility of a scar of a germinal tumour cannot be excluded and should be taken in conjunction with the presence or absence of tumour markers. These were negative in this case and therefore only simple follow-up ultrasound was necessary. Scans at one year and two years showed no change, but this does not always eliminate the possibility of a tumour scar

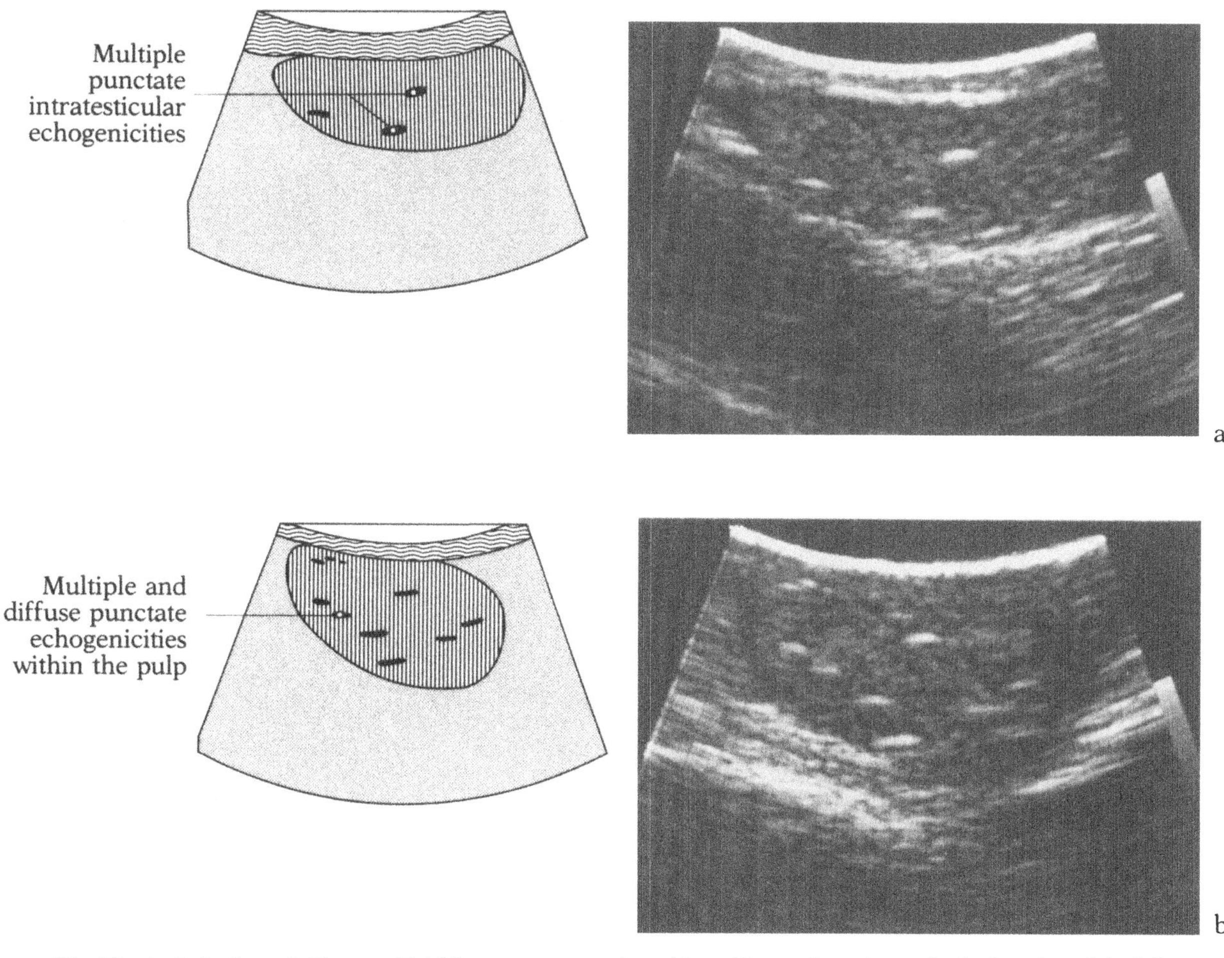

Fig. 23a, b. ***Infections.*** A 29 year old African man, presenting with problems of erection. **a** Sagittal section of the left testis. Multiple echogenic areas of about 1 millimetre scattered throughout the testicular parenchyma. **b** Transverse section of the right testis. Same abnormalities giving a "stars at night" appearance to the testis. Conclusion: bilateral diffuse parenchymal abnormalities with a benign appearance; taking into account the ethnic background of the patient, these could represent calcified microparasites in the lymphatic capillary network of the testes

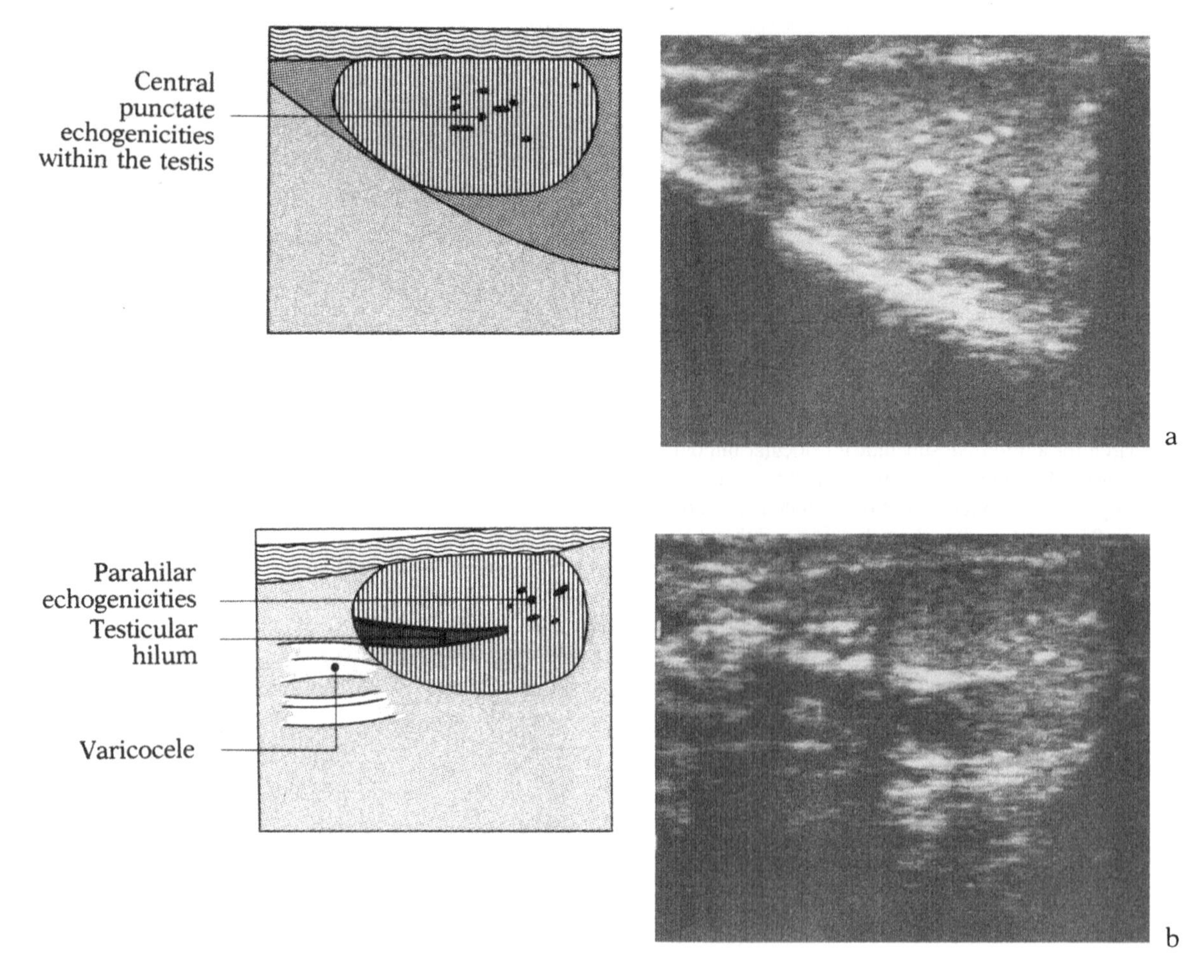

Fig. 24a, b. ***Sterility.*** A 34 year old sterile patient. Severe oligoasthenospermia. Significant bilateral varicocele. **a** Sagittal section. Multiple small echogenicities, finer than in the previous case and grouped in the central portion of the testis. **b** Transverse section. Their perihilar position can be appreciated. Same abnormalities in the other testis. Their bilaterality situation and especially their association with large bilateral varicocele strongly suggest the diagnosis of phleboliths, but the diagnosis of arteriolar occlusion due to reduced blood flow cannot be rule out

Cystic structures of the scrotal contents

These are generally benign and require no treatment. In the majority of cases, they are asymptomatic and are detected by clinical palpation or as an incidental finding during an ultrasound examination performed for another reason.

The majority of cysts occur in or around the epididymis.

The most essential feature is to confirm the purely cystic nature of the lesion, thus differentiating it from pseudo cystic, sometimes neoplastic, masses which require surgical exploration.

Ultrasound appearances of an intra-scrotal cystic lesion

Criteria of a simple cyst

It is essential to fulfill all the criteria of an uncomplicated simple cyst: rounded structure, transonic, well-defined with no wall thickening and with posterior acoustic enhancement.

If all these criteria are not present, it cannot be a simple cyst but must be either a complicated cyst

Table 1. ***Principal cystic and pseudocystic structures of the scrotum***

Origin	Nature
Epididymis (head)	Congenital cysts (derived from embryonic vestiges) Acquired cysts (inflammatory, distal obstruction)
Testis	Pseudocystic masses : + Necrotic germinal tumours, embryonic carcinoma + Epidermoid cyst → **Surgical verification** + Haemangioma + Post-infectious neocyst → **Observe** Leydig cyst Congenital cyst (distended tubule, distal obstruction) "Idiopathic"cyst; ?post-traumatic, ?post-purulent necrosis, ?male menopause (andropause)
Tunica albuginea	Rare cysts
Tunica vaginalis	Dystrophic cyst (inflammatory; hydrocele) = mesothelial inclusions Mesothelial cyst: very rare
Spermatic cord	Solitary cyst = encysted funicular hydrocele (failure of closure of the middle part of the peritoneo-vaginal canal)

(haemorrhage, superinfection, infarction following torsion) or a pseudo-cystic mass, possibly neoplastic, which necessitates an exploratory orchidotomy.

Having established this most fundamental point, the cyst must now be localised.

Cysts of/or in the region of the epididymis

These are by far the commonest cysts of the scrotal contents.

Clinically two types can be distinguished, these cannot be differentiated ultrasonically.

Congenital cysts

These form from abnormally distended vestigial structures (cf. Chapter "Embryology; technical notes and ultrasound anatomy").

They can be large, solitary or more often grouped in clusters in the para-epididymal region.

Acquired cysts

These are most commonly epididymal cysts. They are due to an obstruction of the tubules by an inflammatory process. Generally they are small. When full of spermatozoa they are called spermatoceles which mainly occur in the epididymal head. Clearly, ultrasound can only make the diagnosis of a cyst.

During the investigation of sterility, the presence of several cysts within an enlarged epididymal head is very suggestive of distal obstruction (cf.Chapter "Male infertility").

Cysts of the tunica vaginalis

These are always small, sometimes multiple and occur in the parietal layer of the tunica vaginalis. Their mechanism of formation is usually post-inflammatory; inclusion islets of mesothelium in an inflamed hyperplastic parietal layer which form small vesicles.

This is why there is often an associated, sometimes large, hydrocele. This mechanism also explains the cysts which occur after scrotal surgery. By contrast a true mesothelial cyst is rare.

Cysts of the spermatic cord

Even though they only become apparent in adulthood, they are always congenital. They are formed secondary to non-obliteration of the middle portion of the peritoneo-vaginal canal whereas the proximal and distal portions have closed normally. Thus, this constitutes a true pocket, of variable size, in the centre of the spermatic cord. Given the peritoneal origin of this pocket, some prefer to call it an *"encysted funicular hydrocele"*.

Cysts of the tunica albuginea

These are very rare. It is very difficult to differentiate them from fibromata of the tunica albuginea, also extremely hypoechoic. In both cases, there are small nodules of a few millimetres which are always benign. They are easily recognised by ultrasonic examination which excludes any possibility of an underlying tumour. The patient can therefore be totally reassured.

Cysts of the testicular parenchyma

For a long time, these were essentially restricted ultrasonically to the *epidermoid cyst of the testis*. This entity ,however, should really be considered separately as its ultrasonic appearances indicate it is a pseudocystic mass of the testis (cf.Table) which must be confirmed surgically. It is a rare lesion (1% of testicular tumours), always benign and of ectodermal origin. The wall is composed of a stratified keratinising epithelium. The cyst is filled with a kerato hyaline substance which may contain cartilage, bone, hair and even teeth. The ultrasound appearances are non-specific but sometimes quite suggestive of this lesion: often a small mass with hypoechoic contents punctuated by echogenic areas of variable size, sometimes attenuating, bordered by an echogenic line.

The true cysts of the testis until recently, were considered to be very rare and were infrequently diagnosed. In fact, nowadays they are being recognized more often due to the more frequent use of high frequency probes. Generally they are small, a few millimetres to a centimetre. They may be solitary or in groups and occur in all age groups. The aetiology of these cysts in unknown, probably several mechanisms contribute to their formation. In the context of sterility and distal obstruction, the presence of microcysts in the testis corresponds to dilated tubules. This is not the case for solitary cysts, discovered incidentally, which perhaps are formed from vestigial rests of the Wolffian or Mullerian systems.

Finally, the very rare Leydig cyst should be mentioned, often large (several centimetres), seen in a young adult. It is lined with Leydig cells and can be associated with gynaecomastia due to a hyperplasia of the Leydig cells.

All these cysts are benign and no surgery is indicated unless the cyst is large or in cases of infertility.

Cystic structures of the scrotal contents

Epididymis and para-epididymis

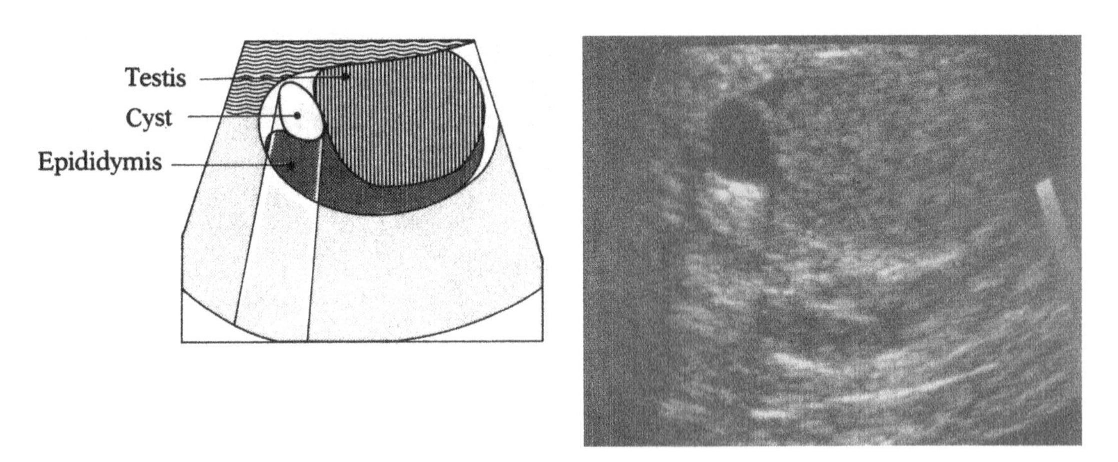

Fig. 1. ***Epididymal or para-epididymal cysts. Inflammation.*** Subacute epididymitis. Little clinical improvement on medical treatment. Control ultrasound examination. Sagittal section. Normal testis. Enlarged and echogenic epididymis with a purely cystic structure in the head: acquired cyst formed above an inflammatory obstruction to the efferent cones

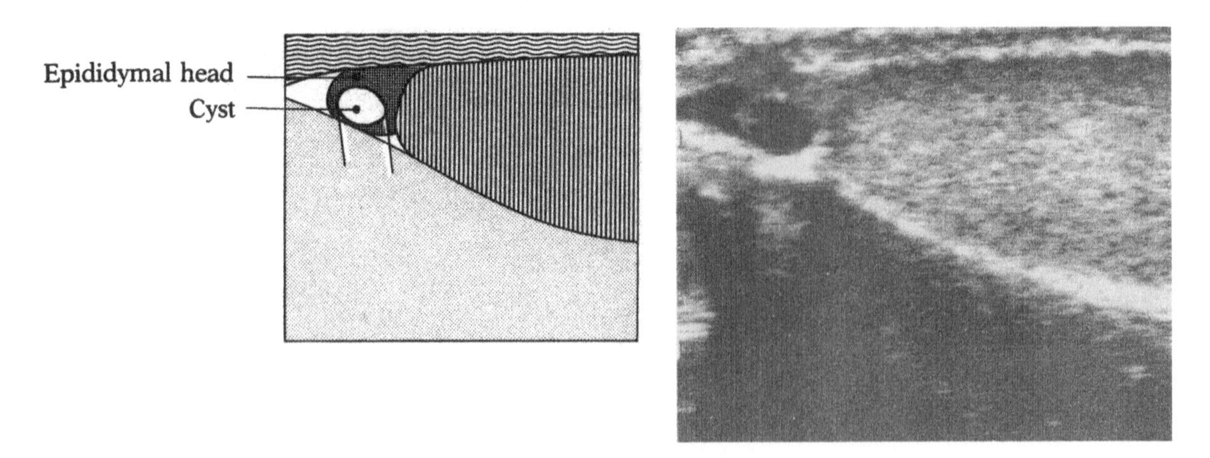

Fig. 2. ***Epididymal or para-epididymal cyst.*** Empty left side of the scrotum. Ultrasound failed to localise a testis which turned out to be cryptorchidism. No previous history of infection. Sagittal section of the right side of the scrotum: incidental finding of a simple cyst (less than 1 cm), developed in or beside the epididymal head. Probably congenital in origin

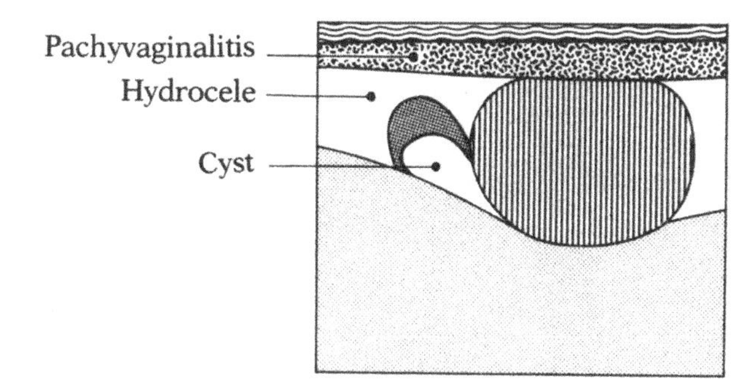

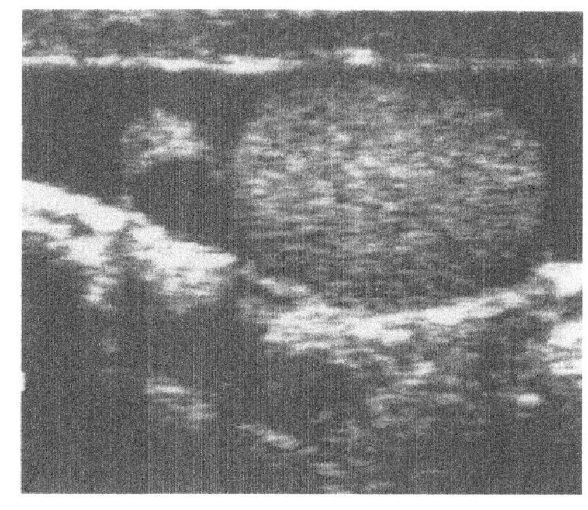

Fig. 3. ***Epididymal or para-epididymal cyst.*** Investigation of a painless enlarged scrotum. Sagittal section: the cyst adjacent to the epididymal head should not be misinterpreted as a hydrocele extending into the interepididymo-testicular recess. Its convexity, rounded appearance and junctional angles with the head indicate an expansive process, a benign cyst. Its aetiology may be congenital or acquired, post-inflammatory in view of the hydrocele and associated pachyvaginalitis

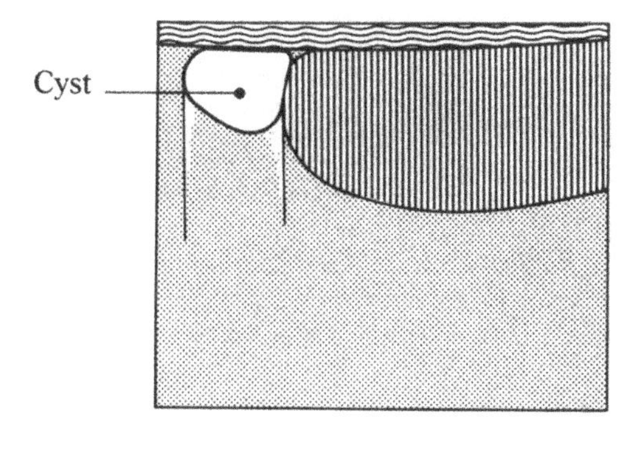

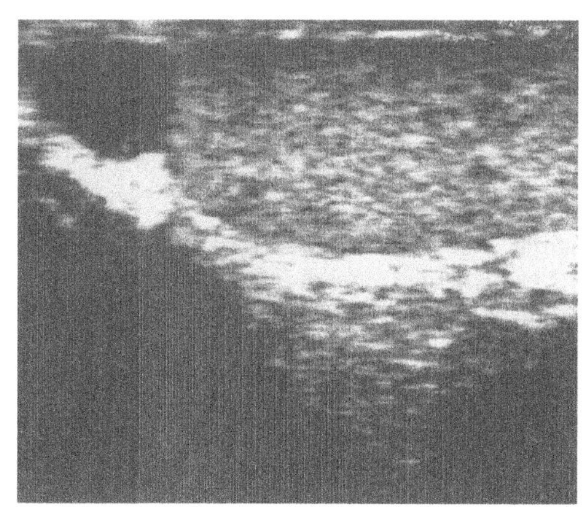

Fig. 4. ***Epididymal or para-epididymal cyst.*** Palpable mobile nodule at the superior pole of the testis. Sagittal section. Solitary, large, uncomplicated cyst in place of the epididymal head: benign appearance of the palpable nodule

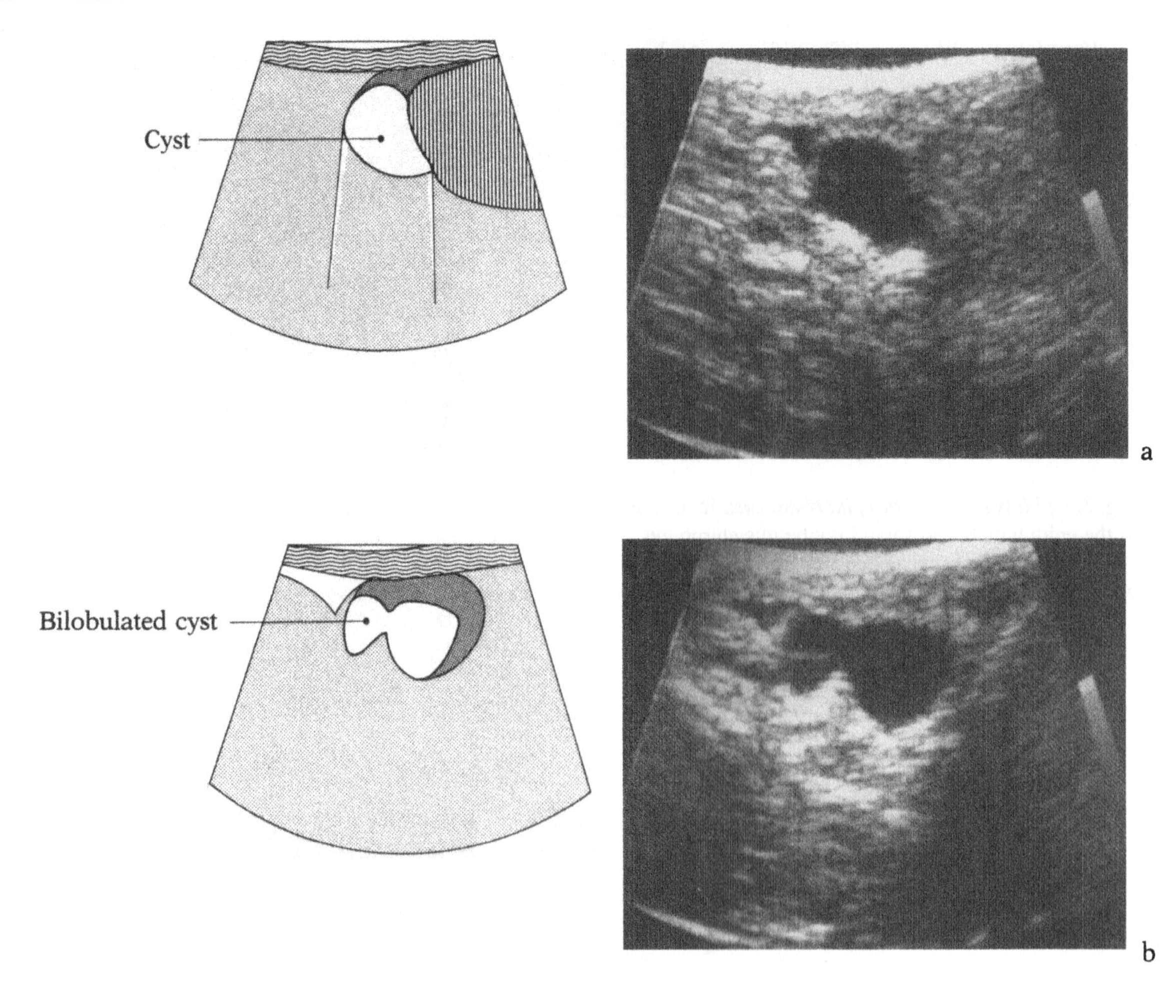

Fig. 5a, b. ***Dystrophic para-epididymal cyst.*** Painless tumefaction of the scrotal sac superiorly. **a** Sagittal section: large cyst overlying the testis. **b** Transverse section : the cystic structure is, in fact, bilobulated with two communicating fluid pockets. A dystrophic congenital cyst formed from the vestigial remnants (hydatid or paradidymal)

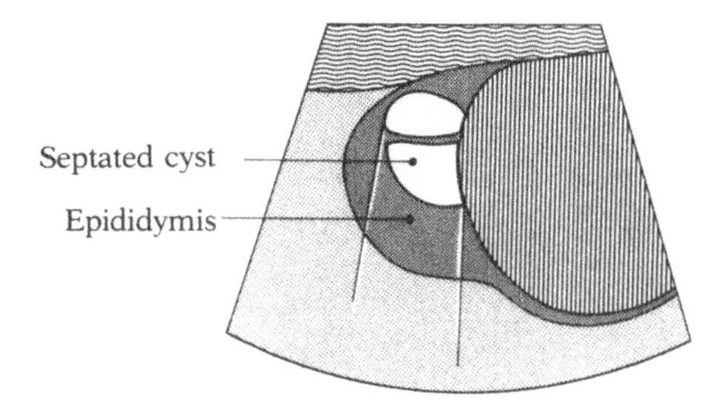

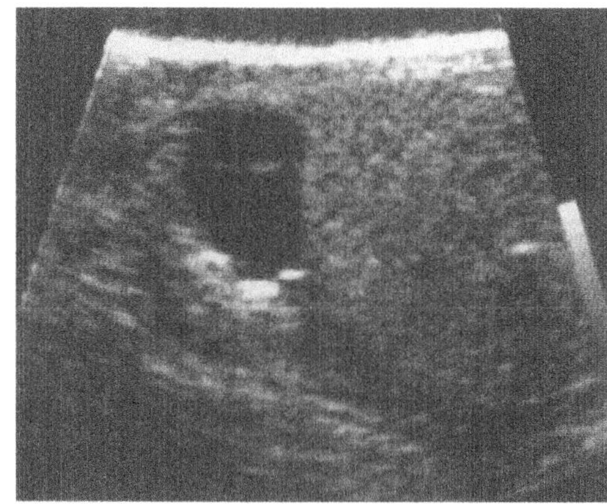

Fig. 6. ***Para-epididymal cystic mass.*** Same clinical picture. High sagittal section. Between the epididymal head and the testis is a cystic mass with a fine central septum: acquired cyst, post-inflammatory, atypical because septated. The possibility of a hydatid cyst should be considered

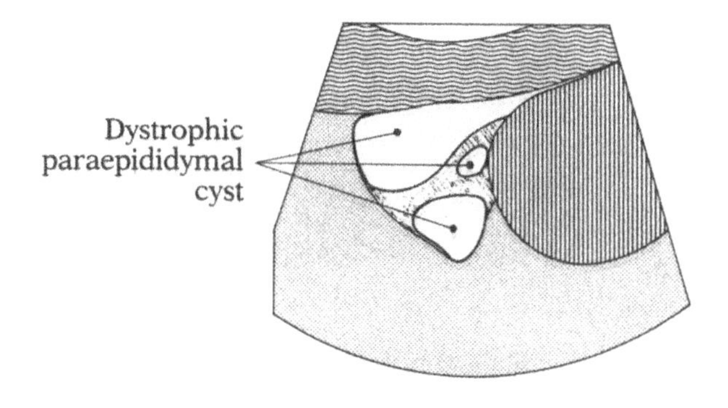

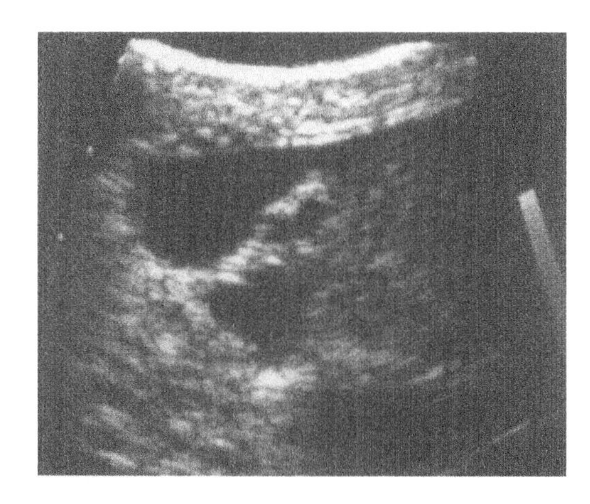

Fig. 7. ***Dystrophic para-epididymal cyst.*** High sagittal section: several cystic masses in a cluster overlying the testis: ectatic tubules of vestigial origin (paradidymis) on histopathological examination of the excised specimen

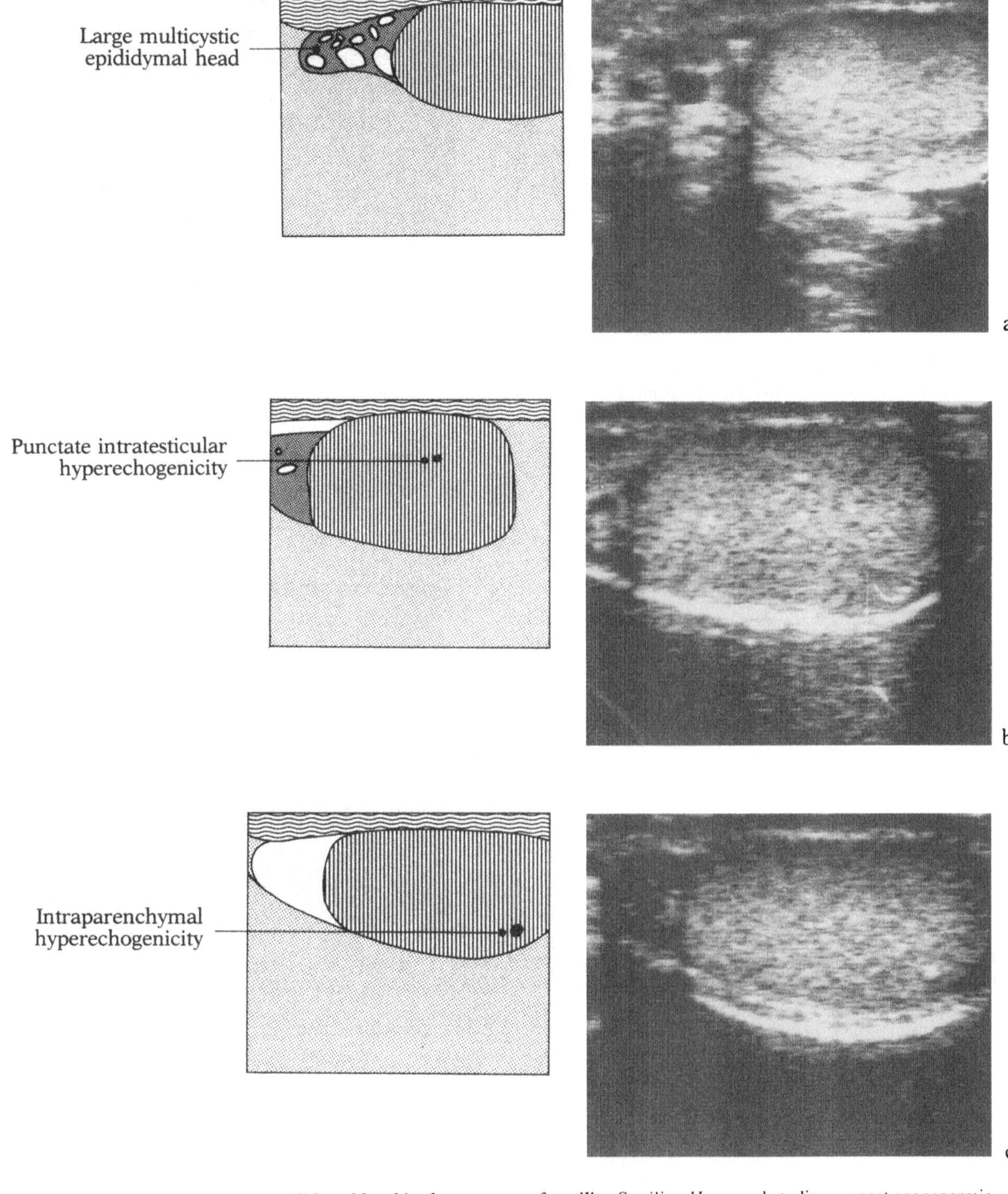

Fig. 8a-c. ***Large multi-cystic epididymal head in the presence of sterility.*** Sterility. Hormonal studies suggest azoospermia of an excretory type. **a** Sagittal section. Enlarged epididymal head (almost 2 cm) made up of several cysts: further evidence suggesting distal obstruction causing tubular distension (epididymis and efferent cones). **b, c** Paramedial sections of the testis: evidence of small punctate intra-parenchymal echogenicities at the limits of the resolution of the scanner: their aetiology is yet to be determined

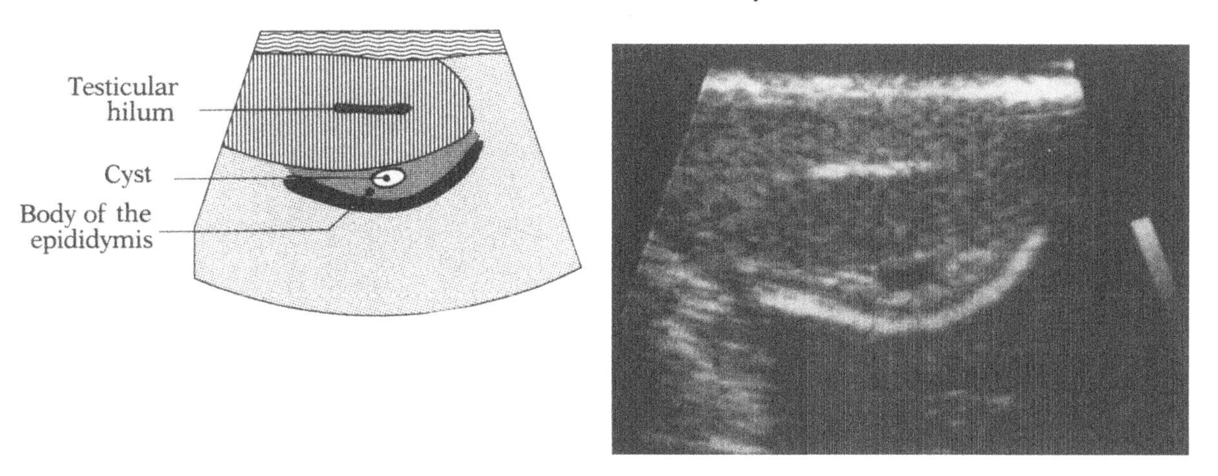

Fig. 9. ***Epididymal or para-epididymal cyst.*** Sagittal section: Posterior to a normal testis in which the hilum is well visualised is a small cyst of a few millimetres in the body of the epididymis or,more likely,in the aberrant canals (organ of Haller)

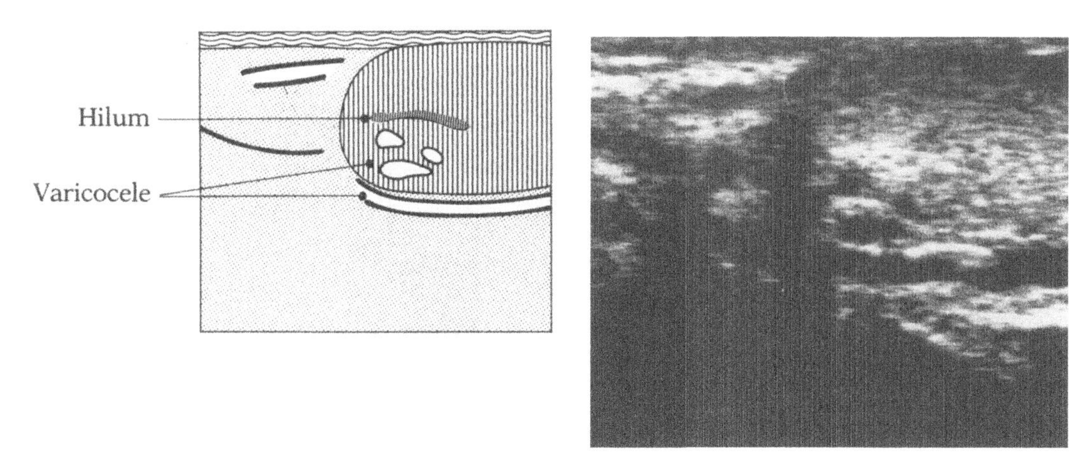

Fig. 10. ***Epididymal or para-epididymal cyst; differential diagnosis*** . Painful swelling of the testis. Sagittal section: postero-inferior to the testis are groups of transonic structures of which some are rounded and others tubular indicating that this is a varicocele which should not be mistaken for a dystrophic cyst. If in doubt, dynamic manoeuvres should be performed which will demonstrate the venous nature of the abnormalities (stand the patient up, Valsalva manoeuvre)

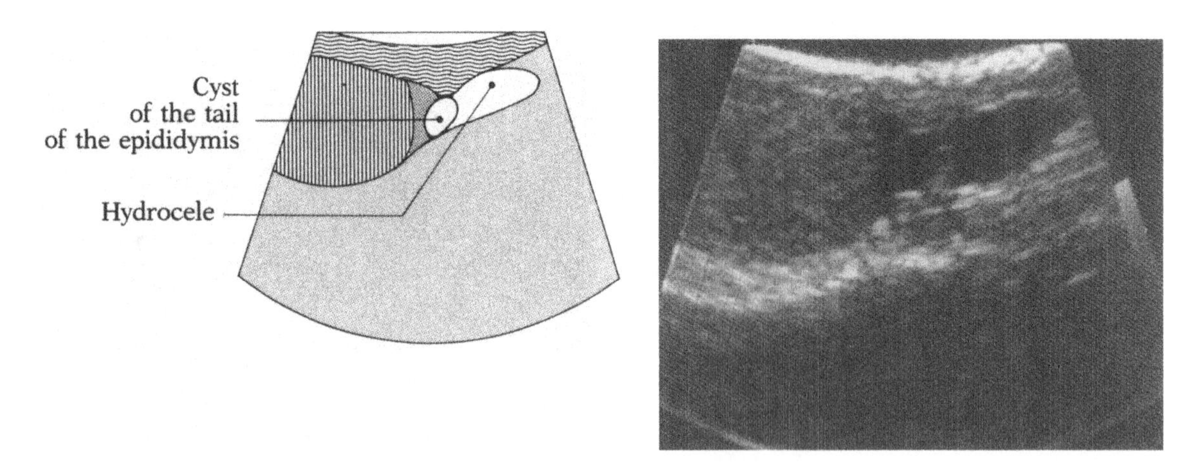

Fig. 11. ***Cyst of the epididymal tail.*** Small tense mass at the inferior pole of the scrotal sac. Sagittal section of the inferior pole: cystic rounded structure with a thin regular wall surrounded by a small hydrocele: cyst of the epididymal tail. In the absence of associated multi-cystic enlargement of the head, cystic distension secondary to obstruction is very unlikely, particularly without the clinical setting of sterility

Tunica vaginalis

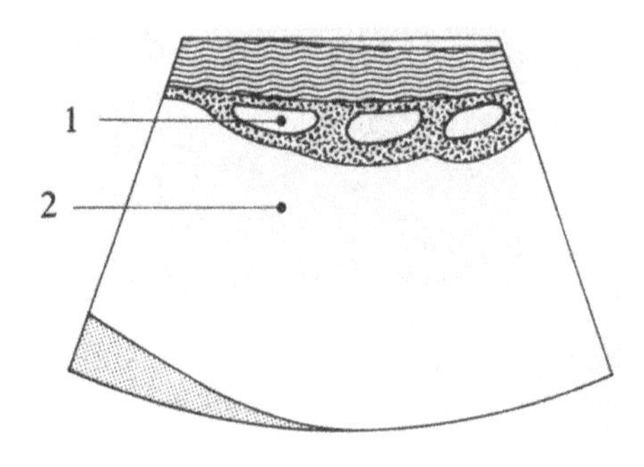

1. Dystrophic cyst of the serous layer of the tunica vaginalis
2. Hydrocele

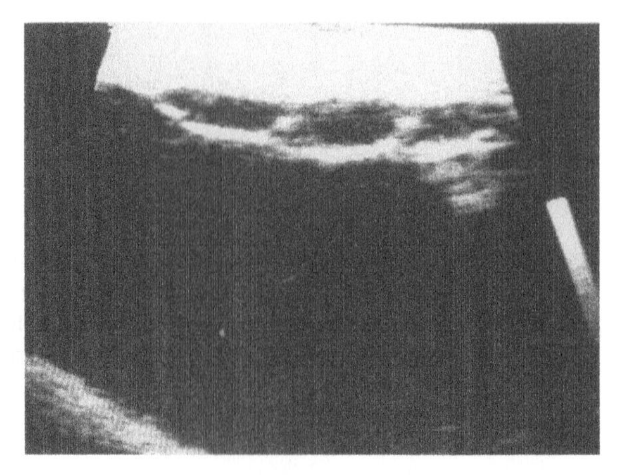

Fig. 12. ***Acquired dystrophic cyst of the tunica vaginalis.*** Enlarged hard painless testis. Transverse section of the superior pole: large hydrocele associated with a string of several cystic structures developed in the parietal layer of the tunica vaginalis: true dystrophic cysts, benign and acquired since they are formed from mesothelial islets resulting from inflammatory lesions

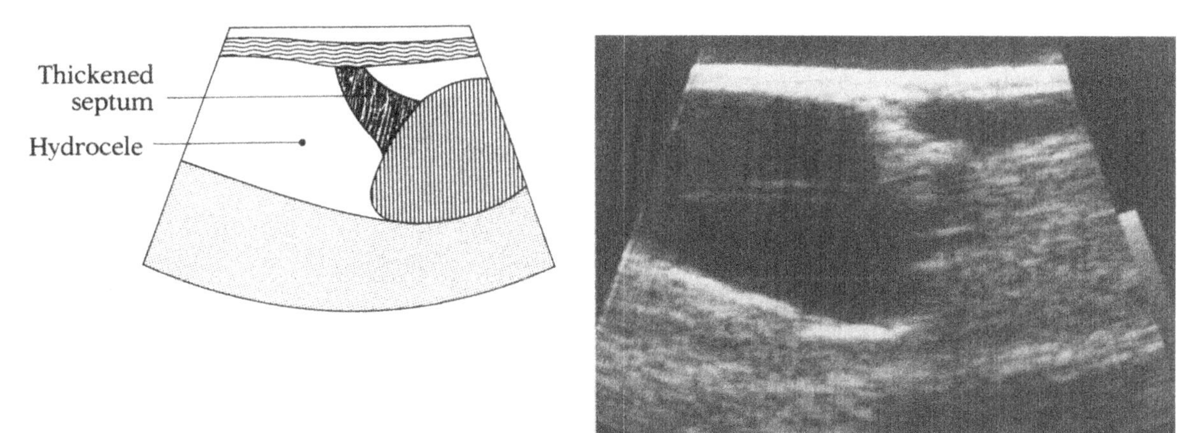

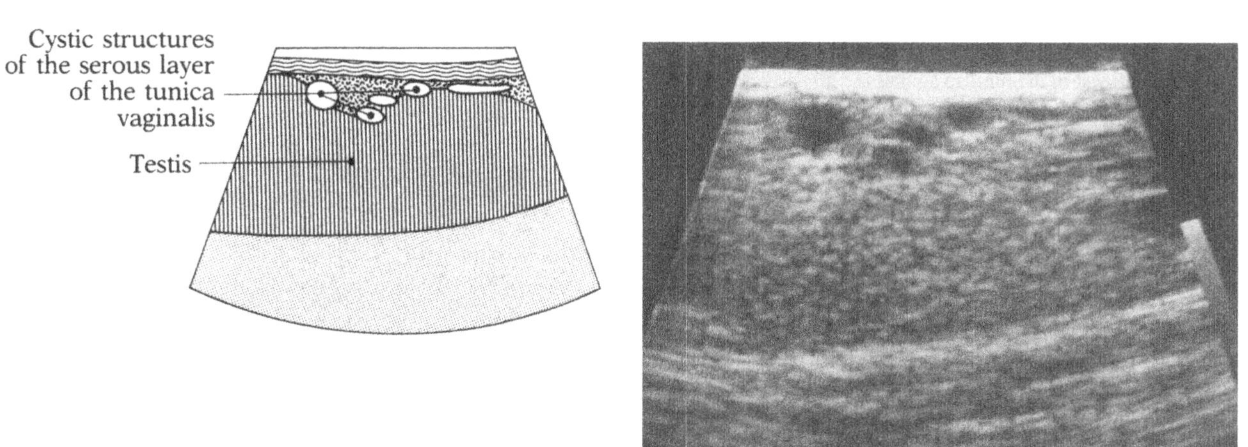

Fig. 13a, b. ***Acquired dystrophic cyst of the tunica vaginalis.*** Same clinical picture. **a** Sagittal section of the superior pole: large septated hydrocele of the superior pole. **b** Sagittal section. The hydrocele is associated with several small cystic structures situated anterior to the testis. These are certainly benign due to the same mechanism as that in Fig. 12; sometimes the septa between the cysts appear thicker and then curative surgery for the hydrocele is justified to confirm that this is simply due to hyperplasia and not to the extremely rare mesothelioma

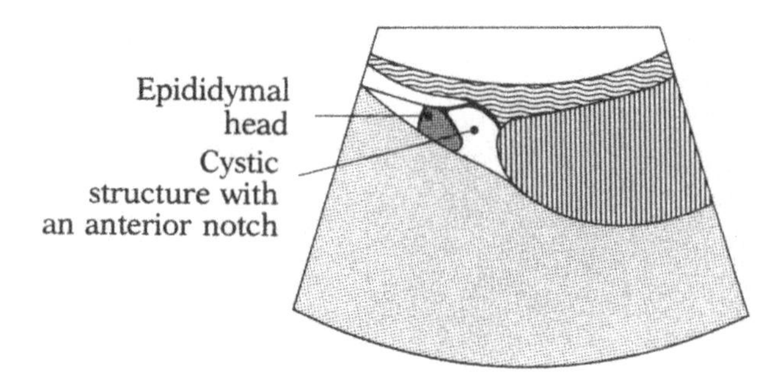

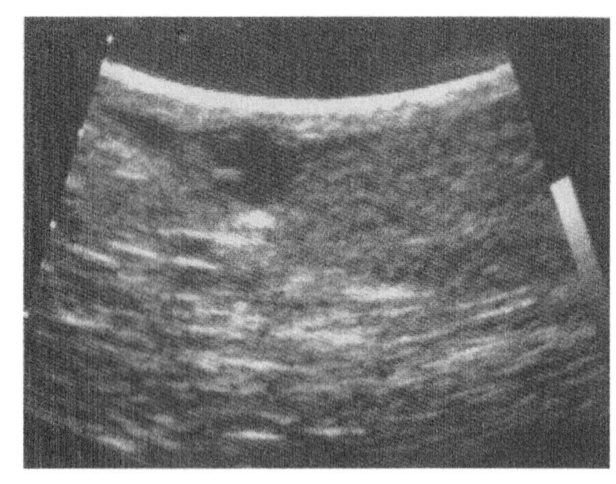

Fig. 14. ***Cyst of the tunica vaginalis.*** Perceptible swelling of the superior pole of the scrotal sac. Sagittal section: small cystic mass situated between the epididymal head and the superior pole of the testis. Its origin from the parietal layer of the tunica vaginalis is confirmed by a notch anteriorly. No change from the original scan two years later: almost certainly a mesothelial cyst of the tunica vaginalis

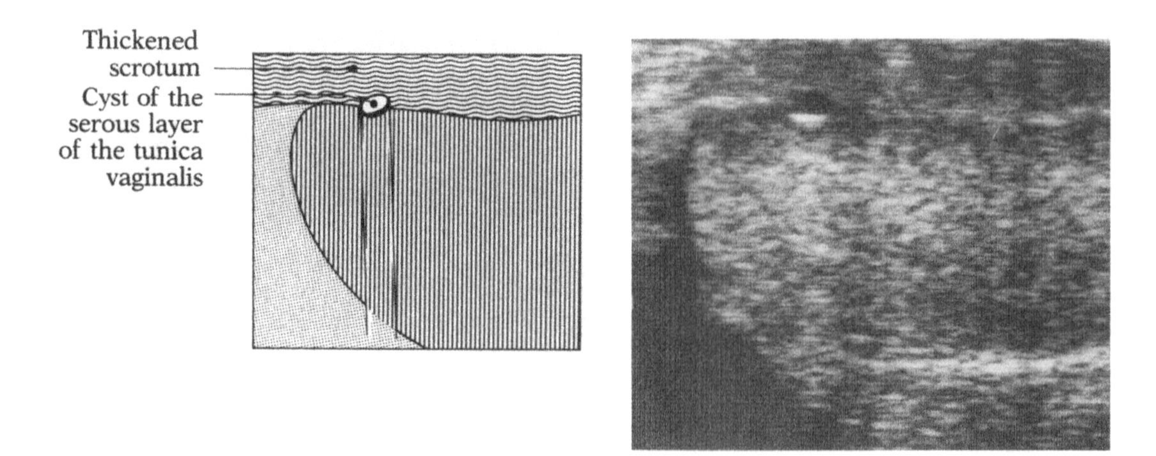

Fig. 15. Cyst of the tunica vaginalis. Investigation of sterility in a 26 year old man with a previous history of cryptorchidism corrected surgically in childhood. Sagittal section: cyst several millimetres in size of the tunica vaginalis, very likely to be due to a mesothelial inclusion at the time of the orchidopexy

Spermatic Cord

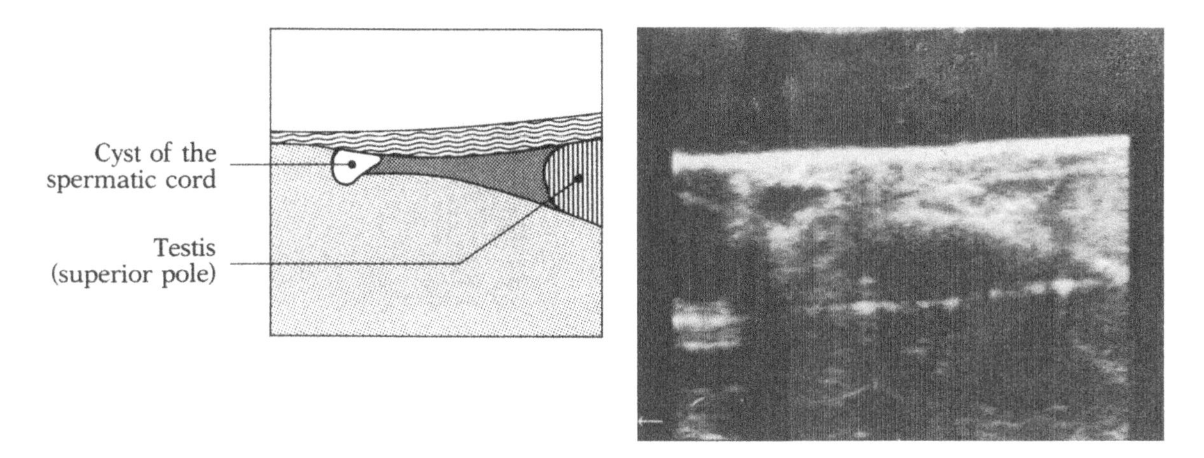

Fig. 16. ***Cyst of the cord.*** Sagittal section of the inguino-scrotal region. The cyst is seen as a small lenticular shaped fluid filled pocket in the pedicle of the spermatic cord. It is due to non-obliteration of the middle portion of the peritoneo-vaginal canal

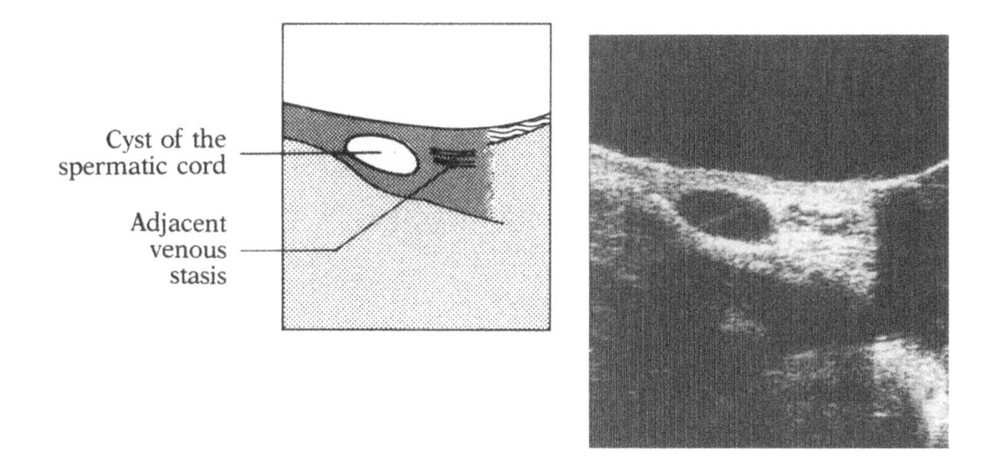

Fig. 17. ***Cyst of the cord.*** Perceptible swelling in the inguinal region in a 24 year old man. Section of the same level (image courtesy of Dr. Ahmad). A perfectly regular cyst is overlying a small varicocele, possibly enlarged due to compression on the spermatic venous plexus by the fluid collection

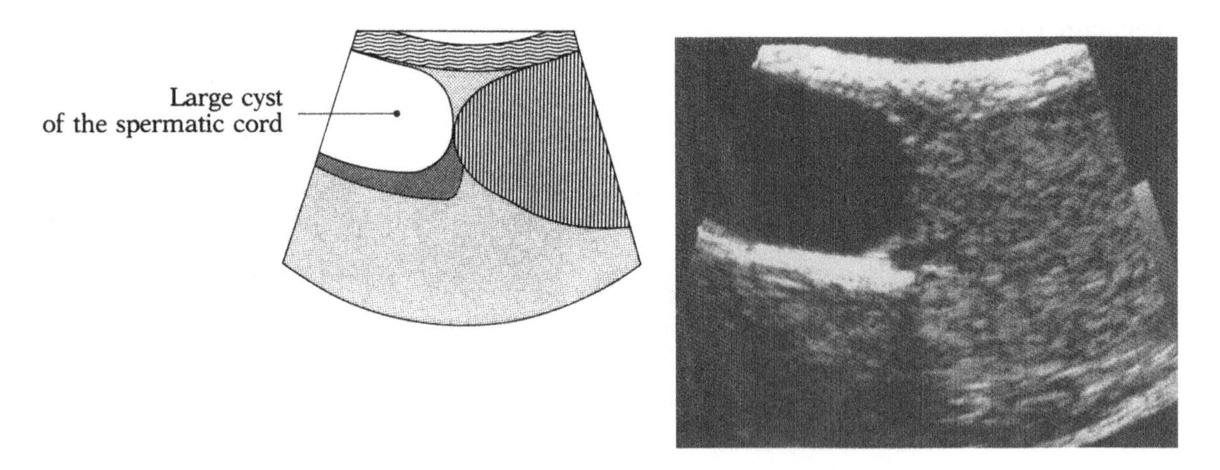

Fig. 18. ***Cyst of the cord.*** Sagittal section of the inguino-scrotal region. Large cyst whose more proximal position could suggest a diagnosis of an isolated encysted hydrocele in the absence of any pachyvaginalitis

Testis

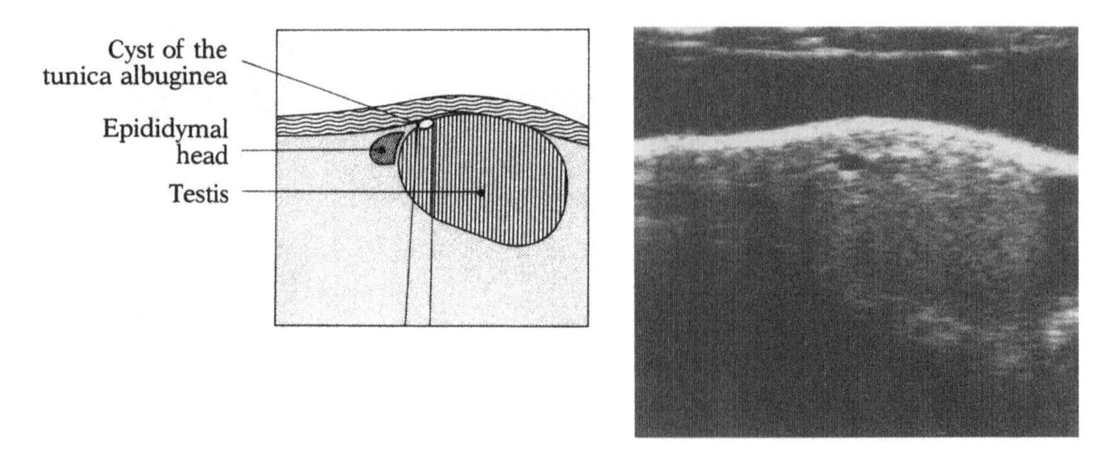

Fig. 19. ***Cyst of the tunica albuginea.*** Palpable solid nodule in the testis of a young man. Sagittal section. Microcyst on the anterior surface of the testis with posterior acoustic enhancement: benign cyst of the tunica albuginea confirmed definitively by the absence of any subsequent change clinically or ultrasonically

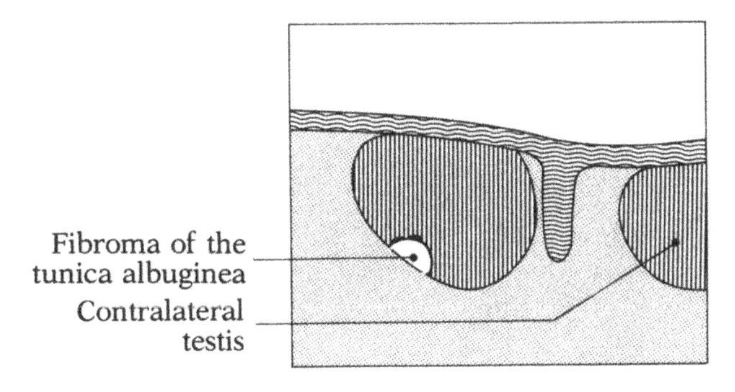

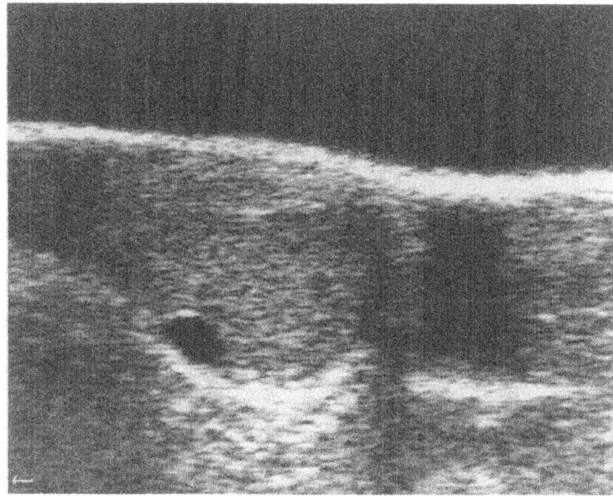

Fig. 20. ***Pseudocyst of the tunica albuginea: fibroma.*** An 85 year old patient with localised painful area in the left testis on palpation. Sagittal section. Small, oval, anechoic mass in the posterior periphery of the testis with some adjacent echoes: fibroma of the tunica albuginea. Its size could possibly explain the pain due to compression of the testicular parenchyma (seen as the internal echogenic rim) and irritation of a branch of the spermatic plexus

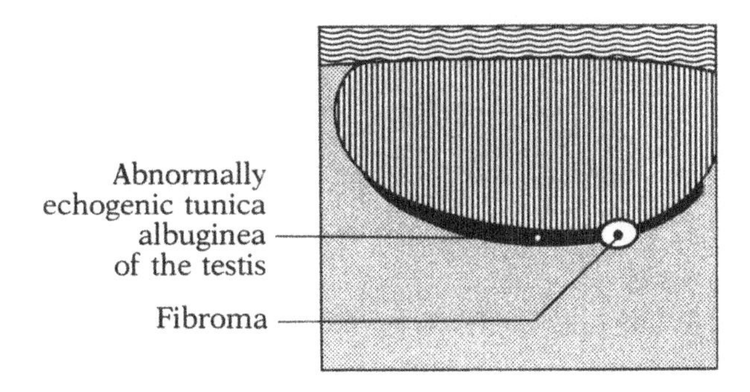

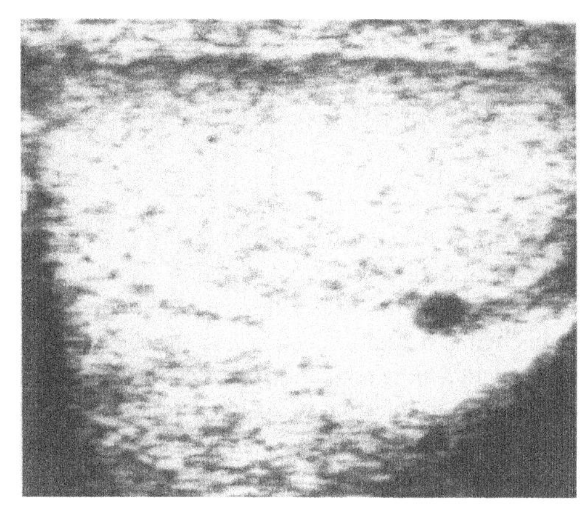

Fig. 21. ***Pseudocyst of the tunica albuginea: fibroma.*** Solid nodule of the testis in a man in his 30's. Sagittal section. The development of the fibroma from the tunica albuginea is particularly clear since it is situated astride the echogenic line of the testicular capsule. No treatment necessary provided if there is no change on clinical and ultrasonic follow-up

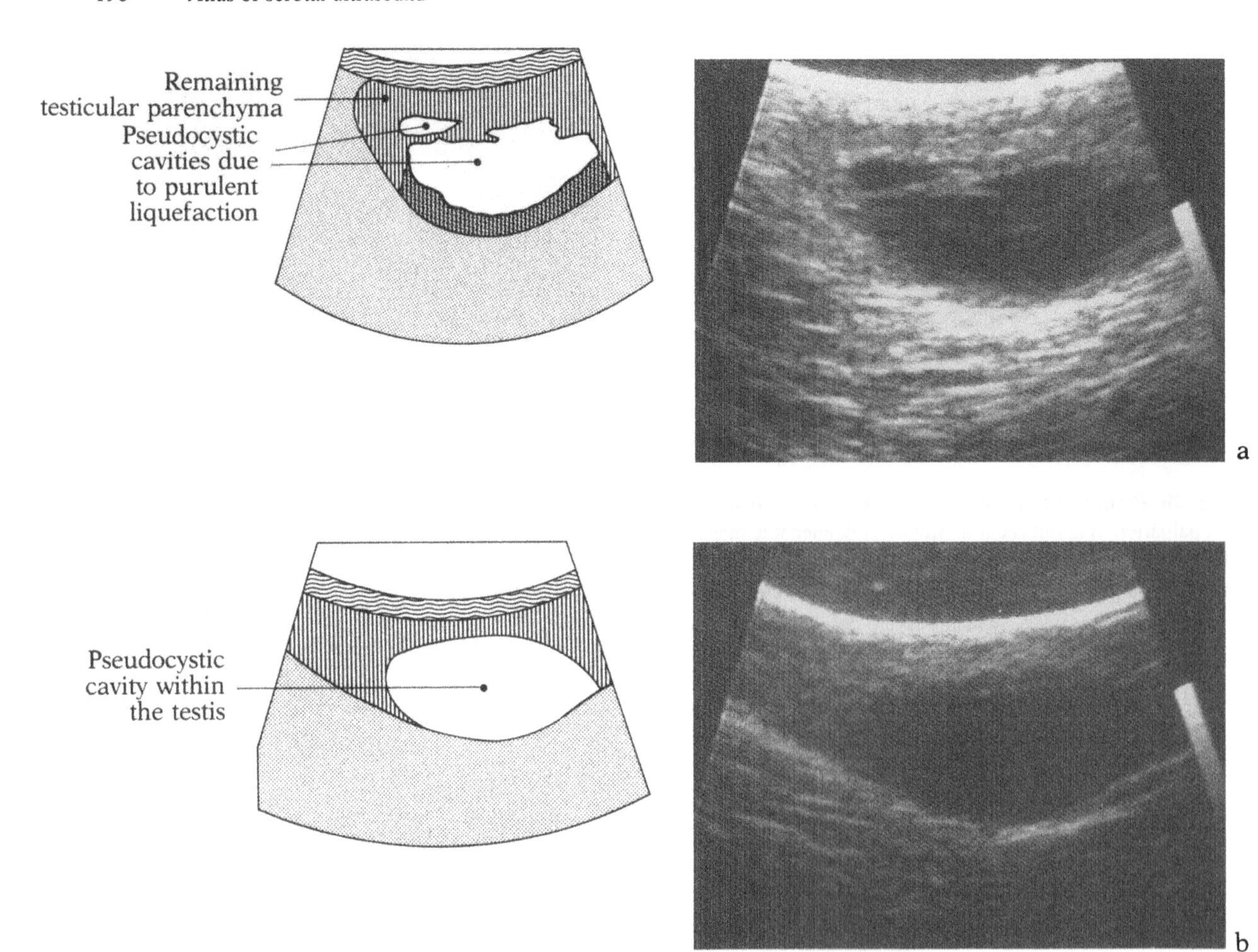

Fig. 22a, b. ***Pseudocystic cavity of the testis.*** A 37 year old patient. Untreated painful orchitis. Soft testis with pyrexia developing over *3 weeks*. **a** Transverse section. Almost the whole testis is replaced by an extremely hypoechoic and irregular area, almost fluid since there is some posterior enhancement: testicular pseudocyst due to purulent liquefaction of the parenchyma. **b** Sagittal section *1 month* later following a course of medical treatment. Frankly transonic appearance of the cavity with a more regular border, clearly separated from the rim of the remaining normal testicular parenchyma: secondary neocyst due to infection or acquired spermatocele. These two entities can only be differentiated by demonstrating the presence of spermatozoa in the fluid which would indicate a spermatocele. They cannot be distinguished ultrasonically

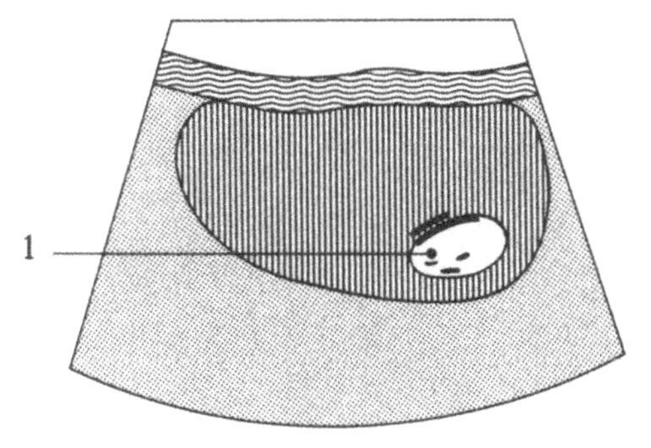

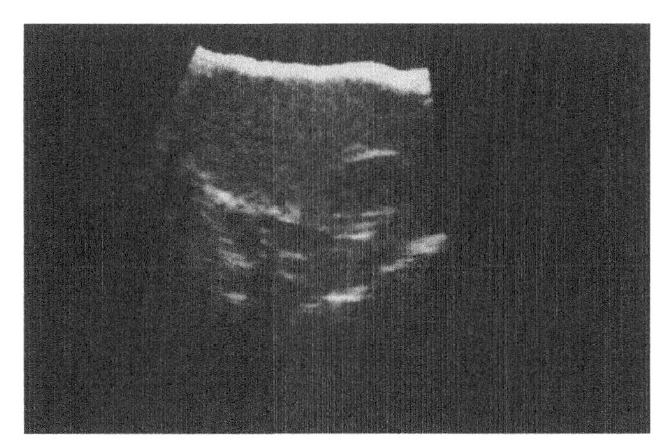

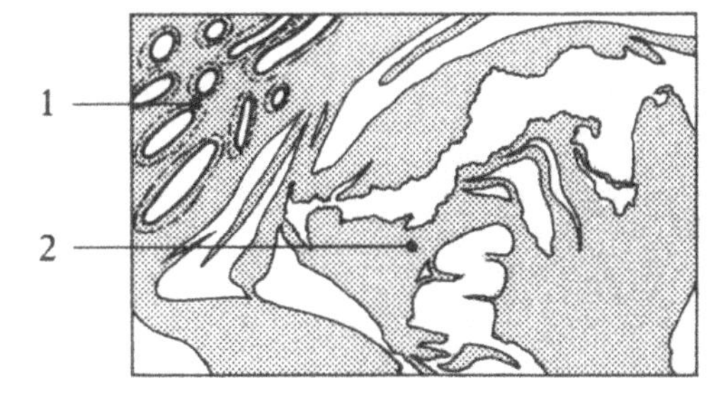

Fig. 23a, b. ***Epidermoid cyst of the testis.*** Painful induration of the testis in a young man. **a** Sagittal section. Intra-testicular abnormality, not purely cystic and therefore a tumour must be considered initially. Mainly anterior hypoechoic zone, with no posterior enhancement, punctuated by small echogenic areas and surrounded by an echogenic line. Orchidotomy. **b** Histological section of the excised specimen: epidermoid cyst of the testis. The cyst was filled with a kerato-hyalin material and lined by a stratified keratinising epithelium. No specific ultrasonic features. The benign nature of the lesion can only be confirmed histopathologically

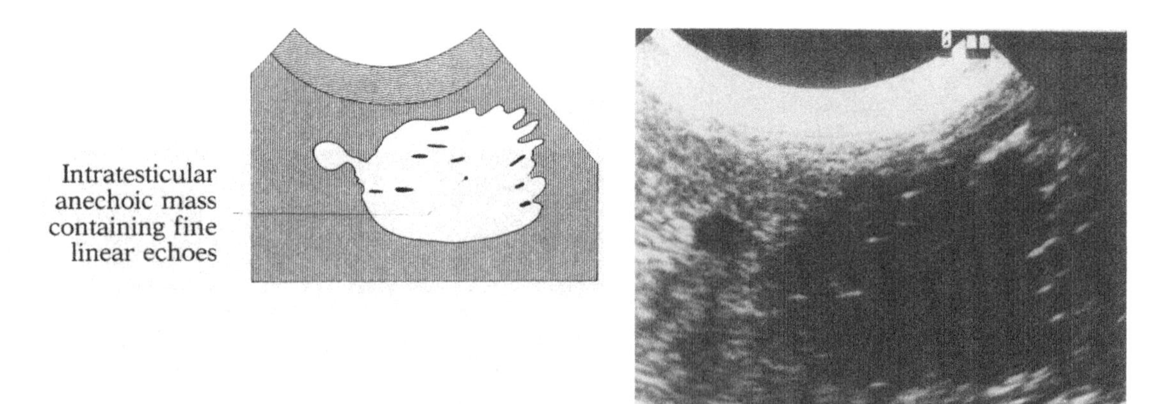

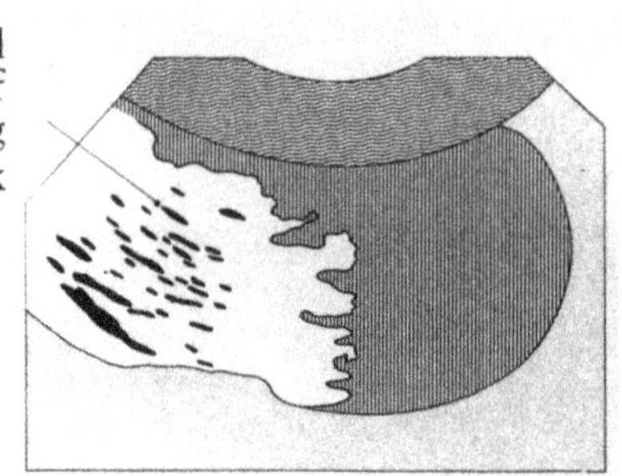

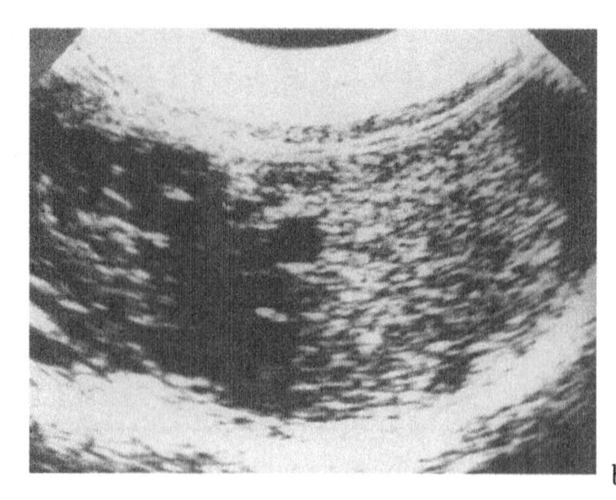

Fig. 24a, b. ***Pseudocystic structure of the testis: haemangioma*** (images courtesy of Dr. C. Kratzik). Painful enlargement of the testis in a man who had several years earlier undergone an operation for a cystic haemangioblastoma of the cerebellum. **a** Sagittal section of the symptomatic testis. Almost all of the testis is replaced by an anechoic mass containing fine linear echogenic structures. **b** Sagittal section of the contralateral testis. Same abnormality but smaller seen in the perihilar region. The appearance of the dilated vessels is more apparent. Appearances unchanged 9 months later. Given the previous history of a cerebellar haemangioblastoma and despite the absence of histopathological proof, the agreed diagnosis is that of bilateral haemangioblastoma of the testes in a case of Von Hippel Lindau disease

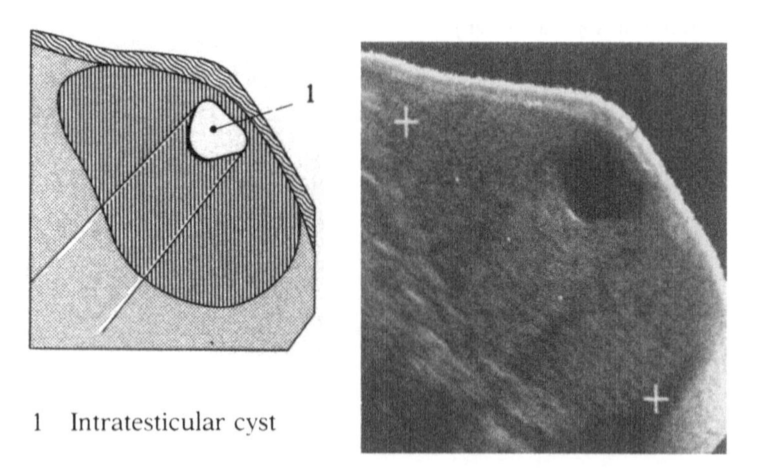

Fig. 25. ***Cyst of the testis.*** A 65 year old patient investigated for a hydrocele. Violent scrotal trauma not investigated forty years earlier. Sagittal section of the supposedly normal testis. A simple cyst fulfilling all the necessary criteria (completely transonic contents, well defined margins, definite posterior acoustic enhancement) of 1 cm diameter in the anterior part of the mid portion of the testis. Its position in the more exposed area supports the proposed diagnosis of a spermatocele secondary to previous trauma. No treatment but a follow-up ultrasound in three months in order to confirm that the appearances are unchanged

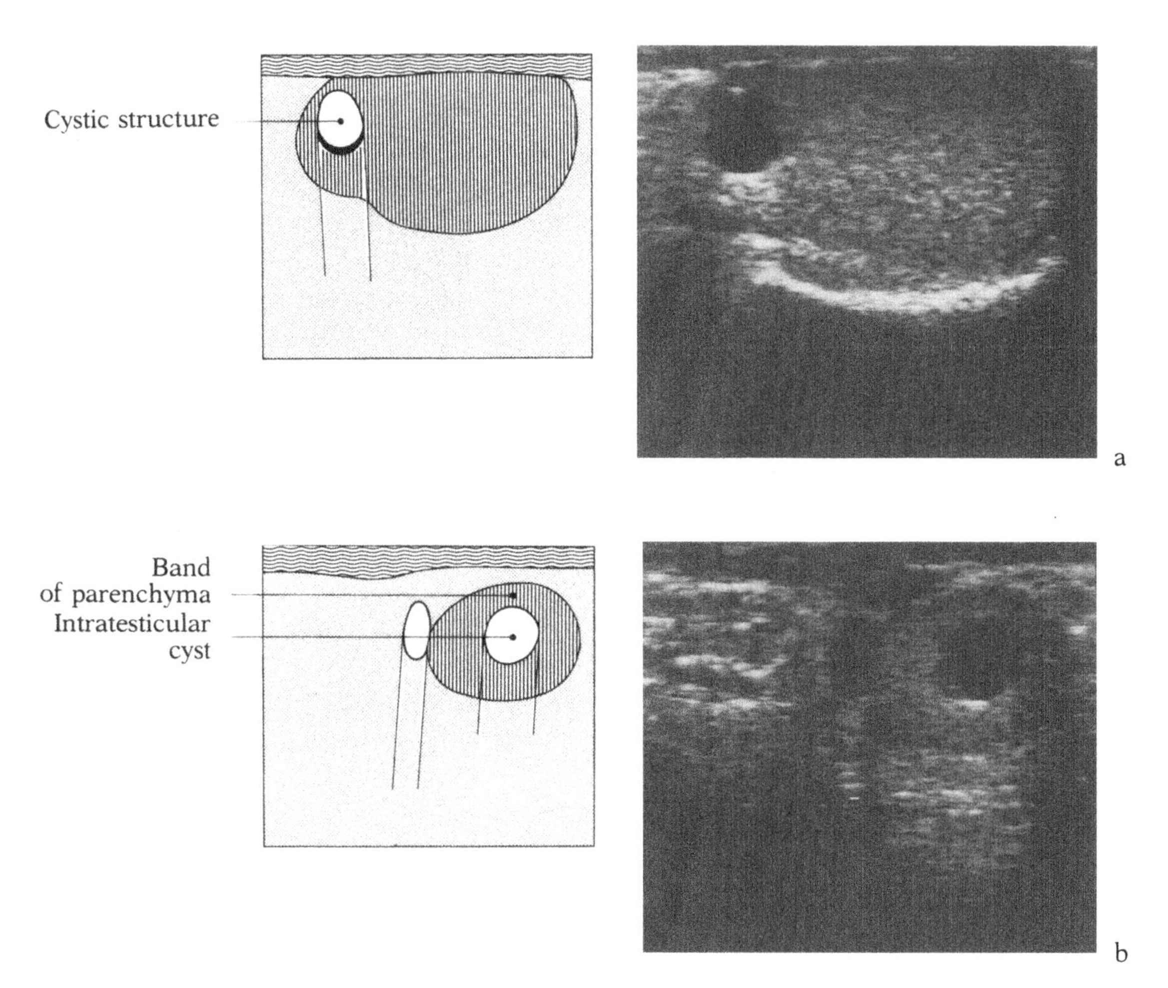

Fig.26a, b. ***Cyst of the testis.*** A 42 year old patient who detected himself a painless intra scrotal nodule. **a** Sagittal section. Large cyst apparently intra-testicular at the superior pole of the testis. **b** Transverse section. The cyst is surrounded by testicular parenchyma confirming that it is definitely intra-glandular. No previous history of trauma or infection: benign idiopathic cyst

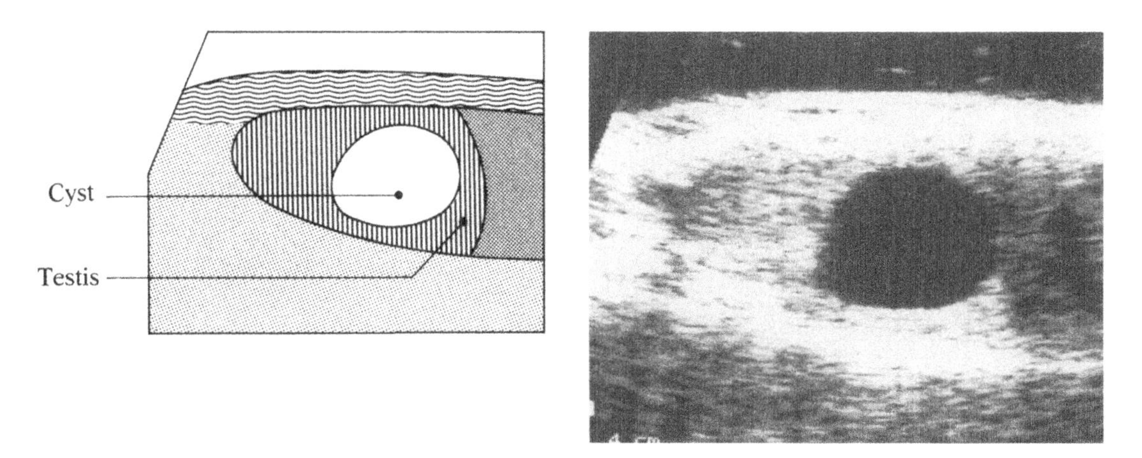

Fig. 27. ***Leydig cyst of the testis*** (image courtesy of Dr. B. Noblinski). A 41 year old patient. Very sensitive left testis. Palpable intra-testicular nodule. Sagittal section: large cyst of 4 cm. in the inferior half of the testis. In view of the pain, an orchidotomy and cystectomy were performed. Histopathologically confirmed to be a Leydig cyst by the presence of Leydig cells in the fibrous wall of the cyst

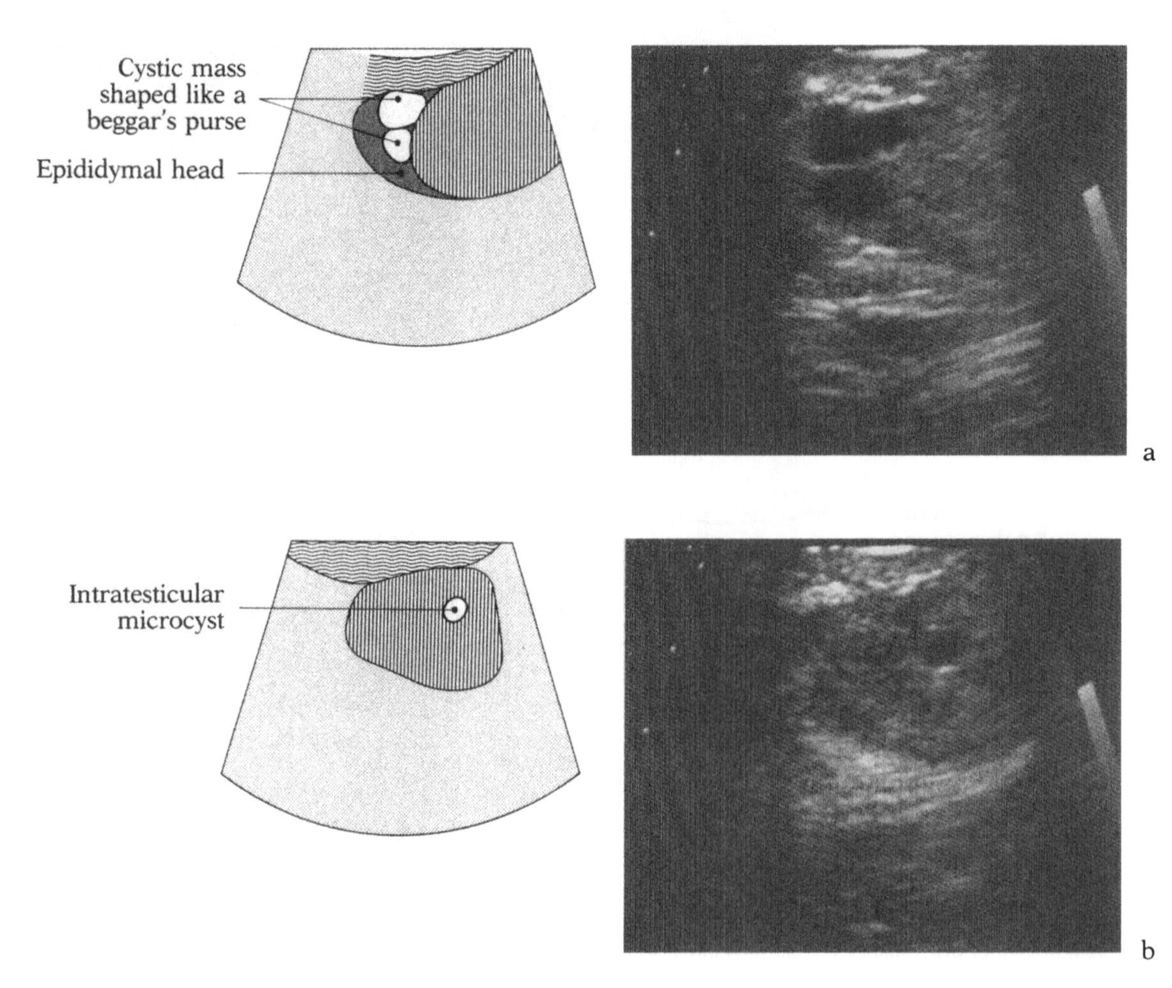

Fig. 28a, b. ***Ectatic pseudocyst of the testis; sterility.*** Crossed anastomosis of the epididymis and vas deferens for excretory azoospermia. **a** High sagittal section. Biloculated cystic mass along the anastomosed epididymal head. **b** Transverse section of the contralateral testis. Several intra-testicular microcysts are seen: in fact due to microcystic dilatation of the seminiferous tubules. The two abnormalities indicated non-functioning anastomosis causing cystic dilatation proximal to the obstruction

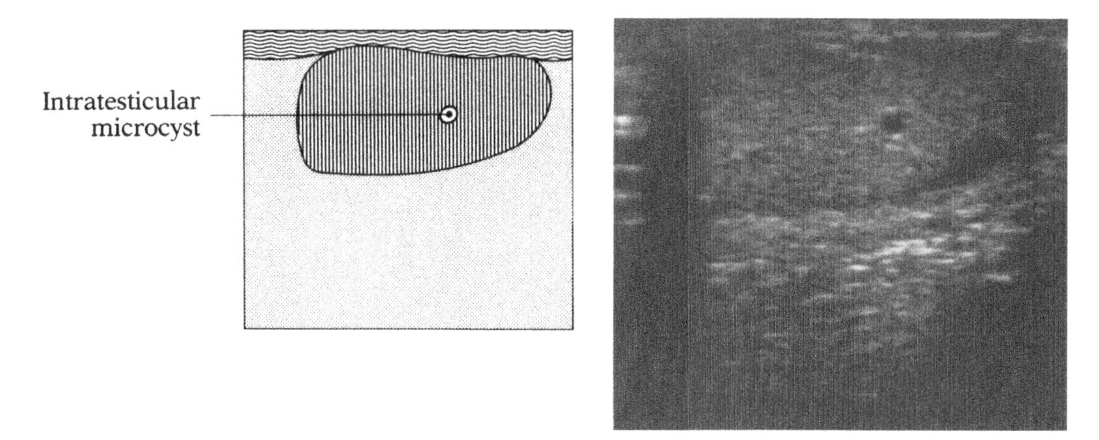

Fig. 29. ***Testicular microcyst; sterility.*** A young man of 28 operated on for bilateral cryptorchidism when aged 12 (testes fixed into the scrotum). Sterility. Sagittal section. Solitary microcyst in the testis. No associated enlargement of the epididymal head. Pseudocyst due to obstruction distally (?accidental ligation of the vas deferens). Appearances need to be taken in conjunction with the FSH levels and the type of abnormality on the sperm analysis

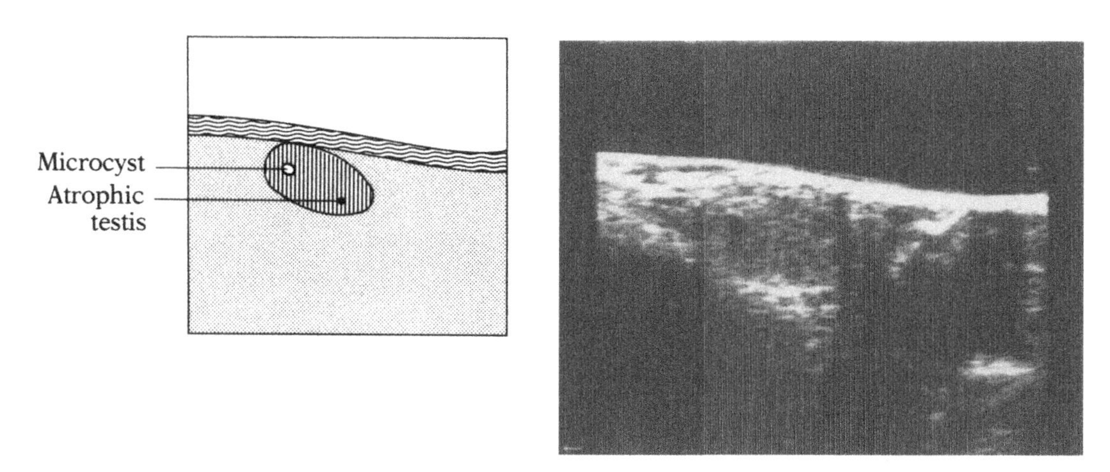

Fig. 30. ***Testicular microcyst; sterility.*** Same clinical context. Bilateral testicular atrophy. Sagittal section of the right testis. Microcyst in the middle of an atrophic gland

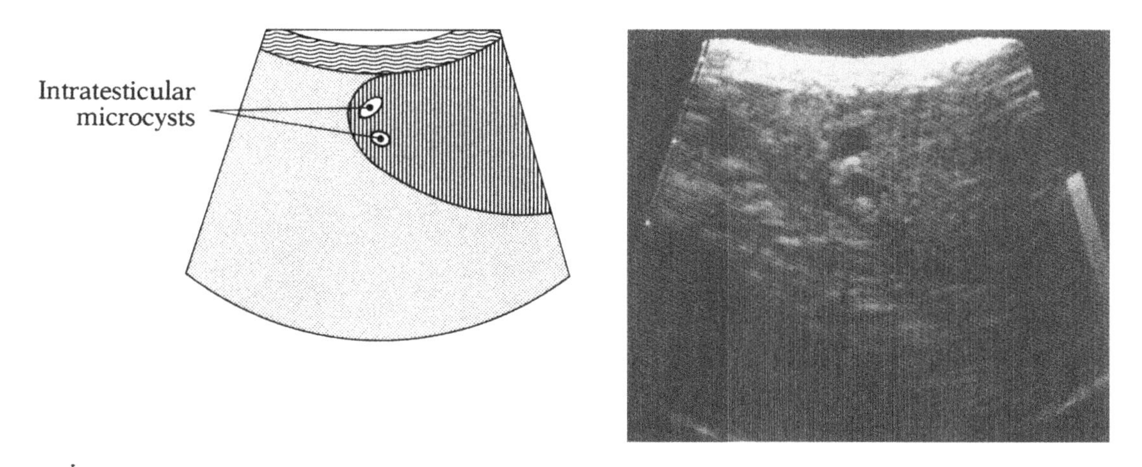

Fig. 31. ***"Degenerative" testicular microcysts.*** Sagittal section: incidental finding of two adjacent microcysts in a 50 year old man with no relevant previous history: this type of cyst is usually in middle-aged patients: degenerative cysts possibly relating to the changes of ageing in the testicular parenchyma

Alphabetical index

Achevé d'imprimer sur les presses
de l'Imprimerie de l'Indépendant
53200 Château-Gontier
N° d'éditeur : 294 - Dépôt légal : juillet 1992

CPSIA information can be obtained at www.ICGtesting.com
Printed in the USA
LVOW02s1927141114

413759LV00001B/1/P

9 783642 85683